Psychiatry

Psychiatry

Second edition

Neel Burton

BSc, MBBS, MRCPsych, MA (Phil), AKC
Green Templeton College
University of Oxford, Oxford, UK

WILEY-BLACKWELL

A John Wiley & Sons, Ltd., Publication

Library of Congress Cataloging-in-Publication Data
Burton, Neel L.
  Psychiatry / Neel Burton. – 2nd ed.
    p. ; cm.
  Includes bibliographical references and index.
  ISBN 978-1-4051-9096-1
  1. Psychiatry. I. Title.
  [DNLM: 1. Psychiatry–methods. 2. Mental Disorders. 3. Mental Health
Services.   WM 30 B974p 2010]
  RC454.B844 2010
  616.89–dc22

                                                                2009021670

ISBN: 9781405190961

A catalogue record for this book is available from the British Library.

Set in 9.5 on 11.5 pt Minion by Toppan Best-set Premedia Limited
Printed and bound in Singapore by Fabulous Printers Pte Ltd

2   2012

Contents

C20045572

True, we love life, not because we are used to living, but because we are used to loving. There is always some madness in love, but there is also always some reason in madness.

Friedrich Nietzsche, *Thus Spake Zarathustra*

Preface to the second edition

This second edition of *Psychiatry* is the product of extensive feedback from students and lecturers, both from the UK and other English-speaking countries. Whilst I have made a large number of changes and additions, I have also tried to preserve what was most liked about the original edition: its clear style and presentation, its appropriate balance of breadth and depth, and its strong 'character'.

Psychiatry continues to include a fair bit of material from the arts and humanities. This material aims to help the student engage with the subject; better understand human emotions, behaviours, and thoughts; and question commonly held assumptions about mental disorders and the people who suffer from them. This is important, first, because students (and the professionals that they eventually become) often stigmatise people with a mental disorder; and second, because this stigma extends to psychiatry and to psychiatrists, and has a deleterious effect on the recruitment of talent into the profession.

Of the medical specialties, psychiatry is by far the most fascinating, the most challenging, and the most obviously relevant to us as thinking and feeling human beings who, in reality, aim at nothing more than happiness. Students often tell me that this book stops them from falling asleep: if so, this has little to do with me, and much to do with the subject matter of psychiatry – namely, human life.

Neel Burton
Oxford, August 2009
neelburton@yahoo.com

Preface to the first edition

Art is long, and Time is fleeting,
And our hearts, though stout and brave,
Still, like muffled drums, are beating
Funeral marches to the grave.

Henry Wadsworth Longfellow,
A Psalm of Life

'Psychiatry' derives from the Ancient Greek, *psyche* and *iatreia*, and means 'healing of the soul'. Just like philosophy differs from other academic disciplines, so psychiatry differs from other medical specialties. Psychiatrists train medically because an understanding of the body is integral to the practice of psychiatry, but psychiatry is about more than just an understanding of the body. It is, indeed, about the very essence of what it means to be human.

Like philosophy then, psychiatry faces empirical and conceptual challenges that hinder its progress and leave it exposed to criticism. Yet it is precisely these challenges that make psychiatry such a satisfying and meaningful pursuit. For in psychiatry each patient is unique, and each patient has something unique to return to the psychiatrist.

Having been a medical student not long ago, I have tried to make this book as readable as possible: clear and concise yet comprehensive and detailed. I have emphasised important areas such as suicide risk assessment but have also included a fair bit of material from the arts and humanities that is not on the core curriculum. In so doing my aim has been to make psychiatry 'come alive' by highlighting some of its more interesting or challenging aspects, and to challenge the stigmatisation of mental disorders that continues to prevail even amongst healthcare professionals.

I hope that you enjoy reading this book, and that it inspires you to get the most out of your necessarily short rotation. *Art is long, and Time is fleeting.*

Neel L. Burton
Oxford, August 2005

Foreword

Welcome to Neel Burton's fascinating and beautifully put together book and, even more importantly, welcome to the world of psychiatry. Perhaps you are approaching the subject with excitement and enthusiasm – as a chance to put into practice what you've learned about communication skills and rapport or to see the reality of how neuroscience maps onto feeling and thinking. Alternatively, psychiatry might be something you are dreading. Will the patients be frightening and dangerous? Will the psychiatrists be only a little better?

Spend a little time browsing this book – stop and read the sections that seem most interesting to you – and you'll have picked up a roadmap to psychiatry. When you've seen a patient with a particular diagnosis, skim the section that relates to him or her. Ask yourself what you learned from the patient that wasn't in the book. For this is what psychiatry is all about – extending the boundaries of understanding of people and conditions beyond the very patchy written knowledge base. I have found a lifetime of fascinating learning and discovery in psychiatry and that the stories of my patients are better than going to the theatre.

So, surprise yourself. Allow yourself to enjoy your placement in psychiatry. You'll get out more or less exactly what you put into it. You'll probably also find out some interesting things about yourself. What could be more fascinating?

If you think you want to train as a GP, consider psychiatry as a specialty within which you will really get to know your patients and become involved in their lives by spending hours with them rather than the regulation four minutes. For those of you who think you want to become neurologists, think of psychiatry as a career where your patients get better and where neuroscience advances are going to make the biggest impact within your working lifetime. For those of you who want to become psychiatrists, stick with it. You have a fabulous opportunity to join the best club in medicine with a career that guarantees fascination, reward and challenge.

Professor Robert Howard
Dean of the Royal College of Psychiatrists

Part 1

'In that direction,' the Cat said, waving its right paw round, 'lives a Hatter: and in that direction,' waving the other paw, 'lives a March Hare. Visit either you like: they're both mad.'
'But I don't want to go among mad people,' Alice remarked.
'Oh, you can't help that,' said the Cat: 'we're all mad here. I'm mad. You're mad.'
'How do you know I'm mad?' said Alice.
'You must be,' said the Cat, 'or you wouldn't have come here.'

Lewis Carroll, *Alice's Adventures in Wonderland*

Lewis Carroll was the pen name of Charles Dodgson (1832–1898), a lecturer in mathematics at Christ Church College, Oxford, who suffered from classic migraine. Classic migraine is sometimes associated with Lilliputian hallucinations, in which objects, animals, and people appear smaller than they really are. It is possible that Dodgson found the inspiration for his Alice stories in Lilliputian hallucinations, which have since acquired the quixotic sobriquet of 'Alice in Wonderland syndrome' (AIWS).

A brief history of psychiatry

Key learning objectives

- To understand that, to a large extent, the history of psychiatry reflects major paradigmal shifts in the history of ideas
- To appreciate that historical constructions of 'madness' have helped to shape current perceptions of mental disorders and psychiatric practice
- To learn a bit about the most famous of all psychiatrists, Freud and Jung

Ancient Greece: the birth of psychiatry

In antiquity, people used the term 'madness' to refer indiscriminately to both the psychosis of schizophrenia and to the 'affective' psychoses of mania and depression. In those days, they did not think of 'madness' in terms of mental disorder, but in terms of divine punishment or demonic possession. For example, the Old Testament relates that Saul became mad after failing in his religious duties and angering God, and nothing is more revealing of Saul's madness than the story of his senseless slaughter of the 85 priests at Nob. The fact that David used to play on his harp to make Saul better suggests that, even in antiquity, people believed that psychosis could be successfully treated.

> But the spirit of the Lord departed from Saul, and an evil spirit from the Lord troubled him.
>
> And it came to pass, when the evil spirit from God was upon Saul, that David took an harp, and played with his hand: so Saul was refreshed, and was well, and the evil spirit departed from him.
>
> 1 Samuel 16.14, 16.23 (King James Version)

In Greek mythology and the Homerian epics, madness is similarly thought of as a punishment from God, or the gods. Thus, Hera punishes Hercules by 'sending madness upon him', and Agamemnon confides to Achilles that 'Zeus robbed me of my wits'. It is in actual fact not until the time of the Greek physician Hippocrates (460–377 BC) that madness first became an object of scientific speculation. Hippocrates thought that madness resulted from an imbalance of four bodily humours. Depression, for instance, resulted from an excess of black bile (*melaina chole*) and could be cured by restoring the balance of humours by such treatments as special diets, purgatives,

Psychiatry, 2e. By Neel Burton. Published 2010 by Blackwell Publishing.

1

and blood-lettings. To modern readers Hippocrates' ideas may seem far-fetched, perhaps even on the dangerous side of eccentric, but in the fourth century BC they represented a significant advance on the idea of madness as a punishment from God. Aristotle (384–322 BC) and later the Roman physician Galen (129–216 AD) expanded on Hippocrates' humoural theories, and both men played an important role in establishing them as Europe's dominant medical model.

> It is interesting to note that not all minds in Ancient Greece invariably thought of 'madness' as a curse or illness. In the *Phaedrus*, Plato quotes Socrates as saying:
>
> *Madness, provided it comes as the gift of heaven, is the channel by which we receive the greatest blessings ... the men of old who gave things their names saw no disgrace or reproach in madness; otherwise they would not have connected it with the name of the noblest of arts, the art of discerning the future, and called it the manic art ... So, according to the evidence provided by our ancestors, madness is a nobler thing than sober sense ... madness comes from God, whereas sober sense is merely human.*
>
> Plato, *Phaedrus*

The Roman Empire

In Ancient Rome, the physician Asclepiades (106–43 BC) and the statesman and philosopher Cicero (106–43 BC) rejected Hippocrates' humoural theories, asserting, for example, that melancholy resulted not from an excess of black bile but from emotions such as rage, fear, and grief. Cicero's questionnaire for the assessment of mental disorders bore remarkable similarities to today's psychiatric history and mental state examination (see Chapter 2). Used throughout the Roman Empire, it included, amongst others, sections on *habitus* (appearance), *orationes* (speech), and casus (significant life events). Unfortunately, around the time of Jesus Christ, the influence of Asclepiades and Cicero declined and the influential Roman physician Celsus (25 BC –50 AD) reinstated the idea of madness as a punishment from the Gods.

The Middle Ages

The fall of the Roman Empire and the rise of Christianity represented important setbacks to the natural progression of thought, and the Church promoted the idea of madness as divine punishment or demonic possession. Accordingly, religion became central to cure and, alongside the mediaeval asylums such as the Bethlehem (an infamous asylum in London that is at the origin of the contemporary expression, *like a bad day at Bedlam*), some monasteries transformed themselves into centres for the treatment of mental disorder. This is not to say that the humoral theories of Hippocrates had been supplanted, but merely that they had been incorporated into the prevailing Christian dogma. Indeed, older treatments such as blood-letting and purgatives continued alongside the prayers and confession.

During the Middle Ages classical ideas had been kept alive in non-Christian centres such as Baghdad and Damascus, and their re-introduction by Saint Thomas Aquinas (1224–1274) and others in the 13th century once again resulted in an increased separation of mind and soul, and in a shift from the Platonic metaphysics of Christianity to the Aristotelian empiricism of science. This movement laid the foundations for the Renaissance and, later, for the Enlightenment.

The Renaissance

The burning of the so-called heretics began in the early Renaissance and reached its peak in the 14th and 15th centuries. First published in 1563, *De Praestigiis Daemonum* (The Deception of Demons) argued that the madness of heretics resulted not from divine punishment or demonic possession, but from natural causes. Perhaps unsurprisingly, the Church proscribed the book and accused its author, Johann Weyer, of being a sorcerer.

From the 15th century scientific breakthroughs such as Galileo's (1564–1642) heliocentric system began challenging the authority of the Church. Man, not God, became the centre of attention and study, and it is also around this time that Vesalius (1514–1564) published his landmark *De humani corporis fabrica libri septem* (The Seven Books on the Structure of the Human Body). The *Fabrica* represented the first serious challenge to Galenic anatomy and brought its author considerable fame and fortune. By the age of 28 Vesalius had become physician to the Holy Roman Emperor (neither Holy nor Roman, but actually the Emperor of Germany), Charles the Quint.

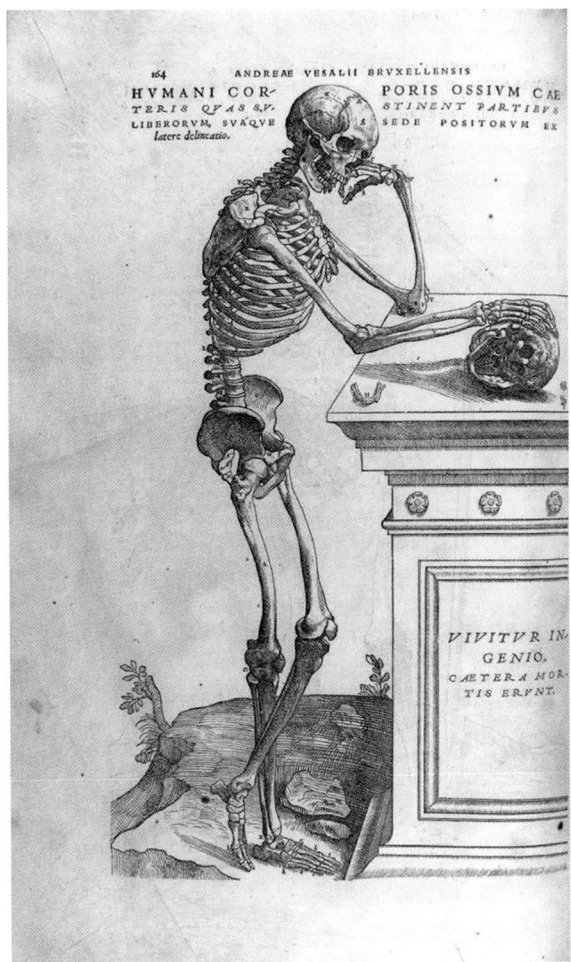

Figure 1.1 An illustration from the Fabrica, by Vesalius.

The Enlightenment

Despite the scientific developments of the Renaissance, Hippocrates' humoral theories persisted into the 17th and 18th centuries to be mocked by Molière (1622–1673) in his plays (notably *Le Malade imaginaire* and *Le Médecin malgré lui*). Empirical thinkers such as John Locke (1632–1704) in England and Denis Diderot (1713–1784) in France challenged this *status quo* by postulating that the psyche arose from sensations to produce reason and emotions. Also in France, Philippe Pinel (1745–1826) began to regard mental disorder as the result of exposure to social and psychological stresses and, to a lesser extent, of heredity and physiological damage. A landmark in the history

of psychiatry, Pinel's *Traité Médico-philosophique sur l'aliénation mentale ou la manie* (Medico-Philosophical Treatise on Mental Alienation or Mania) called for a more humane approach to the treatment of mental disorder. This 'moral treatment', as it had already been dubbed, included respect for the patient, a trusting and confiding doctor–patient relationship, decreased stimuli, routine activity and occupation, and the abandonment of old-fashioned treatments such as special diets, purgatives, and blood-lettings. At about the same time as Pinel in France, the Tukes (father and son) in England founded the York Retreat, the first institution 'for the humane care of the insane' in the British Isles.

The Modern Era

In the 19th century, hopes of successful cures lead to the burgeoning of mental hospitals in North America, Britain, and many of the countries of continental Europe. Unlike the medieval asylums, these hospitals treated the 'insane poor' according to the principles of moral treatment. Like Pinel before him, Jean-Etienne-Dominique Esquirol (Pinel's student and successor as physician-in-chief at the Salpêtrière Hospital in Paris) attempted a classification of mental disorders, and his resulting *Des maladies mentales, considérés sous les rapports médical, hygiénique, et médico-légal* is considered to be the first modern treatise on clinical psychiatry. Half a century later Emil Kraepelin (1856–1926) attempted another classification of mental disorders, and divided them into exogenous, curable disorders and endogenous, incurable disorders. Kraepelin is notable for having distinguished 'dementia praecox' (schizophrenia) from the affective psychoses, and for having further distinguished three clinical presentations of schizophrenia: paranoia, dominated by delusions and hallucinations; hebephrenia, dominated by inappropriate emotional reactions and behaviour; and catatonia, dominated by extreme agitation or immobility and odd mannerisms and posturing. His classification, *Compendium der Psychiatrie*, is the forerunner of modern classifications of mental disorders such as the *Diagnostic and Statistical Manual of Mental Disorders 4th Revision* (DSM-IV) and the *International Classification of Diseases 10th Revision* (ICD-10, see Chapter 2).

In the early 20th century, Karl Jaspers (1883–1969), a German psychiatrist and existentialist philosopher, brought the methods of phenomenology – the direct investigation and description of phenomena as consciously experienced – into the field of clinical psychiatry.

This so-called *descriptive psychopathology* (see Chapter 2) created a scientific basis for the practice of psychiatry, and emphasised that psychiatric symptoms should be diagnosed according to their form rather than according to their content. This means, for example, that a delusion is a delusion not because it is deemed implausible by a person in a position of authority, such as a doctor, but because it is 'an unshakeable belief held in the face of evidence to the contrary, and that cannot be explained by culture or religion'.

Sigmund Freud (1856–1939) and his disciples influenced much of 20th century psychiatry, and by the second half of the century a majority of psychiatrists in the USA (but *not* in the UK) believed that mental disorder resulted from unconscious conflicts originating in childhood. As a director of the US National Institute of Mental Health put it, 'From 1945 to 1955, it was nearly impossible for a non-psychoanalyst to become a chairman of a department or professor of psychiatry'. In the latter part of the 20th century, neuroimaging techniques, genetic studies, and pharmacological breakthroughs such as the first antipsychotic chlorpromazine reversed this psychoanalytical model of mental disorder and prompted a return to a more biological, so-called 'neo-Kraepelinian', model of mental disorder.

> There are more ideas on earth than intellectuals imagine. And these ideas are more active, stronger, more resistant, more passionate than 'politicians' think. We have to be there at the birth of ideas, the bursting outward of their force: not in books expressing them, but in events manifesting this force, in struggles carried on around ideas, for or against them. Ideas do not rule the world. But it is because the world has ideas … that it is not passively ruled by those who are its leaders or those who would like to teach it, once and for all, what it must think.
>
> Michel Foucault (1926–1984): philosopher, social anthropologist, and author of *Madness and Civilisation*, *The Birth of the Clinic*, and other books

One of Foucault's central arguments is that 'madness' is a social construct dating back to the Enlightenment, and that its 'treatment' is nothing more than a disguised form of punishment for the sort of thinking and behaviour that society finds unacceptable. He is one of the principal forerunners of the antipsychiatry movement (see Chapter 2).

At present psychiatrists recognise that several factors are involved in the aetiology of mental disorder and that different approaches to treatment should be seen not as competing but as complementary.

An introduction to Freud

> I do not break my head very much about good and evil, but I have found little that is 'good' about human beings on the whole. In my experience most of them are trash, no matter whether they publicly subscribe to this or that ethical doctrine or to none at all.
>
> S. S. Freud, from a letter to Oskar Pfister

People with a high level of anxiety have historically been referred to as 'neurotic'. The term 'neurosis' derives from the Ancient Greek *neuron* (nerve) and loosely means 'disease of the nerves'. The core feature of neurosis is anxiety, but neurosis can manifest as a range of other problems such as irritability, depression, perfectionism, obsessive–compulsive tendencies, and even personality disorders such as anankastic personality disorder. Although neurosis in some form or other is very common, it can prevent us from enjoying the moment, adapting usefully to our environment, and developing a richer, more complex, and more fulfilling outlook on life. The most original, influential, and yet contentious theory of neurosis is that of Sigmund Freud.

Freud attended medical school at the University of Vienna from 1873 to 1881, carrying out research in physiology under the German scientist Ernst von Brücke and later specialising in neurology. In 1885–1886 he spent the best part of a year in Paris, and returned to Vienna inspired by the French neurologist Jean-Martin Charcot's use of hypnosis in the treatment of 'hysteria', an old-fashioned term referring to the conversion of anxiety into physical and psychological symptoms. Freud opened a private practice for the treatment of neuropsychiatric disorders but eventually gave up the practice of hypnosis, instead preferring the method of 'free association' which involved asking patients to relax on a couch and say whatever came into their minds. In 1895, inspired by the case of a patient called Anna O, he published the seminal *Studies on Hysteria* with his friend and colleague Josef Breuer. After publishing *The Interpretation of Dreams* in 1899 and *The Psychopathology of Everyday Life* in 1901, both public successes, Freud obtained a professorship at the University of Vienna where he began to gather a devoted following. He remained a prolific writer throughout his life, publishing (afmongst others) *Three Essays on the Theory of Sexuality* in 1905, *Totem and Taboo* in 1913, and *Beyond the Pleasure Principle* in 1920. After the Nazi annexation of Austria in 1938, he fled to London, where he died the following year of cancer of the jaw. His daughter, Anna Freud, became a distinguished psychoanalyst who developed the concept of ego defence mechanisms (see Chapter 8).

In *Studies on Hysteria*, Freud and Breuer formulated the psychoanalytical theory according to which neuroses have their origins in deeply traumatic and consequently repressed experiences. Treatment requires the patient to recall these repressed experiences into consciousness and to confront them once and for all, leading to a sudden and dramatic outpouring of emotion (catharsis) and the gaining of insight. This can be achieved through the methods of free association and dream interpretation, and a relative lack of direct involvement by the psychoanalyst so as to encourage the patient to project his or her thoughts and feelings onto him or her – a process called 'transference' (by contrast, in 'countertransference' it is the psychoanalyst who projects his or her thoughts and feelings onto the patient). In the course of analysis, the patient is likely to display 'resistance' in the form of changing the topic, blanking out, falling asleep, or coming late to or missing an appointment; such behaviour merely suggests that he or she is close to recalling repressed material but is afraid of doing so. Other than dream interpretation and free association, other recognized routes into the unconscious are parapraxes (slips of the tongue) and jokes. For this reason, Freud famously noted that 'there is no such thing as a joke'.

In *The Interpretation of Dreams* (1899), Freud developed his 'topographical model' of the mind, describing the conscious, unconscious, and a layer between the two called the preconscious which, though not conscious, could be readily accessed. Freud later became dissatisfied with the topographical model and replaced it with a so-called 'structural model' according to which the mind is divided into the id, ego, and superego (Figure 1.2). The id is fully unconscious and contains our drives and repressed feelings and emotions. It is dominated by the 'pleasure principle' and so seeks out immediate gratification. The id is opposed by the partly conscious superego, a sort of moral judge arising from the internalisation of parental figures and, by extension, of society itself. In the middle

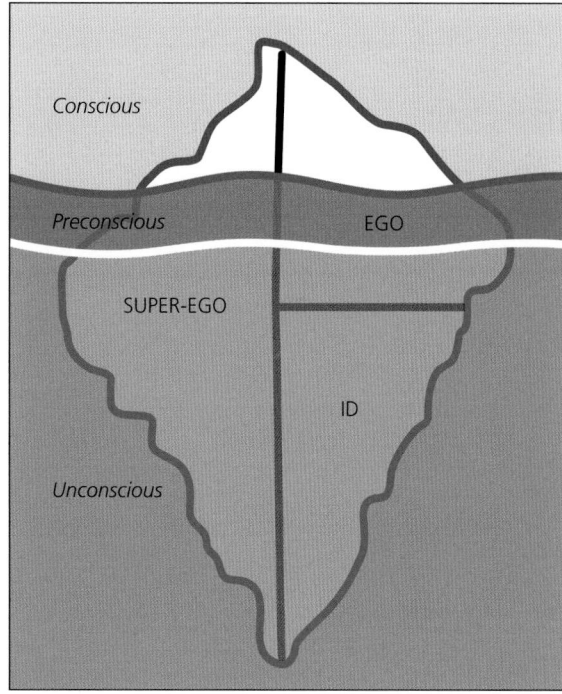

Figure 1.2 Freud's topographical and structural models of the mind.

sits the mostly conscious ego. Dominated by the 'reality principle', the function of the ego is to reconcile the id and the superego and thereby enable us to engage with reality. Neurotic anxiety arises when the ego is overwhelmed by the demands made upon it by the id, the superego, and reality. To cope with these demands, the ego employs defence mechanisms to block or distort impulses from the id, and so to make them more acceptable and less threatening. A broad range of ego defence mechanisms have since been recognised (see Chapter 8).

For Freud, the drives or instincts that motivate human behaviour ('life instinct') are primarily driven by the sex drive or *libido* (Latin, 'I desire'). This life instinct is counterbalanced by the 'death instinct', the unconscious desire to be dead and at peace (the 'Nirvana principle'). Even in children the libido is the primary motivating force, and children must progress through various stages of psychosexual development before they can reach psychosexual maturity. Each one of these stages of psychosexual development (except the latent stage) is focused on the erogenous zone – the mouth, the anus, the phallus, or the genitals – that provides the greatest pleasure at that stage.

Name	Age	Principal task
Oral stage	Birth to 18 months	Weaning
Anal stage	18 months to 3–4 years	Toilet-training
Phallic stage	3–4 years to 5–7 years	Sexual identity
Latent stage	5–7 years to puberty	Learning
Genital stage	From puberty on	Genital intercourse

Table 1.1 Freud's stages of psychosexual development.

For Freud, neuroses ultimately arise from frustrations encountered during a stage of psychosexual development, and are therefore sexual in nature. Freud's stages of psychosexual development are summarised in Table 1.1.

The Oedipus/Electra complex is arguably the most controversial of Freud's theories, and can be interpreted either literally (as Freud intended it to be) or metaphorically. According to Freud, the phallic stage gives rise to the Oedipus complex, Oedipus being a mythological King of Thebes who inadvertently killed his father and married his mother. In the Oedipus complex, a boy sees his mother as a love-object, and feels the need to compete with his father for her attention. His father becomes a threat to him and so he begins to fear for his penis ('castration anxiety'). As his father is stronger than he is, he has no choice but to displace his feelings for his mother onto other girls and to begin identifying with his father/aggressor – thereby becoming a man like him. Girls do not go through the Oedipus complex but through the Electra complex, Electra being a mythological Princess of Mycenae who wanted her brother Orestes to avenge their father's death by killing their mother. In the Electra complex, a girl this time sees her father as a love-object because she feels the need to have a baby as a substitute for the penis that she is lacking. As she discovers that her father is not available to her as a love-object, she displaces her feelings for him onto other boys and begins to identify with her mother – thereby becoming a woman like her. In either case, the main task in the phallic stage is the establishment of sexual identity.

Although much derided in his time and still today, Freud is unquestionably one of the deepest and most original thinkers of the 20th century. He is credited with discovering the unconscious and inventing psychoanalysis, and had a colossal influence not only on his field of psychiatry but also on art, literature, and the humanities. He may have been thinking of himself when he noted that, 'The voice of intelligence is soft, but it does not die until it has made itself heard' (*Die Stimme des Intellekts ist leise, aber sie ruht nicht, ehe sie sich Gehör verschafft hat*).

An introduction to Jung

To be normal is the ideal aim of the unsuccessful.
C. G. Jung (1875–1961)

Carl Gustav Jung was born in 1875 in the canton of Thurgau to Paul Jung, a poor rural pastor in the Swiss Reformed Church, and to Emilie Preiswerk, a melancholic woman who claimed to be visited by spirits at night. His paternal grandfather, Carl Gustav Jung, after whom he was named, was a physician who was rumoured to be the illegitimate son of Goethe, and who rose to become Rector of Basel University and Grand Master of the Swiss Lodge of Freemasons. His maternal grandfather, Samuel Preiswerk, was an eccentric theologian who had visions, conversed with the dead, and devoted his life to learning Hebrew in the belief that it was the language spoken in heaven. He used to make his daughter Emilie sit behind him whilst he composed his sermons, so as to prevent the devil from peering over his shoulder.

When Jung was three years old, his mother had a nervous breakdown for which she needed to spend several months in hospital. In his autobiography, *Memory, Dreams, Reflections*, he wrote, 'From then on, I always felt mistrustful when the word 'love' was spoken. The feeling I associated with 'woman' was for a long time that of innate unreliability'. His father was kind but weak-willed, and all too accepting of the religious dogma in which he had long lost all faith.

Jung was a solitary and introverted child who imagined that he had two personalities, that of a typical schoolboy of his time (Personality No 1), and that of a dignified, authoritative and influential man from the past (Personality No 2). He once carved a tiny mannequin into the end of a wooden ruler, which he kept together with a painted stone in a pencil case in his attic. He periodically returned to the mannequin, bringing to it scrolls inscribed in a secret language of his invention. Perhaps unsurprisingly, he was not popular at school. At the age of 12, he received a blow to the head and for a moment was unconscious. He lay on the ground for much longer than necessary and thought, 'Now you won't have to go to school anymore'. For the next 6 months he avoided school by fainting each time he was made to go, an experience which gave him an early insight into hysteria.

Inspired by a dream, Jung entered the University of Basel in 1895 to study natural science and medicine. His father's premature death a year later prompted his mother to comment, rather eerily, that 'He died in time for you'. During his early years at the University of Basel, Jung had a dream in which he was making painful headway through dense fog, with a tiny light in the cup of his hands and a gigantic black figure chasing after him. When he awoke he realised that the black figure was his own shadow, brought into being by the light that he was carrying, '...this light was my consciousness, the only light that I have. My own understanding is the sole treasure I possess, and the greatest'. After presenting a paper on *The Limits of the Exact Sciences*, he spent 2 years attending and recording the séances of a young medium, his cousin, Hélène Preiswerk. He submitted his observations in the form of a doctoral thesis entitled *On the Psychology and Pathology of So-Called Occult Phenomena*.

Towards the end of his studies, a reading of Krafft-Ebing's textbook of psychiatry led Jung to choose psychiatry as a career. The Preface alone had such a profound effect on him that he had to stand up to catch his breath, 'Here alone the two currents of my interest could flow together and in a united stream dig their own bed. Here was the empirical field common to biological and spiritual facts, which I had everywhere sought and nowhere found'. Jung was taken on at the renowned Burghölzli Psychiatric Hospital in Zürich as an assistant to Eugen Bleuler, who went down in history as the man who coined the term 'schizophrenia'. Bleuler set Jung to work on Galton's word-association test, and in 1906 Jung published *Studies in Word Association* which provided hard evidence for the existence of unconscious complexes. He sent a copy to Freud, and on their first meeting in Vienna the two men conversed without interruption for 13 hours.

Jung needed a father as much as Freud needed a son, and Freud formally anointed Jung his 'son and heir'. However, as time passed, it became increasingly clear that Jung was unable to accept Freud's assumptions that human motivation is exclusively sexual, or that the unconscious mind is entirely personal. For Jung, sexuality was but one aspect or mode of expression of a broader 'life force', and beneath the personal unconscious there lay a deeper and more important layer that contained the entire psychic heritage of mankind. The existence of this 'collective unconscious' had been hinted at by Jung's childhood dreams and experiences, and confirmed by the delusions and hallucinations of psychotic patients, which contained symbols and images that occurred in myths and fairy-tales from all around the world. In *Transformations and Symbols of the Libido*, Jung replaced Freud's concept of libido with a much broader concept of undifferentiated psychic energy, arguing that undifferentiated psychic energy could 'crystallise' into the universal symbols contained in dreams and myths, for example, into the hero's slaying of the dragon, which represents the struggle of the adolescent ego for deliverance from parental dominance. For Jung, the purpose of life was 'individuation', which involved pursuing one's own vision of the truth and, in so

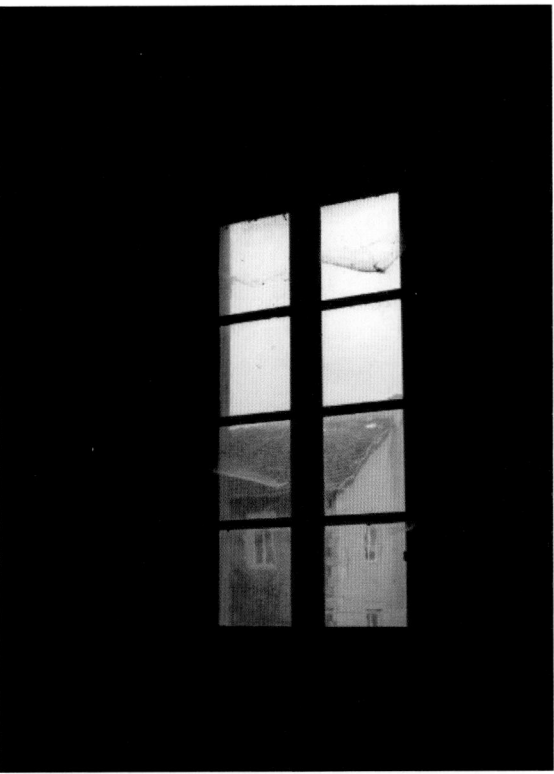

Figure 1.3 According to Jung, beneath the personal unconscious there is a deeper and more important layer called the collective unconscious, which contains the entire psychic heritage of mankind. Photo by Neel Burton.

doing, fulfilling one's fullest potential as a human being. If this meant disagreeing with Freud, then so be it. In 1913, on the eve of the First World War, Jung and Freud broke off their relationship.

Once again Jung was alone, and he spent the next few years in a troubled but highly creative state of mind that verged on psychosis and led him to a 'confrontation with the unconscious'. By then Jung had had five children with his wife Emma Rauschenbach, the daughter of a rich industrialist. Despite being happily married, he felt that he needed a muse as well as a home-maker, observing that 'the pre-requisite of a good marriage … is the licence to be unfaithful'. The marital strife that resulted from his affairs, and particularly from his affair with a former patient called Toni Wolff, contributed to his troubled state of mind, and Emma accepted Toni as much from a concern for Jung's sanity as from a desire to save her marriage.

During his confrontation with the unconscious, Jung gained first-hand experience of psychotic material in which he found a 'matrix of mythopoeic imagination which has vanished from our rational age'. Like Gilgamesh, Odysseus, Heracles, Orpheus, and Aeneas before him, he travelled deep down into an abyssal under-world where he conversed with Salome, a beautiful young woman who was the archetype of the feminine, and Philemon, an old man with a white beard and the wings of a kingfisher who was the archetype of the wise old man. Although Salome and Philemon were products of his unconscious, they had a life of their own and said things that he had not previously thought. In Philemon, Jung had at long last found the father-figure that both Freud and his own father had singularly failed to be. More than a father-figure, Philemon was a guru, and the projection of what Jung himself was later to become: the 'wise old man of Zürich'. At the end of the First World War, Jung re-emerged into sanity, and considered that he had found in his madness 'the prima materia for a lifetime's work'.

Recommended reading

The Meaning of Madness (2009) Neel Burton. Acheron Press.

Madness: A Brief History (2003) Roy Porter. Oxford University Press.

Madmen: A Social History of Mad-houses, Mad-doctors and Lunatics (2001) Roy Porter. Tempus Publishing Ltd.

A History of Psychiatry: From the Era of the Asylum to the Age of Prozac (1998) Edward Shorter. John Wiley & Sons.

What Freud Really Said (1997) David Stafford-Clark. Schocken Books.

Patient assessment

2

Key learning objectives

- To be able to carry out a psychiatric history and mental state examination
- To understand the function of the mental state examination and its relationship to the psychiatric history
- To understand the function of the formulation and its relationship to the psychiatric history and mental state examination
- To learn about the signs and symptoms of mental disorder (descriptive psychopathology)
- To learn about the key features of the ICD-10 and DSM-IV classifications of mental disorders

Descriptive psychopathology

Much of the difficulty we face in mental health, whether as users or providers of services, whether as psychiatrists, psychologists, nurses or advocates, arises from the stigmatisation of our discipline as being, somehow, an inadequate also-ran to general medicine. Well, it is easier to run up a small hill than a mountain! The scientific mountain of psychiatry is, partly, the empirical challenge of developing methods for investigating the brain. Psychiatry shares this empirical challenge with neurology. But psychiatric science, in being concerned with the higher functions (of emotion, belief, volition, and so forth), has conceptual challenges as well. These challenges start with the structure of experience and of the disturbed experiences that are the subject matter of descriptive psychopathology.

B. Fulford, T. Thornton, and G. Graham,
Oxford Textbook of Philosophy and Psychiatry

Psychiatry, 2e. By Neel Burton. Published 2010 by Blackwell Publishing.

Descriptive psychopathology brings a common language to define and recognise the signs and symptoms of mental disorder and, notably by emphasising form over content (see Chapter 1), can be seen as a scientific basis for the practice of psychiatry.

The pioneer of descriptive psychopathology was Karl Jaspers (1883–1969), a German psychiatrist and existentialist philosopher, and his *Allgemeine Psychopathologie* (General Psychopathology) of 1913 still provides the most complete account of the subject. The philosopher Edmund Husserl inspired the thought of Karl Jaspers. Husserl believed that the direct investigation and description of phenomena as consciously experienced, without theories about their causal explanation, could lead to greater insight into the essence of things.

Accordingly, one of the most important principles of descriptive psychopathology is *not* to make assumptions about the causes or consequences of signs and symptoms of mental disorder, but merely to define, differentiate, and inter-relate them. This chapter upholds this principle, and leaves the causes and consequences of mental disorder to subsequent chapters.

Etymology for descriptive psychopathology

Etymon is Ancient Greek for 'literal meaning'. Etymology helps us to understand and remember the terms used in descriptive psychopathology; most of these terms are derived from Ancient Greek, but a minority are derived from Latin, and some are French or even German. The short list provided in Table 2.1 is by no means exhaustive.

Introduction to patient assessment

Patient assessment in psychiatry is usually carried out in two parts:
1. Gathering information: the psychiatric history and mental state examination
2. Assessing and acting upon that information: the formulation.

An example of a psychiatric assessment is provided at the end of the chapter.

Table 2.1 Etymology for descriptive psychopathology.

Root term	Meaning of root term	Example of derived psychopathological term (see Tables 2.2–2.7 for definitions)
Agora	Assembly, market place	Agoraphobia
Alucinor (Latin)	To journey in the mind or dream	Hallucination
Ambi-	Both, around, about	Ambitendence
Athetos	Unfixed	Athetosis
Athron	Joint	Dysarthria
Campus (Latin)	Field	Extracampine hallucination
Choreia	Dance	Choreiform movements
Cryptos	Hidden	Cryptolalia
Eidos	Form, shape	Eidetic image
Eu	Good, easy	Euthymia
Horama	View (from *horan*, to see)	Panoramic hallucination
Hypnos	Sleep	Hypnogogic hallucination
Kinesis	Motion	Akinesia
Laleo	Talk	Echolalia, cryptolalia
Logos	Word	Neologism, logoclonia
Nihil (Latin)	Nothing	Nihilistic delusion
Opsia	Sight	Palinopsia
Palin	Again	Palinopsia, palilalia
Pathos	Emotion	Apathy
Phasis	Speech	Aphasia
Phonia	Sound, voice	Dysphonia
Praxis	Acting, doing	Dyspraxia
Pseudo-	False	Pseudohallucination
Rheos	A stream (from *rhein*, to flow)	Logorrhoea
Soma	Body	Somatic delusion
Stereos	Solid	Stereotypy
Stupere (Latin)	To be numbed or stunned	Stupor
Thumos	Temper	Euthymia, cyclothymia

The psychiatric history

In psychiatry the history is of special importance as physical examination and investigations are seldom of diagnostic value. Mention of the psychiatric history often prompts deep sighs from medical students, but **the psychiatric history is actually not very different from any other medical or surgical history**: its structure is the same, except that 'past medical history' is divided into 'past psychiatric history' and 'past medical history', and that there is an additional section for 'personal history'. 'Drug history', 'family history', 'social history', and 'personal history' are accorded a lot of importance in the psychiatric history because of their strong bearing on the aetiology, treatment, and prognosis of mental disorders.

Thus, the psychiatric history can be carried out under 10 main headings:

1. Introductory information
2. Presenting complaint and history of presenting complaint
3. Past psychiatric history
4. Past medical history
5. Drug history/current treatments
6. Substance use
7. Family history
8. Social history
9. Personal history
10. Informant history

Keep in mind that the aim of the psychiatric history is not so much to rattle through a long list of headings, as it is to facilitate the patient's telling of his or her story. A rigid and inflexible approach may damage your rapport with the patient, who may perceive you as cold and uninterested, and lacking in tact, judgement, and understanding.

The mental state examination

The mental state examination (MSE) is, strictly speaking, **a snapshot of the patient's behaviour and mental experiences at or around that point in time.** Just as an abdominal examination is used to seek out the signs of gastrointestinal disorders, so the MSE is used to seek out the signs of psychiatric disorders. In addition, the MSE is also used to seek out the **symptoms** of psychiatric disorders, and in this respect it also resembles the functional enquiry of a medical history. Being as it is part examination and part functional enquiry, the MSE relies on a firm grasp of the signs and symptoms of psychiatric disorders (descriptive psychopathology).

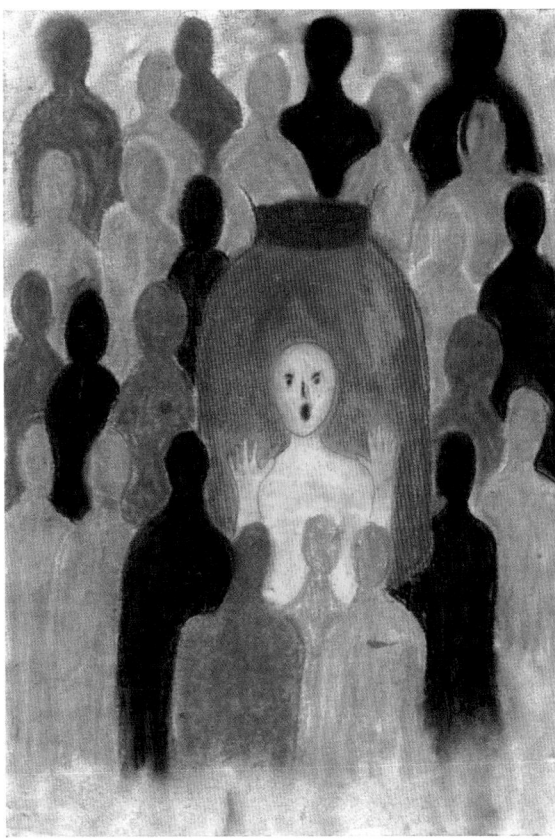

Figure 2.1 A good historian is not one who practises textbook psychiatry, but one who listens for the sake of listening, with interest, respect, and understanding. This is in itself a powerful form of therapy.

The MSE is usually carried out after the psychiatric history. Alternatively, it can be carried out during the psychiatric history, immediately after 'presenting complaint and history of presenting complaint' (an approach that often makes more sense). The MSE can be carried out under seven main headings:

1. Appearance and behaviour
2. Speech
3. Mood, plus anxiety and risk assessment
4. Thoughts
5. Perception
6. Cognition
7. Insight

The MSE's role is to ensure that all important signs and symptoms of mental disorder are screened for and fully explored. It can be considered as a 'core and module' questionnaire: simple screening questions about important psychiatric symptoms are asked, with any positive responses prompting further, in-depth questioning around the symptom(s) in question. If there are no signs or symptoms of mental disorder or if these have already been explored in the psychiatric history, the MSE is usually quick and easy to administer.

The formulation

The formulation is not just a summary of the psychiatric history and MSE, but also an assessment of the case. Like the MSE, it can be carried out under seven headings:

1. Case summary or synopsis
2. Further information required
3. Differential diagnosis
4. Risk assessment
5. Aetiology
6. Management
7. Prognosis

! Your safety

Psychiatric patients are a vulnerable group of people and, by and large, are no more likely to be violent than the average person. Nevertheless, a small minority may pose a threat to safety (see Table 2.9), and some simple precautions need to be taken. Before seeing a patient, ask a qualified member of staff if it is safe for you to do so. If the answer is yes:

- Tell the member of staff where and how long you will be
- Ask to be accompanied, e.g. by another medical student
- Carry portable alarms
- Familiarise yourselves with the interview room's alarm system (if any)
- Configure the interview room so that you are sitting closest to the exit
- At the same time, ensure that you are not blocking the patient's escape route.

Think of the bigger picture and trust your instinct. If you feel unsafe in any given situation, calmly and politely excuse yourself from it: **never feel obliged to put yourself at risk.**

Clinical skills: Open, closed, and leading questions

Open question: *How are you feeling?*
Closed question: *Are there times when you feel tearful?*
Leading question: *You're depressed, aren't you?*

Note: Closed questions are sometimes necessary, but leading questions should never be asked.

The psychiatric history

Introductory information

Before introducing yourself to the patient, note his or her:

- Age, sex, occupation, ethnic/cultural background
- Mode of referral and the reason for the referral
- Mental Health Act status if detained under a Section of the Mental Health Act (see Chapter 3).

Presenting complaint and history of presenting complaint

- After putting the patient at ease, begin with an open question such as,
  Why have you come to see me today?
  How are you?
  What's going on?
  In general, try to use open questions rather than leading questions or closed questions. Then listen. Never underestimate the power of listening. In normal conversation people tend to talk at each other, or past each other, but rarely if ever *to* each other.
- Record the patient's principal complaints verbatim. For example,
  I have a feeling of unreality, that people are conspiring to make life seem normal when in actual fact it's unreal,
  is much better than,
  The patient complains of derealisation.
- Establish the precise nature of the symptoms, including:
  – Onset and progression
  – Possible precipitating and perpetuating factors
  – Effect on everyday life
  – Treatments so far.
- Use the logico-deductive approach rather than the exhaustive approach to history taking: that is, instead of asking about everything under the sun, form a diagnostic hypothesis in your mind and try to validate or falsify it by asking discriminating questions. For example, if you think that a patient might be depressed because he lost his job three months ago and complains of feeling tired all the time, ask about other symptoms of depression such as low mood, loss of interest, poor concentration, poor self-esteem, guilt, pessimism, sleep disturbance, loss of appetite or weight, and loss of libido.

Past psychiatric history

- Nature, date, and duration of previous episodes of mental disorder
- Names of doctors and hospitals
- Nature, date, and duration of any treatments received
- Dates of any hospital admissions (specify if voluntary or under a Section of the Mental Health Act)
- Outcomes
- History of self-harm
- History of harm to others

Past medical history

- Current comorbid illness:
  - Acute illness
  - Chronic illness
  - Epilepsy
  - Head injury
  - Vascular risk factors
- Past and childhood illnesses
- Surgery
- Menstrual and obstetric history (in the context of the presenting complaint)

Drug history/current treatments

- Psychological treatments
- Prescribed medication: dosage, regimen, route, side-effects and longer term complications, compliance
- Recent changes in prescribed medication (an important and often overlooked factor)
- Over-the-counter or alternative remedies, e.g. St John's wort (*Hypericum perforatum*, for depression), kava (*Piper methysticum*, for anxiety), valerian (*Valeriana officinalis*, for insomnia), or *Ginkgo biloba* (for memory)
- Allergies and adverse reactions

Substance use

- Alcohol
- Tobacco
- Illicit drugs, such as cannabis, LSD, ecstasy, amphetamines, cocaine or heroin

Further questioning to elicit the features of dependence syndrome is required if alcohol or drug use is high (see Chapter 11).

Family history

- Determine if anyone in the family is suffering from or has suffered from mental disorder or alcohol or drug dependency. Did they respond to treatment? Start with a question such as,
  Has anyone in the family ever had problems like the ones you've been having?
  Has anyone in the family ever had a nervous breakdown?
- Partners: age or age at death, occupation, health
- Children: age or age at death, occupation, health
- Quality of relationships and atmosphere at home
- Recent events in the family

Use an annotated family tree or genogram if the family history is both complex and relevant (Figure 2.2).

Social history

- Self-care
- Family and social support
- Housing
- Finances
- Typical day
- Interests and hobbies
- Predominant mood and premorbid personality

Clinical skills: Assessment of premorbid personality

Information about premorbid personality can be gained from:

- General questions about personality,
  How would you describe your normal self?
  How would others describe you?
- 'Situational' questions about personality,
  Do you prefer being alone or surrounded by other people?
  How do you cope in a difficult situation? (Use examples from the history so far)
- Social history/personal history
- Informant histories
- Personality inventories: personality inventories such as the 16 Personality Factor Questionnaire (16PF) and the Minnesota Multiphasic Personality Inventory (MMPI) are seldom used in routine clinical practice

NB: It is important to focus on the patient's personality before he or she became ill, and to tease this apart from his or her current mental state.

You can try out a number of personality tests at http://similarminds.com. Remember to be as honest as possible in your responses.

2

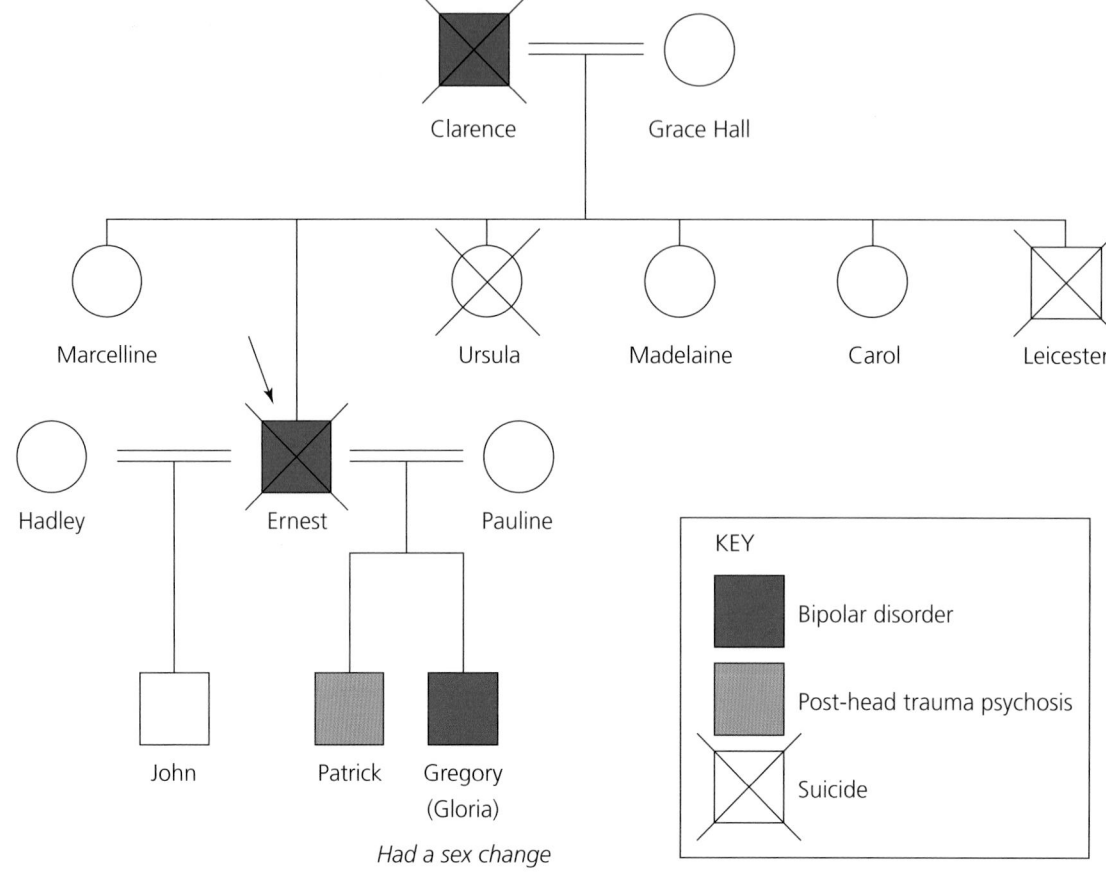

Figure 2.2 Family tree for Ernest Hemingway. (Adapted from Kay Redfield Jamison (1996) *Touched with Fire: Manic Depressive Illness and the Artistic Temperament.* Simon and Schuster.)

Personal history

- Pregnancy and birth
- Developmental milestones
- Childhood: emotional problems, serious illnesses, prolonged separation from parents, bullying
- Educational achievement: academic record, learning disabilities, special education classes. Did the patient enjoy school?
- Occupational history: jobs in chronological order, reasons for changes, current job satisfaction, military service
- Psychosexual history: past and present partners (including same-sex partners), quality of relationships, frequency of sexual intercourse, sexual problems, contraception, physical and sexual abuse

- Forensic history: charges, convictions, imprisonment. A good question to ask is,
  Have you ever had problems with the police?
- Religious orientation and mores. Good questions are,
  Do you believe that there is something beyond us, like God?
  Is religion important to you?

Before closing, use an enjoinder such as,
You've told me a lot about yourself, thank you. Is there anything else that you'd like to mention?

Informant history

If possible, the history from the patient should be supplemented by information from (usually) a close relative or carer. Such informant histories are particularly useful if the patient is unable to give a clear or full history, is lacking in insight, is cognitively impaired, or is under the influence of drugs or alcohol. Informant histories are also opportunities for assessing the attitudes of relatives and carers to the patient and to involve them in the treatment plan. Remember to seek consent from the patient before taking an informant history.

The mental state examination

In this section, descriptive psychopathology is integrated into the MSE in an effort to encourage direct reference to its subject: the signs and symptoms of mental disorder. Note that common and important signs and symptoms are in *italics*; the rest are included mainly for interest.

Recall that the MSE can be carried out under seven main headings:
1. Appearance and behaviour
2. Speech
3. Mood, plus anxiety and risk assessment
4. Thoughts
5. Perception
6. Cognition
7. Insight.

Appearance and behaviour

How are you? You have been in Afghanistan, I perceive.
Sherlock Holmes, *A Study in Scarlet*

Note the following:
- Level of consciousness, e.g. hyperalert/vigilant, alert, somnolent
- Appearance: body build, posture, general physical condition, grooming and hygiene, dress, physical stigmata such as scars, piercings, and tattoos. Remember that scars result not just from accidents and surgical operations, but also – and importantly – from deliberate self-harm
- Behaviour and attitude to the examiner. In particular note: facial expression, degree of eye contact, quality of rapport
- Motor activity/disorders of movement (Table 2.2). Disorders of movement that affect induced movements and posture tend to be associated with catatonic schizophrenia, which is relatively rare.

Clinical skills: Differentiating between catatonia, catalepsy, and cataplexy

Catatonia A motor syndrome diagnosed by the presence of two or more of the following:
- Motor immobility
- Motor excitement
- Negativism or mutism
- Posturing, stereotypies or mannerisms
- Echolalia or echopraxia.

Catalepsy A feature of catatonia in which the limbs can be placed in any posture and maintained thereafter for unusually long periods of time. Catalepsy is also referred to as waxy flexibility or *cerea flexibilitas*.

Cataplexy A sudden loss of muscle tone that leads to collapse. Cataplexy is a feature of the sleep disorder narcolepsy, and is thus completely unrelated to either catatonia or catalepsy.

Speech

Guard your roving thoughts with a jealous care, for speech is but the dealer of thoughts, and every fool can plainly read in your words what is the hour of your thoughts.
Alfred, Lord Tennyson (1809–1892)

A person's speech mirrors his or her thoughts, but under 'speech' you should limit yourself to recording the technical aspects of speech. The **content** of speech is more appropriately described under 'thoughts'.

Note the following:
- Amount, rate, volume, and tone of speech (Table 2.3)
- **Form** of speech (Table 2.3).

Mood

Record the following:
- Current mood and severity. Good screening questions for depression are,
  Have you been keeping reasonably cheerful?
  Are there times when you feel low-spirited or tearful?
  Good screening questions for mania are:
  Have you been feeling particularly cheerful?
  Have you been feeling on top of the world?
  If there is the suggestion of a mood disorder, this should be explored further (see Chapter 5). Note that it

2

Table 2.2 Descriptive psychopathology: disorders of movement.

Amount of movement

Agitation (hyperkinesia) — Excessive motor activity and restlessness, e.g. fidgeting or pacing

Retardation (bradykinesia) — Lack of motor activity; the opposite of agitation

Stupor — An extreme form of retardation such that the patient is immobile and mute

Abnormalities of movement

Spontaneous movements

Mannerism — Odd, repetitive, and goal-directed movement, e.g. hand brushing hair, pulling up socks (cf. stereotypy)

Stereotypy — Odd, repetitive, but non-goal-directed movement, e.g. body rocking, head banging

Tic — Involuntary, sudden, rapid, recurrent, non-rhythmic, stereotyped movement or vocalisation

Static tremor — Resting tremor that is usually attenuated by deliberate movement.

Dystonia — Spasm of muscle groups most commonly affecting the neck, eyes, and trunk, e.g. tongue protrusion, grimacing, torticollis

Akathisia — Subjective feeling of inner restlessness manifested by fidgety leg movements, shuffling of feet, pacing, etc

Dyskinesia — Involuntary, repetitive, purposeless movements of the tongue, lips, face, trunk, and extremities that may be generalised or affect only certain muscle groups, typically the orofacial muscle groups ('rabbit syndrome')

Athetosis — Slow semi-rotatory and writhing movements of the limbs

Myoclonus — Sudden, jerky, and involuntary movement of a muscle or group of muscles

Chorea — Sudden, jerky, and involuntary movements of several muscle groups that resemble fragments of goal-directed behaviour

Induced movements

Advertence/aversion — Turning towards/away from the examiner in an exaggerated way when talking to him or her

Forced grasping — Repetitive grasping and shaking of the examiner's preferred hand despite requests not to

Echopraxia — Imitation of the examiner's body movements despite requests not to

Perseveration — Repetition of a movement or behaviour requested by the examiner even after it is no longer appropriate

Automatic obedience — Indiscriminate obedience of the examiner's commands regardless of their consequences

Blocking — Interruption of a movement before it can be completed

Obstruction — Irregular blocking of movements

Ambitendence — Alternation of opposite movements, e.g. putting out a hand and then pulling it back again before the action can be fully completed

Mitmachen — In mitmachen the limbs can be placed in any posture, after which they return to their resting position (cf. mitgehen, catalepsy)

Mitgehen — An extreme form of mitmachen: the limbs can be placed in any posture even at a slight touch

Abnormalities of posture

Posturing — Voluntary assumption and maintenance of unusual and uncomfortable body postures, often for hours on end. Includes 'psychological pillow' in which the patient lies prone with the head raised a few centimetres

Catalepsy (waxy flexibility) — In catalepsy the limbs can be placed in any posture and maintained thereafter for unusually long periods of time

Rigidity — Maintenance of a rigid posture against attempts to be moved

Gegenhalten — Involuntary resistance to passive movement

Negativism — Extreme form of gegenhalten involving resistance to instructions or attempts to be moved, or movement in the opposite direction

Table 2.3 Descriptive psychopathology: disorders of speech.

Ability for speech

Dysphonia	Impairment of ability to vocalise speech
Dysarthria	Impairment of ability to articulate speech
Dysphasia	Impairment of ability to comprehend or express language

Amount of speech

Logorrhoea	Increased quantity (but not rate) of speech
Poverty of speech	Decreased quantity (but not rate) of speech

Rate of speech

Pressure of speech	Increased quantity and rate of speech; speech is difficult to interrupt
Speech retardation	Decreased quantity and rate of speech
Mutism	Failure to speak despite the physical ability to do so

Form of speech

Circumstantiality	Speech is organised and goal-oriented but cramped by excessive or irrelevant detail and parenthetical remarks (Figure 2.3)
Tangentiality	Speech is organised but not goal-oriented in that it is only very indirectly related to the questions being asked (Figure 2.3)
Neologism	Use of a new word or condensed combination of words
Metonym	Use of an existing word with a new meaning
Clang association	Linkage of words based on sound rather than meaning
Word salad (schizophasia)	Loss of associations between words, speech is experienced as an incoherent jumble of words
Paragrammatism	Incorrect grammatical construction, e.g. *I eaten have apples four*
Paraphasia	Incorrect selection of words, the production of one word when another is meant
Logoclonia	Repetition of the last syllable of every word
Palilalia	Repetition of a word after it is no longer appropriate
Verbigeration	Senseless repetition of sounds, words, or phrases
Echolalia	Senseless and parrot-like imitation of the examiner's speech (cf. echopraxia)
Coprolalia	Vocal tic involving the shouting of obscenities (!)
Glossolalia	Use of non-speech sounds as a substitute for speech
Cryptolalia	Use of an entire private idiom or language
Pseudologica fantastica (mythomania)	Fluent and plausible lying
Vorbeireden (Ganser symptom)	Approximate answers to the questions being asked, e.g. *How many legs does a chair have? – Three*, thereby demonstrating that the question has been understood

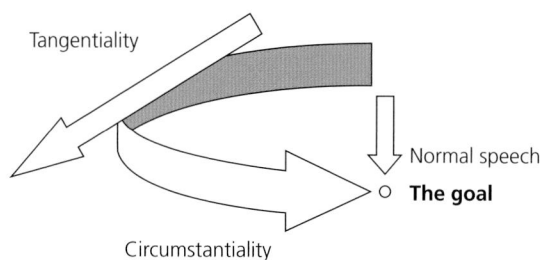

Figure 2.3 Normal speech, circumstantiality, and tangentiality.

is customary to report both '**subjective mood**' (the patient's report of his or her mood) and '**objective mood**' (the examiner's impression of the patient's mood).

- Affect, e.g. expansive, normal, constricted, blunted, flat, inappropriate, labile.
- Ideas of self-harm and suicide. If you haven't done so already, **you must ask about ideas of self-harm and suicide.** This can feel uncomfortable. Use a formulation such as,

People with problems similar to those that you have been describing often feel that life is no longer worth living. Have you felt that life is no longer worth living?

If yes, this should be explored further (see Chapter 6). **Asking about suicide is very unlikely to suggest the idea to the patient**

- Ideas of harm to others.
- Anxiety and anxiety symptoms, e.g. butterflies, giddiness, clamminess, palpitations, difficulty catching breath. A good screening question for anxiety is,

Are there times when you become very anxious or frightened?

If there is the suggestion of an anxiety disorder, this should be explored further (see Chapter 7).

Disorders of mood are listed in Table 2.4.

The philosopher JS Mill on anhedonia

It was the autumn of 1826. I was in a dull state of nerves, such as everybody is occasionally liable to; unsusceptible to enjoyment or pleasurable excitement; one of those moods when what is pleasure at other times, becomes insipid or indifferent … In this frame of mind it occurred to me to put the question directly to myself, 'suppose that all your objects in life were realised; that all the changes in institutions and opinions which you are looking forward to, could be completely effected at this very instant: would this be a great joy and happiness to you?' And an irrepressible self-consciousness distinctly answered, 'No!' At this my heart sank within me: the whole foundation on which my life was constructed fell down.

J. S. Mill, *Autobiography*

Table 2.4 Descriptive psychopathology: disorders of mood.

Mood	A pervasive and sustained emotional state such as anxiety, depression, or euphoria
Affect	Observable *behaviour* that results from changing emotions such as joy, sadness, or fear
	NB: Affect is to mood as weather is to climate
Emotional predispositions	
Euthymia	Normal mood
Dysthymia	A predominantly depressive temperament, chronic mild depression
Hyperthymia	A predominantly euphoric temperament, chronic hypomania
Cyclothymia	Chronic mild bipolar disorder: alternating periods of mild depression and hypomania
Emotional reactions	
Anxiety	A sense of apprehension at a perceived threat
Irritability	A state of reduced control over aggressive impulses
Depression	Depressed mood and other symptoms
Anhedonia	The loss of the capacity to experience pleasure from previously pleasurable activities
Euphoria	Undue cheerfulness and elation
Ecstasy (oceanic experience)	A pantheistic experience that the subject and the universe are one
Apathy	A lack or absence of emotion, interest, or concern
Expression of emotions	
Blunting/flattening of affect	Dulling of normal emotional responses and insensitivity to the emotions of others
Emotional lability	Sudden, rapid shifts in affect. Behaviour appears disproportionate to feelings
Emotional incontinence	Complete loss of control over affect, an extreme form of emotional lability
Dissociation of affect	Affect is inappropriate to thought content, e.g. laughter upon recounting the death of a loved one
Incongruity of affect	Affect is inappropriate to magnitude of events, such that an important event leaves the patient emotionless, but a small and insignificant event produces an emotional outburst
Perplexity	Anxious and puzzled bewilderment

Thought

Record the following:

- Stream of thought
- Form of thought
- Content of thought:
  - Phobias. For a phobia, record the stimulus, its psychological and physiological effects, and the nature and extent of any avoidance behaviour. A good screening question might be,

    Do you have any special fears, like some people are afraid of spiders or snakes?

  - Preoccupations, ruminations, obsessions. For an obsession, determine the underlying fear, the degree of resistance to the intrusive thoughts, and their effect on everyday life. Is the obsession perceived as being senseless? Is it accompanied by compulsive acts? A good screening question for obsessions might be,

    Do certain things keep coming into your mind, even though you try hard to keep them out?

and for compulsive acts,

Do you ever find yourself spending a lot of time doing the same thing over and over again, even though you've already done it well enough?

- Delusions and overvalued ideas. For obvious reasons, you cannot easily ask directly about delusions. Begin with an introductory statement and general questions such as,

  I would like to ask you some questions that might seem a little bit strange. These are questions that we ask to everyone who comes to see us. Is that all right with you?
  Do you have any ideas that your friends and family do not share?

  Then, if you feel that this is necessary, ask specifically about common delusional themes (Table 2.5 and see box, p. 64). For example, for delusions of control ask,

  Is someone or something trying to control you?
  Is someone or something trying to interfere with your thoughts?

Disorders of thought are listed in Table 2.6.

Reflecting upon the definition of a delusion

'... an unshakeable (fixed) belief that is held in the face of evidence to the contrary, and that cannot be explained by culture or religion ...'

There are fictions when the society supports you, there are fictions when nobody supports you. That is the difference between a sane and an insane person; a sane person is one whose fiction is supported by the society. He has manipulated the society to support his fiction. An insane man is one whose fiction is supported by nobody; he is alone so you have to put him in the madhouse.

Reportedly said by Bhagwan Shree Rajneesh (1931–1990), quoted from Anthony Storr, *Feet of Clay: A Study of Gurus* (1997), HarperCollins

The antipsychiatry movement

The antipsychiatry movement took hold in the 1960s and early 1970s. Spearheaded by Thomas Szasz (1920–, author of *The Myth of Mental Illness*) and others, it claimed that severe mental disorder, especially schizophrenia, was little more than an attempt to medicalise and thereby control socially undesirable behaviour. Attractive though it may originally have seemed, this claim has been seriously undermined by the increasing evidence for a biological basis of severe mental disorder.

Table 2.5 Delusional themes.

Delusions of control	Delusions that one's thoughts, feelings, or actions are being replaced by those of an external agency. Types of delusion of control are: ● Thought insertion ● Thought withdrawal ● Thought broadcasting ● Passivity of affect, volition, or actions ● Somatic passivity These are all first-rank symptoms of schizophrenia (see Chapter 4)
Delusions of persecution	Delusions that one is being persecuted, e.g. being spied upon by secret services or being poisoned by aliens
Delusions of reference	Delusions that objects, events, or other persons have a special significance pertaining to the self, e.g. receiving a series of coded messages from the aliens through a radio programme. See 'idea of reference' in Table 2.6
Delusions of misidentification	● Capgras' syndrome is the delusion that a familiar individual has been replaced by an identical-looking imposter ● Fregoli syndrome is the delusion that a familiar individual is disguising as various strangers ● Intermetamorphosis is the delusion that a familiar individual has been transformed into another person ● Reverse intermetamorphosis is the delusion that one has been transformed into another person ● Subjective doubles or *Doppelgangers* is the delusion that there is a double of oneself or *Doppelgangers*: in 'clonal pluralisation', there is more than just one *Doppelganger* ● Reduplicative paramnesia is the delusion that an object, place, or person has been multiplied ● Delusional companions is the delusion that objects are sentient beings, as in children's cartoons
Delusions of grandeur	Delusions of being invested with special status, a special purpose, or special abilities, e.g. being the most intelligent person on earth and being responsible for saving it from the effects of climate change
Religious delusions	Delusions of having a special relationship with God or a supernatural force, e.g. being the next messiah, or being persecuted by the devil
Delusions of guilt	Delusions that one has committed a serious crime, or has sinned greatly, or otherwise deserves punishment, e.g. being personally responsible for an earthquake or a terrorist attack
Nihilistic delusions	Delusions that one no longer exists or that one is about to die or suffer a personal catastrophe. In some cases there may be a belief that other people or objects no longer exist or that the world is coming to an end. The combination of nihilistic and/or somatic delusions in depressive psychosis is sometimes referred to as *délire de négation* or Cotard's syndrome, after the 19th century French psychiatrist Jules Cotard
Somatic delusions	Delusions about the body, e.g. of having a medical condition or deformity. Also referred to as hypochondriacal delusions. (Cf. somatoform disorder, factitious disorder, malingering; see box, p. 128)
Delusions of infestation (delusional parasitosis)	Delusion that one's skin is infested by parasites; in the context of a monosymptomatic delusional disorder, this is referred to as Ekbom's syndrome
Delusions of jealousy	Delusions of the infidelity of a spouse/partner; in the context of a monosymptomatic delusional disorder, this is referred to as Othello syndrome
Delusions of love (amorous delusions)	Delusions of being loved by someone who is inaccessible or with whom one has little contact. Erotomania or De Clérambault's syndrome (named after French psychiatrist Gaëtan Gatian de Clérambault, author of *Les Psychoses Passionelles*) is the delusion of being secretly loved, usually by someone of a higher social status. Delusions of love are more common in women whereas delusions of jealousy are more common in men, hinting that delusional themes may have some basis in human evolution

Table 2.6 Descriptive psychopathology: disorders of thought.

Stream of thought

Pressure of thought	Thoughts arise in unusual variety and abundance and pass through the mind quickly; this is experienced as pressure of speech
Poverty of thought	The opposite of pressure of thought; experienced as poverty of speech
Thought blocking	Sudden loss of the train of thought, often in mid-sentence. There is a subjective experience of the mind just 'going blank'

Form of thought

Flight of ideas	Thoughts move quickly from one idea to another and seem to be only loosely connected (e.g. by clang association, punning, or rhyming)
Loosening of associations	Thoughts move quickly from one idea to another but seem not to be connected at all. This is experienced as muddled or illogical speech
Over-inclusive thinking	An inability to preserve the conceptual boundaries of thought. This is experienced as circumstantiality
Concrete thinking	An inability to understand abstract concepts and metaphorical ideas, e.g. having a literal understanding of sayings and proverbs
Dereistic thinking	Idiosyncratic thinking that is not being falsified by reality, e.g. day-dreaming

Content of thought

Phobia	Persistent irrational fear producing conscious avoidance of the feared object, activity, or situation
Rumination	Repetitive and pointless internal debates that often involve pseudo-philosophical issues
Obsessional thought	A recurrent idea, image, or impulse that is perceived as being senseless, that is unsuccessfully resisted, and that results in marked anxiety and distress
Delusion	An unshakeable (fixed) belief that is held in the face of evidence to the contrary, and that cannot be explained by culture or religion. Although a delusion is not necessarily false, the process by which it arises is bizarre and illogical. A delusion can be primary or secondary: <ul><li>*Primary delusion* (autochthonous delusion, delusional intuition, apophany): fully formed delusion that is unconnected to previous ideas or events and that is psychologically irreducible</li><li>*Secondary delusion*: delusion that arises from, and that is understandable in context of, previous ideas or events</li><li>*Systematised delusions*: a group of delusions organised around a common theme, or multiple elaborations of a single delusion</li></ul>
Delusional perception	The attribution of delusional significance to normal percepts
Delusional memory	The attribution of delusional significance to a memory or false memory
Delusional mood or atmosphere	A delusion arising after a period during which the world seems subtly altered, uncanny, portentous, or sinister
Overvalued idea	An idiosyncratic and firmly held belief which is in itself acceptable and comprehensible but which comes to dominate thinking and behaviour. It differs from a delusion in that the belief is not fixed, and from an obsessional thought in that it is not perceived as being senseless
Idea of reference	The feeling that causal incidents and external events are referring directly to oneself, e.g. the feeling that people on the radio are talking to or about oneself. If this feeling becomes a fixed belief, it is then called a delusion of reference
Magical thinking	An irrational (but not delusional) belief that certain outcomes are connected to certain thoughts, words, or actions, e.g. if I hold my nose, someone will die
Folie à deux	Shared psychotic disorder: one person (the principal) communicates his delusion to another person (the associate) so that he too becomes psychotic

2

Perception

Note the following:

- Sensory distortions. A good screening question is,
  Have you noticed anything unusual about the way things look or sound, or smell, or taste?
- Illusions and hallucinations. Begin by an introductory statement and general questions such as,
  I gather that you have been under quite some stress recently. When people are under stress they sometimes find that their imagination plays tricks on them. Does that ring true for you?
  Have you seen/heard things which are unusual?
  Have you seen things which other people cannot see?
  Have you heard voices when there was no one around?
  If hallucinations are present record their modality, content, and mood congruency. Exclude pseudo-hallucinations and hypnopompic and hypnogogic hallucinations, which can all occur in the absence of a mental illness. For auditory hallucinations of voices, determine if there is more than one voice, and if the voices talk to the patient (second person) or about the patient (third person). Do the voices command the patient to do dangerous things and, importantly, is the patient likely to act on these commands? Patients are sometimes offended by questions about hallucinations so it is important to exercise tact and judgement in asking about them (see box, p. 65).

- Depersonalisation and derealisation. Good screening questions to ask are,
  Have you ever felt distant or unreal?
  Have you ever felt that things around you are unreal?
  Disorders of perception are listed in Table 2.7.

Table 2.7 Descriptive psychopathology: disorders of perception.

Sensory distortions	Sensory distortions include distortions of intensity, colour, form, and proportions
Illusion	A percept that arises as a misinterpretation of a stimulus (Figure 2.4), e.g. hearing voices in rustling leaves
Affect illusion	Illusions that arise during periods of heightened emotion
Completion illusion	Illusions that arise during periods of inattention
Paraidolic illusion	Illusions that arise from poorly defined stiimuli, e.g. seeing 'shapes' in the clouds
Hallucinations	A percept that arises in the absence of a stimulus. The percept is experienced as arising from the sense organs (outer space) and not from the mind (inner space), and is equal in quality to a real perception
Auditory hallucinations	
Simple	Simple sounds
Complex	Complex sounds, e.g. voices, music. Voices may be in the second person (you, addressing the patient directly) or in the third person (he/she, talking about the patient). In a command hallucination (imperative hallucination, teleological hallucination), the voice or voices tell the patient to do something.
Gedankenlautwerden	German for 'thoughts becoming loud': thoughts are 'heard' as they are being formulated (cf. thought broadcasting and *echo de la pensée*)
Echo de la pensée	French for 'thought echo': thoughts are 'heard' shortly after they are formulated
Visual hallucinations	
Simple	Flashes of light
Complex	Images of objects, animals, people
Panoramic hallucination	Images of objects, animals, people – plus the background
Lilliputian hallucination	Images of objects, animals, people that are smaller than in reality (according to Jonathan Swift, the inhabitants of the fictional island of Lilliput are six inches tall)
Eidetic image	Unusually vivid mental image of an object, e.g. flashbacks, 'photographic memory'
Charles Bonnet syndrome	Isolated, complex visual hallucinations, usually secondary to sudden loss of vision
Autoscopic hallucination	Image of the self is projected into external space. Differs from a near-death experience in that it does not involve a feeling of being outside the body
Negative autoscopy	Image of the self cannot be seen in mirrors (!)
Olfactory and gustatory hallucinations	Olfactory and gustatory hallucinations may be difficult to differentiate from each other. They are usually of unpleasant odours/flavours

2

Table 2.7 Continued

Specific types of hallucination	
Hypnopompic hallucination	Visual or auditory hallucinations on awakening
Hypnogogic hallucination	Visual or auditory hallucinations on going to sleep
Extracampine hallucination	Hallucinations outside the limits of the sensory field, e.g. hearing voices from Antarctica
Functional hallucination	A hallucination triggered by an environmental stimulus in the same modality, e.g. hallucinatory voices triggered by the sound of a running tap
Reflex hallucination	A hallucination triggered by an environmental stimulus in a different modality, e.g. a *visual* hallucination triggered by the sound of a running tap
Synaesthesia	In synaesthesia sensations in one mode produce sensations in another mode; for example, a piece of music is experienced as a concert of colours. The French poet Arthur Rimbaud's 'Voyelles' is a poem about synaesthesia. Other artists to experiment with synaesthesia include Charles Baudelaire (poet), Wassily Kandinsky (painter), and Alexander Scriabin (composer)
Palinopsia	The persistence or recurrence of an image long after its stimulus has been removed
Pseudo-hallucinations	A pseudo-hallucination may differ from a true hallucination in that: ● It is perceived to arise from the mind (inner space) rather than from the sense organs (outer space) ● It is less vivid ● It is less distressing ● The patient may have some degree of control over it
Depersonalisation	An alteration in the perception or experience of the self, leading to a sense of detachment from one's mental processes or body processes or body
Derealisation	An alteration in the perception or experience of the environment, leading to a sense that it is strange or unreal

Clinical skills: Speaking to a patient about his psychotic symptoms

In speaking to a patient with psychotic symptoms, you should avoid challenging his or her delusions and hallucinations, but at the same time you should not validate them either. This difficult balance is best achieved by explicitly recognising that the patient's delusions and hallucinations are important to him or her, yet implicitly making it clear that you (personally) regard them as symptoms of mental disorder. For example,

Patient: *The aliens are telling me that they are going to abduct me tonight.*
Doctor: *That sounds terribly frightening.*
Patient: *I've never felt so frightened in all my life.*
Doctor: *I can understand that you feel frightened, although I myself cannot hear the aliens that you speak of.*
Patient: *You mean, you can't hear them?*
Doctor: *No, not at all. Have you tried ignoring them?*
Patient: *If I listen to my iPod then they don't seem so loud, and I don't feel so frightened.*
Doctor: *What about when we talk together, like now?*
Patient: *That's very helpful too.*

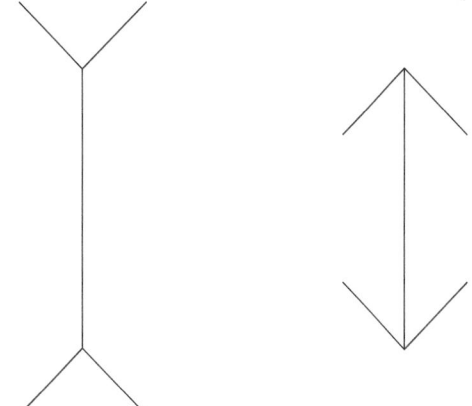

Figure 2.4 The Müller–Lyer illusion arises from the misinterpretation of a stimulus: both lines are in actual fact the same length. In contrast, a hallucination arises in the absence of a stimulus.

2

Cognition

Record the following:
- Orientation in time, place, and person
- Attention and concentration, e.g. serial sevens test (ask the patient to subtract 7 from 100 and to keep on going). Record time taken and number of errors
- Memory:
  - Short-term memory
  - Recent memory
  - Remote memory
  - Grasp, e.g. name the prime-minister and reigning monarch.

If cognitive impairment is suspected, you may carry out the 30-point Folstein Mini-Mental State Examination. Scores of less than 22 out of 30 are indicative of significant cognitive impairment, scores of 22–25 are indicative of moderate cognitive impairment. The result is invalid if the patient is delirious or suffering from an affective disorder.

Insight

To determine degree of insight, ask the patient,
Do you think there is anything wrong with you?
If no,
Why did you come to hospital?
If yes,
What do you think is wrong with you?
What do you think the cause of it is?
Do you think you need treatment?
What are you hoping treatment will do for you?

The formulation

The formulation is not just a synopsis of the psychiatric history and MSE, but an assessment of the case. Like the MSE, it can be carried out under seven headings:
1. Case summary or synopsis
2. Further information required
3. Differential diagnosis
4. Risk assessment
5. Aetiology
6. Management
7. Prognosis

Case summary and synopsis

This should be a short paragraph summarising the salient points of the history and MSE.

Further information required

Consider:
- Full psychiatric history and mental state examination
- Informant history/histories from, for example, relatives, friends, carers, the patient's GP
- Old records, e.g. medical notes, school or employer reports, police record
- Physical examination:
  - To exclude organic causes of the presentation, e.g. endocrine disorder, space-occupying lesion
  - To exclude complications of the presentation e.g. malnutrition, burns, falls, DSH
  - As a baseline for starting psychotropic medication
- Laboratory investigations (at a minimum: FBC, U&Es, LFTs, TFTs, glucose, and lipids) for the same reasons as under Physical examination above
- Brain imaging (CT or MRI head), particularly if the presentation is atypical or if there is evidence of an organic, neurological cause
- Psychological tests and inventories.

Clinical skills: The role of the physical examination in psychiatry

Psychiatrists take responsibility for the physical health of their day- and in-patients, and an integral physical examination (vital signs, examination of the cardiovascular system, examination of the respiratory system, abdominal examination, and neurological examination) should be carried out on all such patients. Medical disorders are more common in psychiatric patients and may arise from a shared aetiology, from a direct or indirect consequence of psychiatric disorder, or from psychotropic drugs. In certain cases, they may actually underlie psychiatric signs and symptoms. For example, depressive symptoms may result from endocrine disorders (e.g. hypothyroidism, Cushing's syndrome), metabolic disorders (e.g. hypercalcaemia, vitamin B_{12} deficiency), infective disorders (e.g. hepatitis, HIV/AIDS), neurological disorders (e.g. stroke, Parkinson's disease), or alcohol and drugs. A physical examination is thus a crucial element of the psychiatric assessment.

Differential diagnosis

List *likely* diagnoses in order of probability, and make a brief note of the evidence for and against each diagnosis. Think about both the psychiatric and the organic differential so that you do not miss anything out:

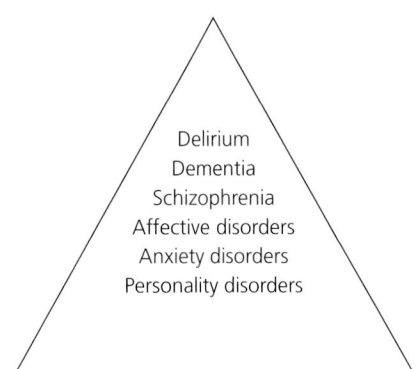

Figure 2.5 Playing trumps: the diagnostic hierarchy.

- Psychiatric differential:
  – Psychotic disorder
  – Mood disorder
  – Anxiety disorder
  – Personality disorder
- Organic differential:
  – Substance misuse
  – Dementia and delirium
  – Medical condition, e.g. endocrine disorder, space-occupying lesion, etc.

Diagnoses that are higher up in the diagnostic hierarchy (Figure 2.5) should take precedence over those that are lower down. For example, if a patient meets the diagnostic criteria for all of schizophrenia, depression, and an anxiety disorder, the diagnosis of schizophrenia takes precedence over the diagnoses of depression and anxiety disorder because affective symptoms and anxiety symptoms are common in schizophrenia and often improve if the schizophrenia is treated.

Risk assessment

Assess the patient's risk in terms of risk to self and risk to others:
- Risk to self:
  – Through self-harm
  – Through neglect
  – Through exploitation
- Risk to others
  See Table 2.8.

Aetiology

Identify precipitating, predisposing, and maintaining factors (Table 2.9). It helps to classify these factors accord-ing to the biopsychosocial model as either biological, psy-chological, or social. You can also identify strengths or positive prognostic factors, e.g. first episode, good pre-morbid functioning, in a supportive relationship, and so on.

Management

The management plan should not focus solely on the bio-logical dimension, but should also include the psycholo-gical and social dimensions. It is useful to subdivide the management plan into short-term and medium/long-term, and to list the 'next steps' (Table 2.10).

Prognosis

Formulate a clear prognosis both for the current episode and for the long-term, and explain your reasoning. You can also list any relevant positive and negative prognostic factors. Examples of important positive prognostic factors are first episode, good premorbid functioning, good response to medication, and good social support. Exam-ples of important negative prognostic factors are strong family history, non-compliance with medication, and substance misuse.

Classification of mental disorders

If any man were bold enough to write a history of psychiatric classifications he would find when he had completed his task that in the process he had written a history of psychiatry as well.
  Robert Kendell, *The Role of Diagnosis in Psychiatry*

Psychiatric disorders such as schizophrenia and affective disorders are concepts that tend to be defined by their symptoms. Compared to concepts that are defined by their aetiology, such as malaria or Cushing's disease, they are more difficult to describe and diagnose, and more open to misunderstanding and misuse. To begin address-ing these problems calls for a classification that contains clearly defined concepts and reliable operational criteria to diagnose them by. It also calls for such a classification to be placed firmly at the centre of psychiatric practice, and for it to be frequently revised in the light of increasing evi-dence and understanding.

Personal factors	Previous violence to self or to others (best predictor) Male sex Young or old age Recent life crisis Unemployed Divorced Socially isolated Socially unstable Victim of physical or sexual abuse Access to victims Access to means
Illness-related factors	Depressive symptoms Psychotic symptoms Substance abuse Treatment resistance Treatment non-compliance
Factors in the mental state	Suicidal ideation Anger Hostility Suspiciousness Expressed intent to harm or take revenge Delusions of persecution Delusions of control Delusions of jealousy Delusions of guilt Commanding second person auditory hallucinations

Table 2.8 Factors that increase a patient's risk to self and/or to others (see also Chapter 6 on suicide and deliberate self-harm).

Table 2.9 Some common aetiological factors for mental disorder.

	Biological	Psychological	Social
Precipitating factors	Genes Family history Substance misuse Organic conditions	Dysfunctional parenting Cognitive distortions Maladaptive behaviours Psychodynamic factors	Childhood abuse Bullying Poor social support Poor housing Unemployment
Predisposing factors	Substance misuse Organic conditions Non-compliance Pattern of sleep	Stress Bereavement/loss	Life events
Maintaining factors	Substance misuse Organic conditions Non-compliance Treatment-resistance Pattern of sleep	Poor insight Cognitive distortions Maladaptive behaviours Psychodynamic factors High expressed emotion Lack of confiding relationships	Stigma Poor coping skills Poor social support Poor housing Unemployment
Strengths	No family history No substance misuse Responsive to medication Compliant with medication	Good insight Motivated Confiding relationships	Good premorbid functioning Good social support Employment

Table 2.10 Some possible measures for the management of mental disorder.

	Biological	Psychological	Social
Short-term	Drugs ECT Detoxification	Counselling Psychoeducation	Family education Carer support
Medium/long-term	Maintenance treatment Depot antipsychotic Mood stabiliser Addictions counseling Genetic counselling	Self-help guides Cognitive behavioural therapy Psychodynamic psychotherapy Family therapy	Patient groups Charities Benefits Housing Rehabilitation Power of attorney

Both clinical experience and research into the aetiology of psychiatric disorders suggest that many of the categorical concepts listed in classifications of mental disorders, such as schizophrenia and affective disorders, may not in fact map onto distinct disease entities, but instead lie at different extremes of a single spectrum of mental disorders.

ICD-10 classification

The ICD-10 Classification of Mental and Behavioural Disorders: Clinical Descriptions and Diagnostic Guidelines, published in 1992, is chapter V of the *Tenth Revision of the International Classification of Diseases* (ICD-10) and is used in all countries. Other than simply listing and coding the names of diseases and disorders like other chapters in ICD-10, Chapter V provides clinical descriptions, diagnostic criteria, and diagnostic criteria for research. These are based on scientific literature and international consultation and consensus. The principal aims of the classification are to serve as a reference for national classifications and to facilitate international comparisons of morbidity and mortality statistics. ICD-10 comes in four different versions: (1) clinical descriptions and diagnostic guidelines; (2) diagnostic criteria for research; (3) primary care version; and (4) multiaspect (axial) systems.

The broad categories of mental and behavioural disorders in ICD-10 are:

F0–F9	Organic, including symptomatic, mental disorders
F10–F19	Mental and behavioural disorders due to psychoactive substance use
F20–F29	Schizophrenia, schizotypal and delusional disorders
F30–F39	Mood (affective) disorders
F40–F48	Neurotic, stress-related and somatoform disorders
F50–F59	Behavioural syndromes associated with physiological disturbances and physical factors
F60–F69	Disorders of adult personality and behaviour
F70–F79	Mental retardation
F80–F89	Disorders of psychological development
F90–F98	Behavioural and emotional disorders with onset usually occurring in childhood and adolescence
F99	Unspecified mental disorder

Note that these are organised in a loose diagnostic hierarchy (see above).

DSM-IV classification

The first classification of mental and behavioural disorders appeared in the sixth edition of *International Classification of Diseases*, published in 1948. The American Psychiatric Association (APA) did not lose much time in publishing an alternative classification, the *Diagnostic and Statistical Manual of Mental Disorders (DSM)*, for use in the USA. The fourth revision of the DSM, published in 1994 (Text Revision in 2000), is broadly similar to the ICD-10 classification. However, unlike the ICD-10 classification, which is available in four different versions, there is only one, multiaxial, version of DSM-IV.

2

Axes of classification in DSM-IV:

Axis I   Clinical disorders and conditions that need clinical attention
Axis II   Personality disorders and mental retardation
Axis III   General medical conditions
Axis IV   Psychosocial and environmental problems
Axis V   Global assessment of functioning

Although some psychiatrists prefer ICD-10 to DSM-IV and *vice versa*, the classifications should be seen as complementary rather than competing. Both are used throughout this book.

Case study: Psychiatric assessment

LD, 22-year-old Caucasian male referred by his GP for hearing voices. Currently a student in architectural engineering at Y University.

Presenting complaint
- LD is hearing voices for about half an hour everyday in the evening:
  - They belong to his three best friends
  - They speak both to him and about him, and are highly critical of him. In particular, they tell him that his parents are going to die because he is failing at university
  - Although he experiences them as coming from outside his head, he does not believe that they are real and tries to ignore them as much as possible
  - They do not tell him to harm himself or anyone else.
- The voices do not stop LD from leading a normal life, but he finds it very difficult to talk about them, and is deeply concerned that he may spiral into a florid psychosis similar to the one he suffered 16 months ago.
- On further questioning, LD reveals that he is also having ideas of reference: although he sometimes feels that people in public places are talking about him, he is able to recognise that this is a product of his mind.
- LD goes to bed in the early hours of the morning to accommodate his busy social life. Yet he gets an average of 7 or 8 hours of uninterrupted sleep every night.

History of presenting complaint
- The voices started about a month ago, whilst LD was revising for his end-of-year exams. Since then they have become more prominent.

Past psychiatric history
- First episode of (?cannabis-induced) psychosis 16 months ago. Prominent auditory hallucinations and delusions of persecution.
- Informally admitted to X hospital under Dr Y for a period of 2 months.

- Started on the atypical antipsychotic risperidone and made a good recovery.
- At the time, Dr Y made a diagnosis of drug-induced psychotic episode.
- No other psychiatric history.

Past medical history
- Mild asthma
- Hay fever
- Uncomplicated appendicectomy at the age of 16
- No history of epilepsy or head injury

Drug history/current treatments
- History of poor compliance on oral medication. Started on risperidone depot.
- Risperidone depot recently increased to 37.5 mg once every 2 weeks by his GP, Dr Z. On this dose he is suffering from troublesome side-effects, including sedation and ejaculatory dysfunction.
- Salbutamol inhaler on an as required basis.
- Allergic to penicillin (rash).

Substance use
- LD used to be a heavy cannabis smoker but denies having used drugs since his first psychotic episode 16 months ago.
- He smokes about 10 cigarettes a day.
- He drinks two to three pints of beer a day in the pub with his friends, although on Friday nights he may drink a bit more than this.

Family history
- LD's maternal grandfather died from complications of catatonic schizophrenia at the age of 43.
- His mother is on an SSRI for panic disorder.
- His parents separated a year ago and since then he has been spending his holidays at his father's place. Although

Continued...

his mother is supportive, his father sometimes finds it difficult to accept that he is mentally ill. Of particular note is the fact that he describes his father as 'a constant nag'.

- He has one elder brother and one elder sister. Both are currently living abroad.

Social history

- During term-time LD lives in university halls of residence.
- His parents are both accountants and are funding him through university.
- He has a busy social life and often goes to bed in the early hours of the morning. As a result, he sometimes misses 2 pm lectures. He finds it difficult to talk to his friends about the voices that he is hearing as he fears that they may mock or reject him.
- He describes himself as socially outgoing despite a natural shyness. He regrets not having achieved his full intellectual potential at school and at university, and at one point asked me what novels he should be reading.

Personal history

- LD has no history of birth complications or of developmental delay.
- He got on well with his parents, but was bullied by his elder brother, who once gave him a black eye.
- He enjoyed school, did rather well, and had a fair number of friends.
- He left school with three good A-Levels and spent a year in the Australian outback, where he was attacked by a koala. He then started a course in architectural engineering at X University but dropped out after his first episode of psychosis. Last October he re-started a similar course at Y University.
- He has never had a girlfriend, which he sorely regrets. Although he is very outgoing, he is not confident with girls.
- When I asked him whether he believes in God, he replied, 'I sometimes go to church, but only to listen to the organ music'.
- He has no history of physical or sexual abuse.
- He has never been in trouble with the police.

Informant history (consent obtained from LD)

LD's mother confirmed LD's history. As far as she knows LD has not smoked cannabis since his first psychotic episode. She is concerned that LD is unable to concentrate on his studies and likely to fail his end-of-year exams.

Mental state examination

Appearance and behaviour

- Tall, slightly stooped
- Well kempt
- Shy, but friendly and cooperative. Good eye contact. Good rapport
- No motor abnormalities

Speech

- No abnormalities of speech

Mood

- Affect is normal
- Mood is objectively and subjectively euthymic
- No suicidal or homicidal ideation
- No anxiety symptoms

Thoughts

- Normal stream and form of thought
- Sometimes feels that people in public places are talking about him, but is able to recognise that this is a product of his mind
- Deeply concerned that he might spiral into a florid psychosis similar to the one he suffered 16 months ago
- Preoccupied about failing his end-of-year exams
- Preoccupied about never having been in a relationship
- No obsessions
- No phobias

Perception

- Although he is not hearing voices at the moment, LD does describe hearing voices for about half an hour everyday in the evening

Cognition

- Fully oriented in time and place. Cognition not formally tested

Insight

- Believes that he is having another episode of psychosis
- Believes that he needs pharmacological treatment to get better

Formulation

Synopsis

- 22-year-old Caucasian male with ideas of reference and second and third person auditory hallucinations for half an hour every evening since starting exam revision one month ago.

Continued...

2

- First episode of drug-induced psychosis with prominent auditory hallucinations and delusions of persecution 16 months ago. Informally admitted under Dr X for a period of 2 months. Started on risperidone and made a good recovery. Has not since used drugs, but has a history of poor compliance with medication.
- Risperidone depot recently increased to 37.5 mg every 2 weeks leading to multiple side-effects.

Further information required
- Physical examination unremarkable
- Urine drug screen negative
- Blood tests normal
- Need to speak to GP and obtain medical notes from X Hospital

Differential diagnosis
- F20.0 Paranoid schizophrenia (ICD-10). Has one first rank symptom of schizophrenia (third person auditory hallucinations) and fulfils the ICD-10 duration criteria. Also has a family history of schizophrenia.
- Drug-induced psychotic disorder. Claims not to have been taking drugs.
- Schizophreniform disorder (DSM-IV). Symptoms for ? more than 1 month but less than 6 months.

Risk assessment
Symptoms are currently mild and have a minimal impact on the patient's functioning. Risk to himself and to others is currently low.

Aetiology

	Biological	Psychological	Social
Precipitating factors	• ?Cannabis • Irregular sleeping pattern	• Exam-related stress	• Parental separation • Going to university
Predisposing factors	• Family history	• High expressed emotion • Lack of a confiding relationship	• Childhood bullying
Perpetuating factors	• ?Cannabis • Irregular sleeping pattern	• High expressed emotion • Lack of a confiding relationship	• Stigma of mental illness

Management

	Biological	Psychological	Social
Short-term	• Change antipsychotic to amisulpiride (less sedating)	• Support the patient and family and educate them about schizophrenia. In particular, advise on importance of drug compliance, regular sleeping pattern, and avoidance of illicit drugs	
Medium-term	• Monitor response to amisulpiride and consider aripiprazole if LD continues experiencing troublesome side-effects • Monitor symptoms	• Schizophrenia support group • Family therapy to address high expressed emotion – to discuss with patient and family	• Schizophrenia support group
Long-term		• Find a confiding relationship (hopefully)	• Find a confiding relationship (hopefully)

Continued...

Next steps:

1. Appointment made with Dr A (SHO) next Monday at 3 pm to monitor response to amisulpiride, monitor symptoms, and support and educate the patient and family
2. Weekly home visits by CPN to monitor symptoms, and support and educate the patient and family
3. CPN to provide the patient with the contact details of a local schizophrenia support group.

Prognosis

In the short-term he is likely to respond to amisulpiride and make a good recovery. In the long-term, he is likely to suffer from further relapses, particularly if he comes under stress, uses drugs, or stops taking his medication. Compliance with anti-psychotic medication is likely to be a major issue.

Positive prognostic factors, at least initially, include acute onset, presence of precipitating factors, florid symptoms, good premorbid occupational/social adjustment, good social support, early treatment, and good response to treatment.

Negative prognostic factors include male sex, family history, history of substance misuse, history of poor compliance with medication, and lack of a confiding relationship.

2

Recommended reading

Symptoms in the Mind: An Introduction to Descriptive Psychopathology (1997) Andrew Sims. W. B. Saunders Co Ltd.
Clinical Psychopathology: Signs and Symptoms in Psychiatry (1985) Frank Fish and Max Hamilton (eds). Butterworth Heinemann.

Psychiatric Interviewing: The Art of Understanding (1998) Shawn Shea. W. B. Saunders Co Ltd.
The Present State Examination (1974) J. K. Wing. Cambridge University Press.
Pocket Guide to the ICD-10 Classification of Mental and Behavioural Diseases (1994) J. E. Cooper. WHO.

Patient assessment: Checklist and summary

Psychiatric history

1. Introductory information.
2. Presenting complaint/history of presenting complaint: use open questions first, record patient's complaints verbatim, use a logico-deductive approach.
3. Past psychiatric history, including previous episodes of mental disorder, treatments, admissions, and history of self-harm and harm to others.
4. Past medical history, including history of epilepsy or head injury and vascular risk factors.
5. Drug history/current treatments, including psychological treatments, recent changes in medication, adverse reactions, and alternative remedies.
6. Substance use: alcohol, tobacco, and illicit drugs.
7. Family history, including quality of relationships and recent events in the family.
8. Social history: self-care, support, housing, finances, typical day, interests and hobbies, premorbid personality.
9. Personal history: pregnancy and birth, developmental milestones, childhood problems, educational achievement, occupational history, psychosexual history, forensic history, religious orientation.
10. Informant history/histories.

Mental state examination

1. Appearance and behaviour: level of consciousness, appearance, behaviour, motor activity/disorders of movement.
2. Speech: especially amount, rate, and form.
3. Mood: subjective and objective mood, affect, ideas of self-harm and suicide, ideas of harm to others, anxiety.
4. Thoughts: stream, form, content: delusions, overvalued ideas, preoccupations, ruminations, obsessions, phobias.
5. Perception: sensory distortions, illusions, hallucinations, depersonalisation and derealisation.
6. Cognition: orientation, attention and concentration, memory, grasp.
7. Insight.

Formulation

1. Case summary or synopsis.
2. Further information required: full psychiatric history and mental state examination, informant histories, old records, physical examination, laboratory investigations, brain imaging, psychological tests and inventories.

Continued...

2

3. Differential diagnosis: psychiatric differential and organic differential, including substance misuse.
4. Risk assessment: risk to self (through self-harm, neglect, or exploitation) and risk to others.
5. Aetiology: precipitating, predisposing, and perpetuating factors; biological, psychological, and social.

6. Management: short-, medium- and long-term; biological, psychological, and social.
7. Prognosis: current episode and long-term.

Self-assessment

Simply answer with true or false. Answers on p. 216.

1. The mental state examination is a snapshot of the patient's mental state at (or around) that time.
2. The mental state examination can be compared to both a physical examination and a functional enquiry.
3. One of the most important principles of descriptive psychopathology is to make assumptions about the causes of signs and symptoms of mental illness.
4. Asking about suicide often suggests it to the patient.
5. Before talking to an informant, consent from the patient is generally required.
6. Scores of less than 22 out of 30 on the MMSE are indicative of significant cognitive impairment, and scores of 22–25 are indicative of moderate cognitive impairment.
7. A stereotypy is an odd, repetitive movement that has a functional significance.
8. Apraxia describes a reduced ability to carry out purposive movements in spite of intact comprehension and motor function.
9. *Mitmachen* is an extreme form of *mitgehen*.
10. *Gegenhalten* describes involuntary resistance to passive movement.
11. Dysphasia describes an impairment of the ability to vocalise speech.
12. Echolalia describes the parrot-like imitation of another person's speech.
13. In incongruity of affect, affect does not reflect content of thought.

14. In circumstantial thinking the normal structure of thought is preserved, but thoughts are cramped by an excess of irrelevant detail.
15. A secondary delusion is one that arises from, and is understandable in context of, previous ideas or events.
16. Delusional perception is the attribution of delusional significance to normal percepts.
17. An overvalued idea differs from a delusion partly in that the person accepts the possibility that the belief may not be true.
18. Fregoli syndrome is the delusion that a familiar individual has been replaced by an identical-looking imposter.
19. A pseudo-hallucination differs from a hallucination in that it is perceived to come from the sense organs and not from the mind.
20. Reflex hallucination describes a hallucination triggered by an environmental stimulus in the same modality, e.g. hallucinatory voices triggered by the sound of a running tap.
21. A patient's level of insight can be assessed independently of the assessor's set of values.
22. In the diagnostic hierarchy, delirium is higher up than dementia and dementia is higher up than schizophrenia.
23. The DSM-IV classification is based on international consultation and consensus.
24. The DSM-IV classification comes in four different versions: clinical descriptions and diagnostic guidelines; diagnostic criteria for research; primary care version; and multiaspect (axial) systems.
25. The DSM-IV classification is multiaxial.

The delivery of mental health care

3

3

Key learning objectives

- Factors involved in the development of community care
- Advantages and disadvantages of community care
- Organisation of mental health services
- Function and implementation of the Care Programme Approach (CPA)

- Civil Sections of the Mental Health Act, especially Sections 5(2), 2, and 3

Introduction: the development of community care

The advent of community care in the 1950s and 1960s resulted from:

- Important social changes and heavy criticism of the institutional model of psychiatric care, epitomised by the so-called 'antipsychiatry' movement
- Better drugs such as the antipsychotic chlorpromazine
- Perceived financial benefits of community care.

By removing patients from the isolation of old Victorian asylums and integrating them into the community under the care of Community Mental Health Teams (CMHTs), policy-makers hoped to improve their social functioning and reduce the stigma of mental illness.

The expansion in community care continued throughout the 1970s and 1980s, but came under heavy criticism in the 1980s after a series of headline-grabbing killings by mentally ill people in the community. (Killings by mentally ill people in the community, although rare, are often

Psychiatry, 2e. By Neel Burton. Published 2010 by Blackwell Publishing.

sensationally reported by the press. For example, the author once spotted an article headed 'Beast freed from prison psycho ward chopped my mum into 16 little pieces'.) This prompted a government inquiry that culminated in the Community Care Act of 1990, a major piece of legislation that is at the origins of the present, more 'fail-safe', model of community care. According to this model, prior to discharge from hospital, each patient should have an agreed care plan and can, in a minority of cases, be placed on a community supervision order (referred to as a 'supervised discharge').

The advantages of community care are clear. By shifting the emphasis from a person's mental illness to his or her strengths and life aspirations, community care promotes independence and self-reliance, while discouraging isolation and institutionalisation and reducing stigmatisation. On the other hand, a lack of mental health staff and resources can in some cases shift the burden of care onto informal carers, such as relatives and friends, and make it especially difficult to care for those most in need, such as the isolated or the homeless. The advantages and disadvantages of community care are summarised in Table 3.1.

Table 3.1 Advantages and disadvantages of community care.

Advantages	Disadvantages/problems
Promotes self-reliance by focusing on strengths and life aspirations, rather than on illness	Poses a (? mainly perceived) threat to the safety of the patient and of the community
Discourages isolation and institutionalisation	Makes it difficult to provide care for those most in need of it, such as the homeless
Promotes relapse prevention	Places a heavy burden on carers
Reduces the stigma of mental illness	Places a heavy burden on staff and resources
Originally thought to be cheaper than providing inpatient care	Has resulted in a shortage of hospital beds as resources are diverted to community services

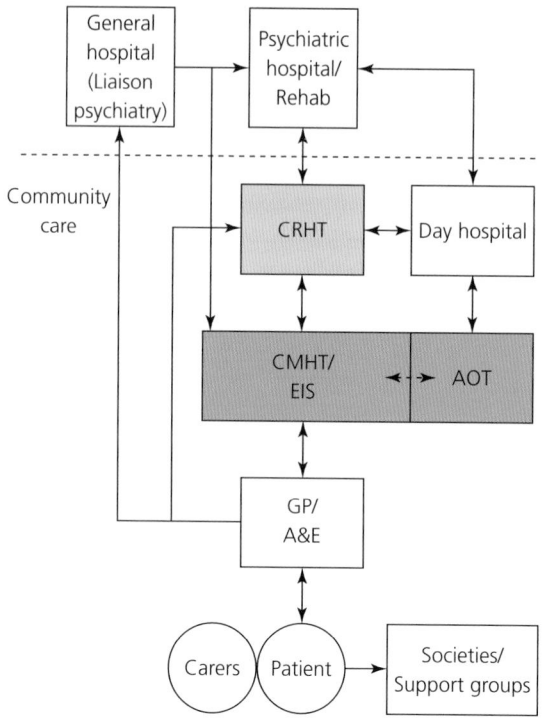

Figure 3.1 Example of organisation of mental healthcare services (local services may differ). Note that mental healthcare services are organised so as avoid unnecessary hospital admissions. All terms used in this figure are explained in this chapter. CRHT, Crisis Resolution and Home Treatment team; CMHT, Community Mental Health Team; AOT or AORT, Assertive Outreach Team; EIS, Early Intervention Service; GP, General Practitioner; A&E, Accident and Emergency department.

The organisation of mental healthcare services

General practice and accident and emergency

The bulk of mental disorder (mild and moderate anxiety or depressive disorders) is treated by GPs. If a referral to secondary care is required, this is usually to the CMHT or, in an emergency or at night, to the Crisis Resolution and Home Treatment Team (CRHT). A minority of cases first present to Accident and Emergency (A&E) rather than to their general practitioner (GP). In this case the patient is usually screened by a casualty doctor, and then referred for further assessment by a psychiatrist. If the psychiatrist forms an opinion that the patient is suffering from a severe mental disorder, he is most likely to refer him to his local CMHT or, in an emergency, to the CRHT.

Community Mental Health Team

The CMHT is at the centre of mental health care provision. It is a multidisciplinary team led by a consultant psychiatrist and operating from a team base in the geographical sector that it covers. Community Psychiatric Nurses (CPNs) and social workers often play a key role in the CMHT, coordinating patient care, monitoring patients in the community, and taking urgent referrals. Other important members of the multidisciplinary team include psychiatrists, clinical psychologists, occupational therapists,

and administrative staff (see Table 3.2 for more information on members of the multidisciplinary team). If a person suffering from a severe mental disorder is referred to a CMHT, he usually undergoes an initial assessment by a psychiatrist, sometimes in the presence of another member of the team, such as a CPN or social worker. The skill mix of the multidisciplinary team means that the different parts of the person's life can be understood – and addressed – from a number of different angles.

Crisis Resolution and Home Treatment Team

The 'Crisis Team' is a 24 hours a day, 365 days a year multidisciplinary team that acts as a gatekeeper to a variety of psychiatric services, including admission to a psychiatric hospital. Patients in a crisis are referred to the Crisis Team from a variety of places and agencies, most commonly GPs, A&E, and CMHTs. A member of the team (often a community psychiatric nurse) promptly assesses the patient in conjunction with a psychiatrist to determine if a hospital admission can be avoided by providing short-term intensive home care. If so, the Crisis Team arranges for a team member to visit the patient's home up to three times a day, gradually decreasing the frequency of visits as the patient gets better. Other than simply providing support, the Crisis Team can assist in implementing a care and treatment plan and in monitoring progress. If a patient has already been admitted to hospital, the Crisis Team can get involved in expediting and facilitating his discharge back into the community. The key features of the Crisis Team are summarised in Table 3.3.

Assertive Outreach Team

Some people with a severe mental disorder are reluctant to seek help and treatment, and as a consequence only appear in times of crisis. Paradoxically, these so-called 'revolving door patients' often have the most complex mental health needs and social problems. For this reason, the responsibility for their care is sometimes transferred to the Assertive Outreach Team (AOT), a specialised multidisciplinary team dedicated to engaging them in treatment and supporting them in their daily activities.

Early Intervention Service

Like the AOT, the Early Intervention Service (EIS) may also operate from the CMHT base. Its role is specifically to improve the short- and long-term outcomes of schizophrenia and other psychotic disorders through a three-pronged approach involving preventative measures, earlier detection of untreated cases, and intensive treatment and support in the early stages of illness.

Hospital and day hospital

If a patient requires admission to a psychiatric hospital, this is usually because care in the community is not an option. Commonly this is because:
- The patient is a danger to himself and/or to others
- The patient requires specialised care or supervised treatment
- The patient is lacking a social structure
- Carers can no longer cope and are in need of respite.

The vast majority of patients who are admitted are done so on an informal, voluntary basis. This is either because they are happy to take the advice of their psychiatrist or carers or because they are frightened of their symptoms and feel that the hospital is a relatively safe place for them

---

One Flew Over the Cuckoo's Nest

Vintery, mintery, cutery, corn,
Apple seed and apple thorn;
Wire, briar, limber lock,
Three geese in a flock.
One flew east,
And one flew west,
And one flew over the cuckoo's nest.

Popular nursery rhyme

The film *One Flew Over the Cuckoo's Nest*, adapted from Ken Kesey's popular 1962 novel of the same name, is directed by Milos Forman and stars Jack Nicholson as the spirited R. P. McMurphy ('Mac') and Louise Fletcher as the chilly but softly-spoken Nurse Ratched. When Mac arrives at the Oregon state mental hospital, he challenges the stultifying routine and bureaucratic authoritarianism personified by Nurse Ratched, and pays the price by being drugged, electro-shocked and, ultimately, lobotomised. Nominated for nine Academy Awards, the film is not only a (belated and contentious) criticism of the institutional model of psychiatric care, but also a metaphor of total institutions – institutions that repress individuality to create a compliant society. It is such criticism of the institutional model of psychiatric care that, in the UK and other countries, led to the development of community care.

It seems that utopias are much more easily achieved than we once thought. Today we are faced with a different and more agonising question: How do we prevent them from being finally achieved?… Utopias can be achieved. Life moves on towards utopia. And perhaps a new age is beginning, an age when intellectuals and cultured people will dream up a way of avoiding utopias, and returning to a society that is not utopian, with less 'perfection' and more freedom.

Nicolas Berdiaeff, translated from the foreword to *Brave New World* by Aldous Huxley, Longman Edition

Table 3.2 Key non-medical members of the CMHT.

Community psychiatric nurse (CPN)	The CPN is the member of the team with whom the patient is likely to come into contact most often. The CPN usually visits the patient's home to facilitate the treatment plan and monitor progress.
Social worker	Sometimes a patient may be allocated a social worker instead of a CPN, in which case the social worker fulfils a role similar to that of the CPN. The social worker can also help to sort out housing and benefits, and to ensure that the patient makes the most of any services and facilities that are available.
Clinical psychologist	A clinical psychologist has expertise of human experience and behaviour. A clinical psychologist may spend a lot of time listening to and trying to understand a patient and his or her relatives and carers, and may deliver talking treatments such as cognitive-behavioural therapy (CBT) and family therapy. *'Clinical psychologist' is often confused with 'psychiatrist', 'psychotherapist', and 'psychoanalyst'. A psychiatrist is a medical doctor specialised in diagnosing and treating mental disorders. A psychotherapist is any person trained in delivering talking treatments – commonly a clinical psychologist or a psychiatrist. A psychoanalyst is a type of psychotherapist trained in delivering talking treatments based on the psychoanalytical principles pioneered by Freud and others, including Alfred Adler, Carl Jung, and Melanie Klein.*
Occupational therapist	The role of the occupational therapist is to help the patient to maintain his or her skills, as well as to develop new ones. This not only helps the patient to get back to work, but also keeps him or her engaged and motivated.
Pharmacist	Patients suffering from a physical illness or who are pregnant or breastfeeding may find it particularly helpful to speak to a pharmacist, who can help with information about medication.
Administrative staff	Administrative staff work at the interface between patients and team members: they are responsible for arranging appointments and are often the first port of call if urgent help is required.

NB: Other forms of support which are available but which do not form part of the CMHT include support groups, telephone helplines, hobby groups, and the Citizen's Advice Bureau.

Table 3.3 Key features of the Crisis Team.

- Gatekeeper to psychiatric services, including admission to a psychiatric hospital
- Prompt assessment of patients in a crisis
- Intensive, community-based, round-the-clock support in the early stages of the crisis
- Continued involvement until the crisis has resolved
- Action to prevent similar crises occurring again
- Partnership with the patient and his relatives and carers

to be. In some cases, attendance at a day hospital during office hours only may provide some patients with a more tolerable alternative to hospital admission.

Rehabilitation

Some patients, especially those suffering from prominent negative symptoms of schizophrenia, may need a period of long-term rehabilitation either in inpatient units or in the community. Areas that need to be considered during rehabilitation are accommodation, activities of daily living, occupational activities, leisure activities, and social skills (see Chapter 4).

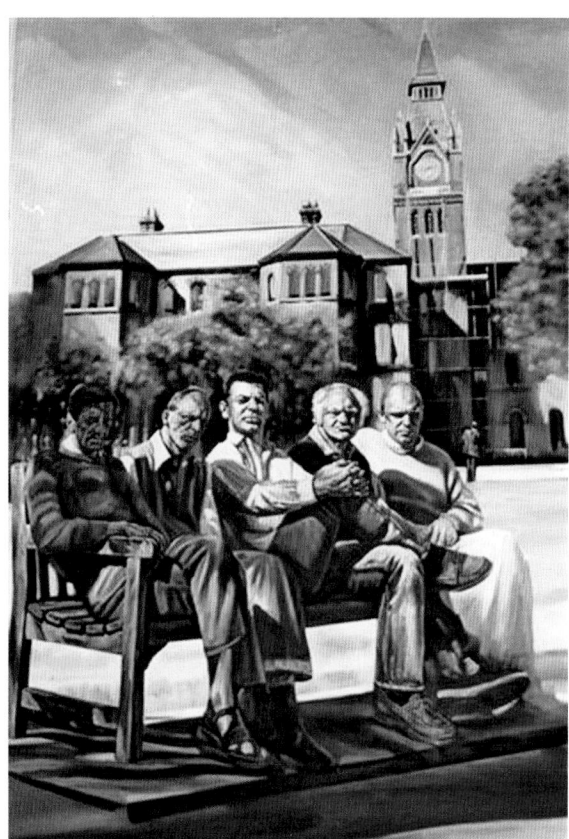

Figure 3.2 'Barmy days' by Paul Lake. Support from the SANE Arts Grant Scheme helped Paul Lake to achieve his ambitions and become a successful artist. 'Barmy days' is a portrait of himself and some friends at the Brookwood Psychiatric Hospital. 'I wanted to show the positive side of the mental hospital and the way it allowed us the time and space to accept our illness.'

General hospital: liaison psychiatry

Liaison psychiatry refers to psychiatric services in the general hospital. Since the 1970s, liaison psychiatry has developed into a recognised sub-specialty of psychiatry which focuses on the overlap between psychiatry and the rest of medicine and surgery. It principally involves providing expert advice and treatment to inpatients and outpatients referred by physicians and surgeons, and assessing patients with suspected psychological or psychiatric complaints in A&E. Cases vary greatly, e.g. self-harm, somatisation disorder, and depression after a mastectomy.

Societies and support groups

Selected societies and support groups relevant to the practice of psychiatry in the UK include MIND, Rethink, SANE, The Mental Health Foundation, Manic Depression Fellowship (MDF), Bipolar Organisation, Depression Alliance, Cruse Bereavement Care, Relate (support with relationships), Anxiety UK, No Panic, OCD Action, b-eat (support with eating disorders), Alzheimer's Society, The Sleep Council, Drinkline, Alcoholics Anonymous, Al Anon, QUIT (support with smoking cessation), Cocaine Anonymous, Narcotics Anonymous, The Samaritans, CRISIS (support with homelessness), Carers UK, and the Royal College of Psychiatrists.

The Care Programme Approach

The management of patients accepted into specialist mental health services is planned at one or several Care Programme Approach (CPA) meetings attended by both the patient and his carers. These meetings are useful to establish the context of the patient's disorder, evaluate his current personal circumstances, assess his medical, psychological, and social needs, and formulate a detailed care programme or care plan to ensure that these needs are met. Other than ensuring that the patient takes his medication and is regularly seen by a psychiatrist or CPN, this care plan may involve a number of psychosocial measures such as attendance at self-help groups, carer education and support, and home help. A care coordinator, most often a CPN or social worker, is appointed to ensure that the care programme is implemented and revised in light of the patient's changing needs and circumstances. **At the outcome of a CPA meeting, the patient should feel that his needs and circumstances have been understood, and that the care plan that he has helped to formulate closely reflects these.**

Ethics and the law

A full discussion of ethical principles in psychiatry is beyond the scope of this book, and this section merely highlights some of the more pertinent ethical principles involved in daily psychiatric practice, as typified by the story of Mr AB. Many countries have professional guidelines overseen by national medical and psychiatric organisations, e.g. those of the General Medical Council and Royal College of Psychiatrists in the UK, and of the American Psychiatric Association in the USA.

The story of Mr AB

Mr AB, a 48-year-old bank manager, arrives in A&E complaining of burning pains in his face and head. He has a letter from his GP in which she opines that he is suffering from an episode of severe depression. He has a history of recurrent depressive disorder and once made an impulsive and almost fatal suicide attempt.

Although Mr AB appears to be depressed, he denies feeling in the least suicidal. He refuses to let the casualty officer call his wife. The casualty officer tries to call his GP but she is out on a home visit. He then obtains Mr AB's telephone number from directory enquiries and calls his wife, who did not know that he was in A&E or even that he had been to see his GP. She says that Mr AB has become increasingly gloomy and preoccupied over the past three or four weeks. She is alarmed to discover that he is complaining of pains in the face and head: the last time he complained of such pains, he tried to take his life. She is adamant that he should not be allowed to leave the hospital or, at any rate, not before she can get there.

The casualty officer calls the duty psychiatrist to see Mr AB. Although initially guarded and suspicious, Mr AB eventually reveals that he has 'advanced brain cancer'. After a careful neurological examination, the psychiatrist finds no evidence of a tumour and explains this to Mr AB, who nevertheless remains completely unconvinced. All he wants is to be given something for the pains, and then to go home.

Mrs AB arrives and tells the psychiatrist that she fears that her husband is planning to kill himself, as he is behaving just as he did prior to his previous suicide attempt. As Mr AB insists that he will not stay in hospital, he is admitted involuntarily under a 'Section' of the Mental Health Act. After some further tests, he is started on antidepressant treatment.

Adapted from Bill Fulford, *Moral Theory and Medical Practice*

Confidentiality

Patient information should not be disclosed and further patient information should not be collected unless the patient has given consent. That having been said, in exceptional circumstances there is an obligation to disclose information if:

- This is in the public interest, e.g. in the prevention, detection, or prosecution of a serious crime or in relation to fitness to drive
- This is in the best interests of the patient, e.g. if the patient is legally incapable because of severe mental or physical illness.

In Mr AB's case, the casualty officer breached confidentiality by letting Mrs AB know that her husband had turned up in casualty, and providing her with some details of his presentation. This could be justified on the grounds of **best interest**, as Mr AB had been deemed to be suffering from a severe mental illness and to have been lacking in capacity. It is interesting to note that in our autonomy-dominated ethic, a breach of confidentiality to Mr AB's family must be 'justified' on certain grounds. But in cultures that value families and communities before individuals, it may be considered entirely natural and appropriate to make every effort to contact Mr AB's family. This reveals that our autonomy-dominated ethic, although often taken for granted, is heavily *values-laden*.

Tarasoff v Regents of the University of California (1976)

In 1969 Prosenjit Poddar was a patient of Dr Lawrence Moore, a psychologist at UC Berkeley's Cowell Memorial Hospital. In August of that year, during his ninth session, he confided to Dr Moore that he was going to kill Tatiana Tarasoff, a fellow student who had spurned his romantic advances. Dr Moore informed the campus police that he felt Poddar was dangerous and should be hospitalised involuntarily, but the police released Poddar after they felt that he had 'changed his attitude'. The psychiatric director, Dr Harvey Powelson, learned of the situation and instructed his staff not to pursue further attempts to hospitalise Poddar. Neither Tarasoff nor her parents were informed of the threat made against Tarasoff's life. Several months later, on October 27, Poddar went to Tarasoff's house and stabbed her to death with a kitchen knife. He then called the police and asked to be handcuffed. When Tarasoff's parents sued Moore and various other members of the University, the California Supreme Court famously ruled that physicians have a duty to breach confidentiality if maintaining confidentiality may result in harm to the patient or to the community.

Mental capacity

Doctors and especially psychiatrists may be called upon to give an assessment of capacity and competence to decide on the ability of a patient to give informed consent or enter into another contract.

The terms 'capacity' and 'competence' are often used interchangeably, but strictly speaking:

- 'Capacity' is a **legal presumption** that adult persons have the ability to make decisions
- 'Competence' is a **clinical determination** of a patient's ability to make decisions about his or her treatment.

Issues about capacity arise in three groups of patients: children and adolescents, patients with learning difficulties, and patients with mental illness. A person has capacity so long as he or she has the ability to understand and retain relevant information for long enough to reach a **reasoned decision, regardless of the actual decision reached.** An adult person should be presumed to have the competence to make a particular decision until a judgement about capacity can be made. This judgement can only be made about present capacity, not about past or future capacity, and it should only be made for a specific decision, as different decisions require different levels of capacity. If capacity is lacking or cannot be established (e.g. in an emergency situation), treatment can be justified under the common law *Principle of Necessity*, as established by the case of *Re F* (1990). The doctor in charge has the responsibility to act in the best interests of the patient and in accordance with a responsible and competent body of opinion, as established by the case of *Bolam v Friern Hospital Management Committee* (1957) (the 'Bolam test'). Nevertheless, it is good practice for him or her to involve colleagues, carers, and relatives in the decision-making. In difficult situations or if there are differences of opinion about the patient's best interests, the doctor should consult a senior colleague or seek expert or legal advice. In England and Wales, the Mental Capacity Act 2005 provides for a Court of Protection to help with difficult decisions. Note that, in some cases, a child (a person under the age of 16) can be competent to consent to treatment if he or she fully understands the treatment proposed. This is sometimes referred to as 'Gillick competency', because it relies on a ruling of the House of Lords in the case *Gillick v West Norfolk and Wisbech Area Health Authority* (1985).

Having deemed Mr AB to be lacking in capacity on the grounds of mental illness, the casualty officer proceeded to act in his best interests by breaking confidentiality and disclosing information to and seeking information from Mrs AB (this information turned out to be of vital importance in Mr AB's assessment and management). Similarly, the psychiatrist proceeded to act in his best interests by admitting him as an involuntary patient and starting him on antidepressant therapy.

Re C (1994)

Mr C was a patient in a psychiatric secure hospital who had chronic paranoid schizophrenia with grandiose delusions of being a world famous doctor. When he developed gangrene in his right foot, he refused to consent to a below-knee amputation, as a result of which he was granted an injunction preventing such an operation. In granting such an injunction, Justice Thorpe held that Mr C sufficiently understood the nature, purpose, and effects of the proposed amputation, and that he retained sufficient capacity to consent to, or refuse, medical treatment. The case of *Re C* helped to establish the 'Re C criteria' or legal criteria for capacity.

Clinical skills/OSCE: Assessing mental capacity and obtaining consent

1. Ensure that the patient understands:
   - What the intervention is
   - Why the intervention is being proposed
   - The alternatives to the intervention, including no intervention
   - The principal benefits and risks of the intervention and of its alternatives
   - The consequences of the intervention and of its alternatives.
2. Ensure that the patient retains the information for long enough to weigh it in the balance and reach a reasoned decision, whatever that decision might be.
3. Ensure that the patient is not subject to coercion or threat. It is important to bear in mind that a patient's capacity can and should be enhanced by, for example:

- Making your explanations easier to understand, e.g. adapting your language, using diagrams
- Seeing the patient at his or her best time of day
- Seeing the patient with a friend or relatives of his
- Improving the patient's environment, e.g. turning off the television, finding a quiet side-room
- Adjusting the patient's medication, e.g. decreasing the dose of sedative drugs.

Adapted from *Clinical Skills for OSCEs*, 3e (2009), by Neel Burton, Scion Publishing

Compulsory admission and treatment

Some people with severe mental disorders pose a risk to themselves or to others but lack insight and refuse the care and treatment that they require. In many countries – and certainly in all developed countries – there are special legal provisions to protect such people and to protect society from the consequences of their mental disorder. In England and Wales, the compulsory admission and treatment of people with a severe mental disorder is enabled by the Mental Health Act 1983, as amended by the Mental Health Act 2007 (see next section). In Scotland it is governed by the Mental Health (Care and Treatment) (Scotland) Act 2003, and in Northern Ireland by the Mental Health (Northern Ireland) Order 1986.

From Mrs AB's account of her husband, there seemed to be good reason for the psychiatrist to think that Mr AB was planning to kill himself. As Mr AB insisted that he would not stay in hospital, the psychiatrist had to weigh Mr AB's right to be at liberty with his need for care and treatment, and decided that he needed to be admitted and treated under the Mental Health Act. This could not have been done had Mr AB not been deemed to be suffering from a mental disorder.

Common law

Common law is the law that is based on previous court rulings (case law, such as *Re C*), in contradistinction to the law that is enacted by parliament (statute law, such as the Mental Health Act). Under common law adults have a right to refuse treatment, even when doing so may result in permanent physical injury or death. If a competent adult refuses consent or lacks the capacity to provide consent, no one can provide consent on his or her behalf, not even his or her next of kin. That having been said, treatment without consent can be given under common law:

- If serious harm or death is likely to occur and there is doubt about the patient's capacity at the time and no advance directive (or 'living will') has been made; and the clinician is able to justify that he or she is acting in the patient's best interests and in accordance with established medical practice ('Bolam's test')
- In an emergency to prevent serious harm to the patient or to others or to prevent a crime.

Mr AB had been deemed to be lacking in capacity on the grounds of severe mental illness. Had he tried to leave A&E before a Mental Health Act assessment could be convened, the casualty officer could have had him temporarily restrained under common law. If he had then become aggressive, the casualty officer could have had him medicated, also under common law. Whilst it is sometimes necessary to restrain or medicate a patient under common law, it is best practice to convene a Mental Health Act assessment as soon as possible so that the patient can benefit from the rights and protection afforded by the Mental Health Act.

The Mental Health Act

In England and Wales, the Mental Health Act is the principal Act governing not only the compulsory admission and detention of people to a psychiatric hospital, but also their treatment, discharge from hospital, and aftercare. People with a mental disorder as defined by the Act can be detained under the Act in the interests of their health or safety or in the interests of the safety of others. To minimize the potential for abuse, the Act specifically excludes as mental disorder dependence on alcohol or drugs. Note that Scotland is governed by the Mental Health (Care and Treatment) (Scotland) Act 2003 and Northern Ireland by the Mental Health (Northern Ireland) Order 1986.

'Section 2'

Two of the most common 'Sections' of the Mental Health Act that are used to admit people with a mental disorder to a psychiatric hospital are the so-called Sections 2 and 3. Section 2 allows for an admission for assessment and treatment that can last for up to 28 days. An application for a Section 2 is usually made by an Approved Mental Health Professional (AMHP) with special training in mental health, and recommended by two doctors, one of whom must have special experience in the diagnosis and treatment of mental disorders. Under a Section 2, treatment can be given, but only if this treatment is aimed at treating the mental disorder or conditions directly resulting from the mental disorder (so, for example, treatment for an inflamed appendix cannot be given under the Act, although treatment for deliberate self-harm might). A Section 2 can be 'discharged' or revoked at any time by the Responsible Clinician (usually the consultant psychiatrist in charge), by the hospital managers, or by the nearest relative. Furthermore, a patient under a Section 2 can appeal against the Section, in which case his or her appeal is heard by a specially constituted tribunal. The claimant is represented by a solicitor who helps him or her to make a case in favour of discharge to the tribunal. The tribunal is by nature adversarial, and it falls upon members of the detained patient's care team to argue the case for continued detention. This can be quite trying for both the claimant and his or her care team, and it can at times undermine the claimant's trust in his or her care team. Section 2 is broadly equivalent to Section 26 of the Mental Health (Care and Treatment) (Scotland) Act 2003, except that Section 26 cannot be used to admit a patient to hospital. Instead, Section 26 tags onto Section 24 (Emergency Admission to Hospital) or Section 25 (Detention of Patients Already in Hospital).

'Section 3'

A patient can be detained under a 'Section 3' after a conclusive period of assessment under a Section 2. Alternatively, he or she can be detained directly under a Section 3 if his or her diagnosis has already been established by the care team and is not in reasonable doubt. Section 3 corresponds to an admission for treatment and lasts for up to six months. As for a Section 2, it is usually applied for by an AMHP with special training in mental health and approved by two doctors, one of whom must have special experience in the diagnosis and treatment of mental disorders. Treatment can only be given under a Section 3 if it is aimed at treating the mental disorder or conditions directly resulting from the mental disorder. After the first 3 months, any treatment requires either the consent of the patient being treated or the recommendation of a second doctor. A Section 3 can be discharged at any time by the Responsible Clinician (usually the consultant psychiatrist in charge), by the hospital managers, or by the nearest relative. Furthermore, the patient under a Section 3 can appeal against the Section, in which case his or her appeal is heard by a specially constituted tribunal, as explained above. If the patient still needs to be detained after six months, the Section 3 can be renewed for further periods. Section 3 is broadly similar to Section 18 of the Mental Health (Care and Treatment) (Scotland) Act 2003.

'Aftercare'

If a patient has been detained under Section 3 of the Mental Health Act, he is automatically placed under a 'Section 117' at the time of his discharge from the Section 3. Section 117 corresponds to 'aftercare' and places a duty on the local health authority and local social services authority to provide the patient with a care package aimed at rehabilitation and relapse prevention. Although the patient is under no obligation to accept aftercare, in some cases he may also be placed under a 'Supervised Community Treatment' or Guardianship to ensure that he receives aftercare. Under Supervised Community Treatment, the patient is made subject to certain conditions. If these conditions are not met, he can be recalled into hospital.

Other civil Sections

Commonly used civil Sections of the Mental Health Act are summarised in Table 3.4.

Police Sections

Section 135 enables the removal of a person from his or her premises to a place of safety, and is valid for 72 hours. Section 136 enables the removal of a person from a public place to a place of safety by a police officer, and is also valid for 72 hours. The person must appear to the police officer to have a mental disorder.

Criminal Sections

The principal criminal Sections are Sections 35 and 36, and Sections 37 and 41.

Sections 35 and 36 mirror Sections 2 and 3 (above), but are used for persons suffering from a mental disorder and awaiting trial for a serious offence. Section 35 can be enacted by a Crown Court or Magistrates' Court on the evidence of a Section 12 approved doctor. Section 36 can only be enacted by a Crown Court on the evidence of two doctors, one of whom must be Section 12 approved. In contrast to Section 36, Section 35 does not enable treatment, and is used solely for the purpose of remanding a person to hospital for a report on his or her mental state. Both Sections 35 and 36 have an initial duration of 28 days, but can be extended for up to 28 days at a time for up to 12 weeks.

Section 37 is used for the detention and treatment of persons suffering from a mental disorder and convicted of a serious offence which is punishable by imprisonment. It is enacted by a Crown Court or Magistrates' Court on the evidence of two Section 12 approved doctors. Section 37 has an initial duration of six months, and can be either discharged or extended. Sometimes a Section 41 or 'restriction order' is added onto a Section 37, such that leave and discharge can only be granted with the approval of the Ministry of Justice.

Consent to treatment

Patients on a long-term treatment order can be treated with standard psychiatric drugs with or without consent for up to three months, after which an additional order is

3

Table 3.4 Commonly used Sections of the Mental Health Act.

Section	Description	Duration	Treatment	Application/ recommendation	Discharge/renewal
2	Admission for assessment	28 days	Can be given, but note that the Mental Health Act only authorizes treatment of the mental disorder itself or conditions directly resulting from the mental disorder	Application by AMHP or nearest relative. Recommendation by two doctors (at least one must be Section 12 approved)	Patient may appeal to tribunal. Can be discharged by RC, hospital managers, or nearest relative. Usually converted to Section 3 if longer period of detention is required
3	Admission for treatment	6 months	Can be given for first 3 months, then consent or second opinion is needed	Application by AMHP or nearest relative. Recommendation by two doctors (at least one must be Section 12 approved)	Patient may appeal to tribunal. Can be discharged by RC, hospital managers, or nearest relative. Can be renewed if needed
4	Emergency admission for assessment (usually used in lieu of a Section 2)	72 hours	Consent needed unless treatment is being given under common law	Application by AMHP or nearest relative. Recommendation by any doctor	Patient cannot appeal. Can be discharged by RC only
5(2)	Emergency holding order (patient already admitted to hospital on an informal basis)	72 hours	Consent needed unless treatment is being given under common law	Recommendation from the doctor or AC in charge of the patient's care or their nominated deputy	Patient cannot appeal. Can be discharged by RC only
5(4)	Emergency holding order (patient already admitted to hospital on an informal basis)	6 hours	Consent needed unless treatment is being given under common law	Recommendation from a registered mental nurse	Patient cannot appeal
117	Automatically applies if a patient has been detained under Section 3. Under Section 117 it is the duty of the local health authority and the local social services authority to provide aftercare. Unlike under Supervised Community Treatment, there is no obligation for the patient to accept it.				

AMHP, approved mental health professional; RC, responsible clinician, usually the consultant in charge; AC, approved clinician. Section 12 approval is usually granted to psychiatrists having obtained Membership of the Royal College of Psychiatrists (MRCPsych) or having more than 3 years of relevant experience.

required for their continued treatment. This additional order is a Section 58, which requires either the patient's consent or a second opinion.

Reform of the Mental Health Act

In July 1998, the Government announced its intention to reform the Mental Health Act 1983, and this culminated nine years later in the Mental Health Act 2007, which amends the Mental Health Act 1983. The Mental Health Act 2007 introduced a number of significant changes, some of the most important being:

- A single definition of mental disorder
- The introduction of a requirement that a person cannot be detained for treatment unless appropriate treatment is available (the 'appropriate medical treatment test'), rather than the previous situation in which a person could not be detained unless he or she could be treated (the 'treatability test')
- A broadening of the range of professionals who can take

on the functions which were performed by the Approved Social Worker (ASW, renamed 'Approved Mental Health Professional') and the Responsible Medical Officer (RMO, renamed 'Responsible Clinician')

- The ability for a person to make an application to displace (or change) his or her nearest relative, and the ability for civil partners to be the nearest relative
- The replacement of supervised discharge with 'Supervised Community Treatment', with a power to recall a person into hospital if he does not comply with certain conditions
- Statutory advocacy for all detained persons
- New safeguards for electroconvulsive therapy, which may no longer be given to a person who has capacity to refuse consent to it, and may only be given to a person without such capacity if it does not conflict with an advance directive, decision of a donee or deputy, or decision of the Court of Protection.

Clinical skills: Mental disorders and driving

The following advice applies to mania, schizophrenia and other schizophrenia-like psychotic disorders, and more severe forms of anxiety and depression.

You should stop driving during a first episode or relapse of your illness, because driving while ill can seriously endanger lives. In the UK, you must notify the Driver and Vehicle Licensing Authority (DVLA). Failure to do so makes it illegal for you to drive and invalidates your insurance. The DVLA then sends you a medical questionnaire to fill in, and a form asking for your permission to contact your psychiatrist. Your driving licence can generally be reinstated if your psychiatrist can confirm that:

- Your illness has been successfully treated with medication for a variable period of time, typically at least 3 months
- You are conscientious about taking your medication
- The side-effects of your medication are not likely to impair your driving
- You are not misusing drugs.

NB: People who suffer from substance misuse or dependence should also stop driving, as should *some* people who suffer from other mental disorders such as dementia, learning disability, or personality disorder.

Further information can be obtained from the DVLA website at www.DVLA.gov.uk. Note that the rules for professional driving are different from those described above.

Introduction to psychological or 'talking' treatments

He [the mystical physician to the King of Thrace] *said the soul was treated with certain charms, my dear Charmides, and that these charms were beautiful words.*

Plato (428–347BC), *Charmides*

Although drug treatments are the most readily available treatment option for mental disorders such as anxiety and depression, psychological or 'talking' treatments can in many cases be more effective. Many people prefer psychological treatments to drug treatments, because they consider (often correctly) that psychological treatments address underlying problems, rather than simply mask superficial symptoms. Of course, drug treatment and psychological treatment are not mutually exclusive and, although psychological treatments can have a role to play in mental disorders such as schizophrenia, bipolar disorder, and severe depression, they are no substitute for treatment with antipsychotic, mood-stabilising, or antidepressant medication. The type of psychological treatment that is chosen, if any, depends not only on the patient's diagnosis but also on his personal circumstances, his preferences, and – sadly all too often – on the funding and human resources that are available in his local area.

At its most basic, psychological treatment involves little more than explanation and reassurance. Such 'supportive therapy' should form an important part of treatment for all mental disorders, and in mild anxiety or depression is often the only treatment that is necessary or, indeed, appropriate. Counselling is similar to supportive therapy in that it involves explanation, reassurance, and support. However, it is more problem-focused and goal-oriented than supportive therapy, and also involves the identification and resolution of current life difficulties.

In contrast to supportive psychotherapy, exploratory psychotherapy such as cognitive-behavioural therapy (CBT) and psychodynamic psychotherapy aims to delve into the person's thoughts and feelings. Although CBT and psychodynamic psychotherapy are both forms of exploratory psychotherapy, CBT is principally based on learning and cognitive theories, whereas psychodynamic psychotherapy is principally based on psychoanalytical theory. Psychodynamic psychotherapy is similar to psychoanalysis but is briefer and less intensive; it aims to bring unconscious feelings to the surface so that they can

3

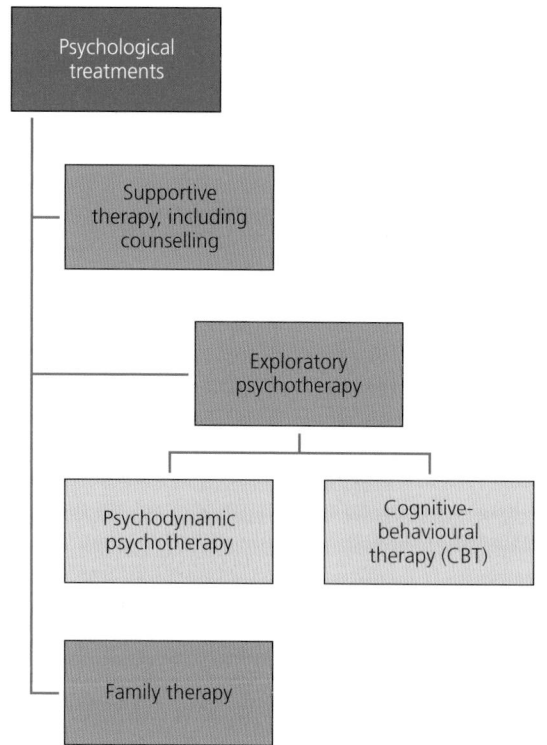

Figure 3.3 The three main forms of psychotherapy are: supportive psychotherapy, exploratory psychotherapy, and family therapy. Exploratory psychotherapy can be divided into dynamic therapies based on psychoanalytical theory and cognitive-behavioural therapies based on learning and cognitive theories. The principal form of the former is psychodynamic psychotherapy, and the principal form of the latter is cognitive-behavioural therapy.

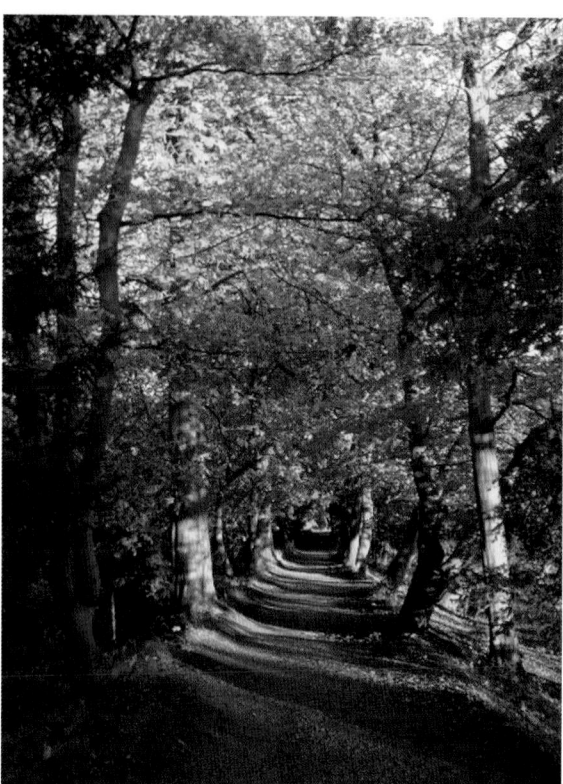

Figure 3.4 Psychodynamic psychotherapy involves a long journey exploring past and childhood experiences. Photo by Neel Burton.

be felt and understood, and so 'dealt with'. In contrast to CBT which focuses exclusively on the 'here and now', psychodynamic psychotherapy also focuses on past and childhood experiences, which can be particularly useful if the person's problems appear to be rooted there.

Developed by the psychiatrist Aaron Beck (born 1921) in the 1960s, CBT is an increasingly popular form of psychological treatment for a range of mental disorders, including anxiety disorders, non-severe depression, eating disorders, and chronic schizophrenia. Compared to psychodynamic psychotherapy, it is more evidence-based and more time-limited, and so more cost-effective. CBT is most often carried out on a one-to-one basis, but can also be offered in small groups. It involves a limited number of sessions, typically between 10 and 20, but principally takes

place outside of sessions through 'homework'. The person and a trained therapist (who may be a doctor, a psychologist, a nurse, or a counsellor) develop a shared understanding of the person's current problems and try to understand them in terms of his or her thoughts (cognitions), emotions, and behaviour, and of how these might be related to one another. This then leads to the identification of realistic, time-limited goals and of cognitive and behavioural strategies for achieving them. For example, in panic disorder these cognitive and behavioural strategies may involve cognitive restructuring (examining, testing, and modifying unhelpful thoughts and beliefs), relaxation training, and graded exposure to anxiety-provoking situations (so-called 'behavioural experiments'). In depression, the principal focus of CBT is to modify automatic and self-perpetuating negative thoughts. These negative thoughts (or 'thinking errors') are considered to be hypotheses that, through gentle questioning and guided discovery, can be examined, tested, and modified. Behav-

ioural tasks might include self-monitoring, activity sched-
uling, graded task assignments, and assertiveness training.
In some cases, there may also be an added focus on medication compliance and relapse prevention.

Clinical skills: Selection criteria for CBT

Selection criteria for CBT (and other forms of psychotherapy)
are:
- 'Psychological-mindedness'
- Adequate 'ego strength'
- Able to form and maintain relationships
- Motivated for insight and change
- Able to tolerate change and a degree of frustration.

Family therapy involves the identification and resolution of negative aspects of couple or family relationships
that may be contributing to mental disorder, such as
deeply rooted conflict or high expressed emotion, and
usually involves the direct participation of all parties
involved. There are also other types of psychological treatment, such as interpersonal therapy (IPT) and dialectical

behavioural therapy (DBT). IPT involves a systematic and
standardised treatment approach to personal relationships and life problems that are contributing to depression. DBT is a psychological method based on Buddhist
teachings for the treatment of borderline personality
disorder and recurrent self-harm.

Recommended reading

Confidentiality: Protecting and Providing Information (2004)
    General Medical Council. http://www.gmc-uk.org/guidance/
    library/confidentiality.asp
Consent: Patients and Doctors Making Decisions Together (2008)
    General Medical Council. http://www.gmc-uk.org/guidance/
    ethical_guidance/consent_guidance/index.asp
Mental Health Act 1983: Code of Practice (2008) The
    Department of Health. The Stationary Office.
In Two Minds: A Casebook of Psychiatric Ethics (2001) Donna
    Dickenson, and Bill Fulford. Oxford University Press.
*Healthcare Ethics and Human Values: An Introductory Text with
    Readings, and Case Studies* (2002) Bill Fulford, Donna
    Dickenson and Thomas Murray (eds). Blackwell Publishing.
Oxford Textbook of Philosophy of Psychiatry (2005) Bill Fulford,
    Tim Thornton, and George Graham. Oxford University
    Press.

3

3

Self-assessment

Simply answer with true or false. Answers on p. 216.

1. According to the Community Care Act of 1990, prior to discharge from hospital each patient should have an agreed care plan.
2. Community care was originally thought to be cheaper than inpatient care.
3. If a GP refers a patient to specialist care, this is usually to the Community Mental Health Team or Assertive Outreach Team.
4. The Crisis Team is a 24 hours a day, 365 days a year multidisciplinary team dedicated to engaging 'revolving door' patients in treatment and supporting them in their daily activities.
5. The case of *Re C* (1994) helped to establish the legal criteria for capacity.
6. A child can be competent to consent to treatment if he or she at least partially understands the treatment proposed.
7. Simple measures such as ensuring that an elderly person has access to his or her spectacles or hearing aid can have a significant impact on level of capacity.
8. Common law can be invoked to restrain and medicate a patient if there are doubts about his capacity.
9. According to the Mental Health Act, immoral conduct is sometimes tantamount to a mental disorder.
10. Section 2, admission for assessment, lasts 28 days, and Section 3, admission for treatment, lasts six months.
11. An application for a Section 2 must be recommended by two doctors, both of whom must have special experience in the diagnosis and treatment of mental disorders.
12. Under a Section 2, treatment cannot be given unless under common law.
13. A patient with a severe mental disorder can be treated for life-threatening diabetic ketoacidosis under the Mental Health Act.
14. Only a psychiatrist can make a recommendation for a Section 5(2).
15. A patient in the A&E department can be detained under Section 5(2).
16. A patient in the A&E department can be detained under Section 2, 3, or 4.
17. Under Section 117, there is an obligation for the patient to accept aftercare.
18. If a person in a public place appears to a police officer to have a mental disorder, the said police officer can remove him or her to a place of safety under a Section 135.
19. The Mental Health Act 2007 replaced the 'treatability test' with the 'appropriate medical treatment test'.
20. The Mental Health Act 2007 replaced supervised discharge with 'supervised community treatment', with a power to recall a person into hospital if he or she does not comply with certain conditions.

Part 2

That he's mad, 'tis true, 'tis true 'tis pity,
And pity 'tis 'tis true – a foolish figure,
But farewell it, for I will use no art.
Mad let us grant him then, and now remains
That we find out the cause of this effect,
Or rather say, the cause of this defect,
For this effect defective comes by cause:
Thus it remains, and the remainder thus.

Shakespeare, *Hamlet*, Act II, Scene 2

Schizophrenia and other psychotic disorders

4

Key learning objectives

- First rank symptoms of schizophrenia
- Aetiological factors in schizophrenia, including the dopamine hypothesis
- Clinical features of schizophrenia: positive symptoms, disorganised symptoms, negative symptoms
- Differential diagnosis of schizophrenia
- Management of schizophrenia
- Prognostic factors in schizophrenia

The story of VL

A 23-year-old female anthropology student of Afro-Caribbean descent, VL, is brought to Accident and Emergency by one of her colleagues. She is very agitated and difficult to assess. The psychiatry SHO on nights is able to make out that she is hearing three or four male voices coming from outside her head. These voices are talking together about her, making fun of her, blaming her for her family's financial problems, and commenting on her thoughts and behaviour. She is convinced that they are the voices of SAS paratroopers engaged by her parents to destroy her. It seems that the paratroopers are trying to put harmful thoughts, such as the thought of cutting off her fingers one by one, into her head. Any further questioning only serves to make her more agitated. When the SHO leaves the interview room she screams, 'I've seen your belt, they've sent you, they've sent you to distract me. I can't... I can't fight them anymore!'

VL's colleague reports that she has been behaving oddly for the past six months, and that she has not been to lectures since the beginning of last term. The SHO phones VL's house and one of her flatmates tells him that she has been locking herself in her room for hours on end. The flatmate thinks that she started hearing the voices about 10 days ago after she discovered that a close childhood friend recently died from leukaemia.

The SHO ascertains that VL hasn't taken any drugs and that she doesn't have a psychiatric or medical history. He makes a provisional diagnosis of acute schizophrenia-like psychosis as, according to ICD-10, her symptoms have not been present for long enough to make a diagnosis of schizophrenia. After speaking to his registrar, he prescribes 1 mg of lorazepam to sedate her and arranges to admit her for further assessment and treatment. Three days later she is started on the antipsychotic drug risperidone by her consultant psychiatrist.

Issues raised by this case history are:

- Was the SHO justified in phoning VL's house to talk to her flatmate?
- Should VL be detained under the Mental Health Act? Can the SHO do this?
- If the patient refuses to take the risperidone, can it be enforced under the Mental Health Act?

Refer back to Chapter 3 for the answers.

Psychiatry, 2e. By Neel Burton. Published 2010 by Blackwell Publishing.

4

A brief history of schizophrenia

If you talk to God, you are praying. If God talks to you, you have schizophrenia.

Thomas Szasz

Although the oldest description of schizophrenia can be traced back to the second millenium before Christ, it is not until 1887 that **Emil Kraepelin** first recognised it as a distinct entity, distinguishing it from manic-depressive psychosis and naming it **dementia praecox** ('dementia of early life') to differentiate it from other forms of dementia such as Alzheimer's disease. Further to his credit, Kraepelin distinguished at least three clinical varieties of schizophrenia: catatonia, hebephrenia, and paranoia. Although he repeatedly stressed the diversity of signs and symptoms occurring in dementia praecox, he found a chronic course and a poor outcome to be its characteristic defining features.

In 1911 **Eugen Bleuler** (1957–1939) coined the term *schizophrenia* (Ancient Greek, 'splitting of the mind') because, unlike Kraepelin, he did not think that the illness inevitably lead to mental deterioration (*dementia*) nor that it inevitably affected young people (*praecox*). Although Bleuler's term of 'schizophrenia' has been upheld by history, it has lead to much confusion about the nature of the illness. The term does *not* refer to 'split personality' but to the splitting of an individual's thinking and feeling processes ('split personality' or multiple personality disorder is a very rare condition classified under dissociative disorders, see Chapter 8). Bleuler's description of schizophrenia put more emphasis on thought disorder and on negative symptoms than on the more florid positive, or psychotic, symptoms. He described the primary symptoms of the illness as **ambivalence**, **autistic behaviour**, **abnormal associations**, and **abnormal affect** (the so-called 'four As').

In 1959 the German psychiatrist **Kurt Schneider** defined the first rank symptoms of schizophrenia, symptoms supposed to be specific to, and therefore pathognomonic of, schizophrenia (Table 4.1). Schneider's first rank symptoms largely consisted of florid psychotic symptoms

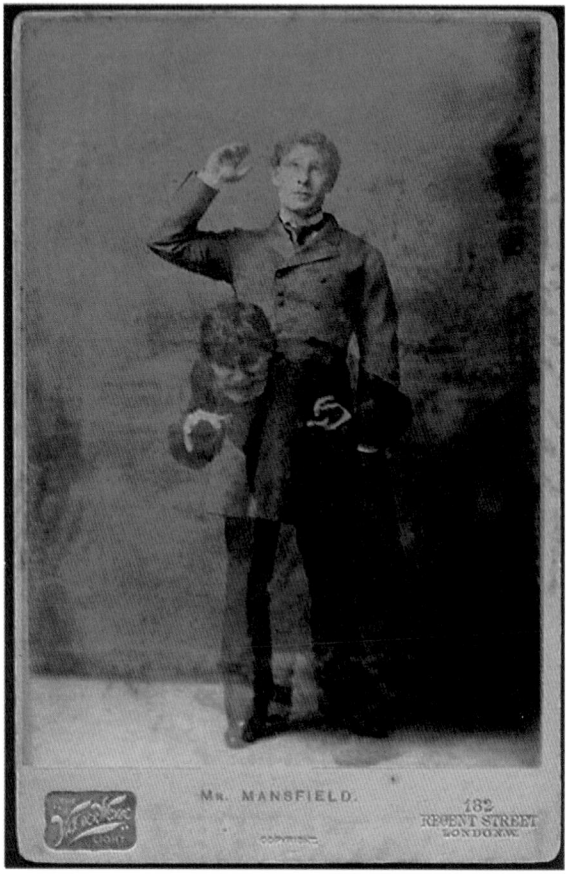

Figure 4.1 Double exposure photograph (1895) of Richard Mansfield, who played the roles of both Dr Jekyll and Mr Hyde. People with schizophrenia do not suddenly change into a different, unrecognisable person.

such as thought insertion, thought broadcasting, and third person auditory hallucinations – symptoms held together by a common theme of loss of control over thoughts, feelings, and the body. Unfortunately these symptoms are common to many psychotic disorders and are therefore not as useful as originally thought at differentiating schizophrenia from other psychotic disorders. They are also absent in about 20% of schizophrenia sufferers.

Case studies of Schneider's first rank symptoms

Echo de la pensée

A 32-year-old housewife complained of a man's voice, speaking in an intense whisper from a point about two feet above her head. The voice would repeat almost all the patient's goal-directed thinking – even the most banal thoughts. The patient would think, 'I must put the kettle on' and after a pause of not more than one second the voice would say, 'I must put the kettle on'. It would often say the opposite, 'Don't put the kettle on'.

Thought insertion

A 29-year-old housewife said, 'I look out of the window and I think the garden looks nice and the grass looks cool, but the thoughts of Eamonn Andrews come into my mind. There are no other thoughts there, only his … He treats my mind like a screen and flashes his thoughts on to it like you flash a picture'.

Thought withdrawal

A 22-year-old woman said, 'I am thinking about my mother, and suddenly my thoughts are sucked out of my mind by a phrenological vacuum extractor, and there is nothing in my mind, it is empty …'

Thought broadcasting

A 21-year-old student said, 'As I think, my thoughts leave my head on a type of mental ticker-tape. Everyone around has only to pass the tape through their mind and they know my thoughts'.

Passivity of affect

A 23-year-old female patient reported, 'I cry, tears roll down my cheeks and I look unhappy, but inside I have a cold anger because they are using me in this way, and it is not me who is unhappy, but they are projecting unhappiness onto my brain. They project upon me laughter, for no reason, and you have no idea how terrible it is to laugh and look happy and know it is not your, but their, emotions'.

Passivity of volition

A 29-year-old shorthand typist described her actions as follows, 'When I reach my hand for the comb it is my hand and arm which move, and my fingers pick up the comb, but I don't control them … I sit there watching them move, and they are quite independent, what they do is nothing to do with me … I am just a puppet who is manipulated by cosmic strings. When the strings are pulled my body moves and I cannot prevent it'.

Passivity of impulse

A 26-year-old engineer emptied the contents of a urine bottle over the ward dinner trolley. He said, 'The sudden impulse came over me that I must do it. It was not my feeling, it came into me from the X-ray department, that was why I was sent there for implants yesterday. It was nothing to do with me, they wanted it done. So I picked up the bottle and poured it in. It seemed all I could do'.

Somatic passivity

A 38-year-old man had jumped from a bedroom window, injuring his right knee which was very painful. He described his physical experience as, 'The sun-rays are directed by a US army satellite in an intense beam which I can feel entering the centre of my knee and then radiating outwards causing the pain'.

Delusional perception

A young Irishman was at breakfast with two fellow-lodgers. He felt a sense of unease, that something frightening was going to happen. One of the lodgers pushed the salt cellar towards him (he appreciated at the time that this was an ordinary salt cellar and his friend's intention was innocent). Almost before the salt cellar reached him he knew that he must return home, 'to greet the Pope, who is visiting Ireland to see his family and to reward them… because our Lord is going to be born again to one of the women… And because of this they [*all the women*] are born different with their private parts back to front'.

C. S. Mellor, First rank symptoms in schizophrenia. *British Journal of Psychiatry* (1970), 117, 15–23

4

Table 4.1 Schneider's first rank symptoms.

Auditory hallucinations	
Third person	Voices discuss or argue about the patient
Running commentary	Voices comment on the patient's thoughts and behaviour
Gedankenlautwerden and *echo de la pensée*	The patient's thoughts are heard as, or shortly after, they are formulated
Delusions of thought control	
Thought insertion	Alien thoughts are put into the patient's mind by an external agency
Thought withdrawal	The opposite; thoughts are removed from the patient's mind by an external agency
Thought broadcasting	The patient's thoughts are overheard by, or otherwise accessible to, others
Delusions of control (passivity phenomena)	
Passivity of affect, volition, and impulses	The patient's affect, impulses, and volition are under the control of an external agency
Somatic passivity	The patient's bodily sensations are under the control of an external agency
Delusional perception	The patient attributes delusional significance to normal percepts

Reminder of some important definitions

Delusion: an unshakeable (fixed) belief that is held in the face of evidence to the contrary, and that cannot be explained by culture or religion.

Hallucination: a percept that arises in the absence of a stimulus, and that is not subject to conscious manipulation.

Gedankenlautwerden: thoughts are 'heard' as they are being formulated.

Echo de la pensée: thoughts are 'heard' shortly after they have been formulated.

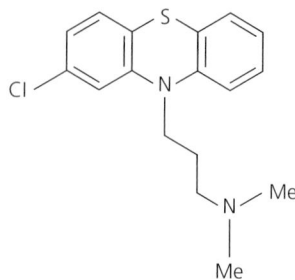

Figure 4.2 Chemical structure of the first anti-psychotic, chlorpromazine, stumbled upon by Henri Laborit in 1952. The French surgeon had been looking for a drug for the treatment of surgical shock.

sulphur or oil. Other popular but unsatisfactory treatments included electroconvulsive treatment, lobotomy, and sleep therapy. The first antipsychotic drug, **chlorpromazine**, first became available in the 1950s. Described as a 'chemical lobotomy', it controlled the positive symptoms of schizophrenia and made patients 'indifferent'. The side-effects of chlorpromazine and related drugs included tremors, restlessness, loss of muscle tone, and postural disorders, and this earned the drug class the name of **neuroleptic** (Ancient Greek, 'nerve seizure').

Although discovered in 1959, the second-generation or 'atypical' antipsychotic **clozapine** did not receive regulatory approval until the 1990s because of its potentially fatal side-effect of agranulocytosis. Like other atypical antipsychotics that came after it, clozapine had, overall, fewer side-effects than chlorpromazine, and controlled both the positive and the negative symptoms of schizophrenia. Today atypical antipsychotics such as risperidone, olanzapine, and quetiapine have become the first line of treatment for schizophrenia. Clozapine, because of its potentially fatal side-effect of agranulocytosis, is reserved for treatment-resistant cases and requires close monitoring (see later).

Epidemiology

- **Prevalence:** figures for the lifetime prevalence of schizophrenia depend on the diagnostic criteria used but are usually quoted at around 1%.
- **Sex ratio:** unlike many other mental disorders such as depression and anxiety disorders, which tend to be more common in women, schizophrenia affects men and women in more or less equal numbers. However, the illness tends to present at a younger age in men, and

Febrile illnesses such as malaria had been observed to moderate psychotic symptoms, and in the early 20th century fever therapy became a popular form of treatment for schizophrenia. Psychiatrists tried to induce fevers in their patients, sometimes by means of injections of

also tends to affect them more severely. Why this should be so is at present unclear.

- **Age of onset:**
  - Any age, but rare in childhood and early adolescence and uncommon after the age of 45 (suspect organic causes)
  - Mean age of onset in men is 28 years
  - Mean age of onset in women is 32 years, with peak incidence in the 20s and 40s (bimodal distribution).
- **Geography:** generally speaking, lifetime prevalence is similar across populations and stable over time, despite the reduced reproductive fitness of affected individuals. Prevalence and severity tend to be greater in urban areas than in rural areas.
  - *Drift hypothesis*: prevalence is higher in urban areas because schizophrenia sufferers drift from rural areas to urban areas as a consequence of their illness or its prodromal symptoms.
  - *Breeder hypothesis*: prevalence is higher in urban areas because the stress of urban living actually plays a part in the aetiology of the illness.
- **Migration:** prevalence is higher in immigrants, and especially in second-generation Afro-Caribbean immigrants to the UK (about a 10-fold increase). This may reflect such factors as poor integration, socioeconomic deprivation, or diagnostic bias amongst

psychiatrists (although recent studies seem to rule out this factor).

- **Seasonality of births:** increased lifetime prevalence (+5–10%) if born from January to April in the northern hemisphere or July to September in the southern hemisphere. Seasonality of births may reflect a viral aetiology.
- **Socioeconomic status:** observed differences are likely accounted for by social drifting, as the socioeconomic status of the fathers of schizophrenia sufferers are normally distributed.

Aetiology

Genetics

Several candidate genes for schizophrenia have been identified, and it seems likely that any given individual has a complement of genetic variations that make him or her more or less vulnerable to developing the disorder. Individual genes identified so far include *dysbindin* (chromosome 6p), *neuregulin 1* (8p), and *G72* (13q). A concordance rate of about 50% in monozygotic twins suggests that genetic and environmental factors are more or less equally involved in the expression of the disorder.

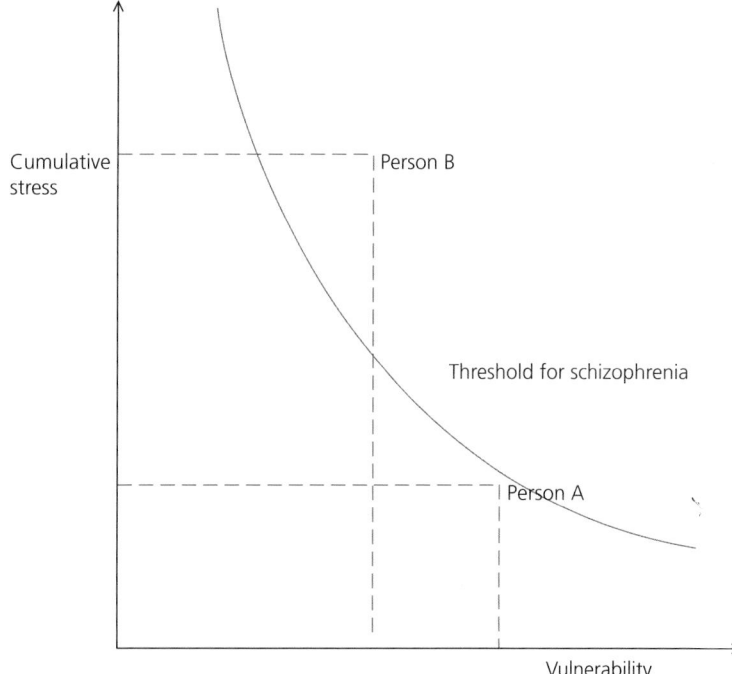

Figure 4.3 The stress–vulnerability or stress–diathesis model for schizophrenia. A person develops schizophrenia when the stress that he or she faces becomes greater than his or her ability to cope with it. Person A is highly vulnerable to developing schizophrenia but does not develop it because he or she is subjected to only moderate amounts of stress. On the other hand, person B is only moderately vulnerable to developing schizophrenia but does develop it because he or she is subjected to unusually high amounts of stress.

4

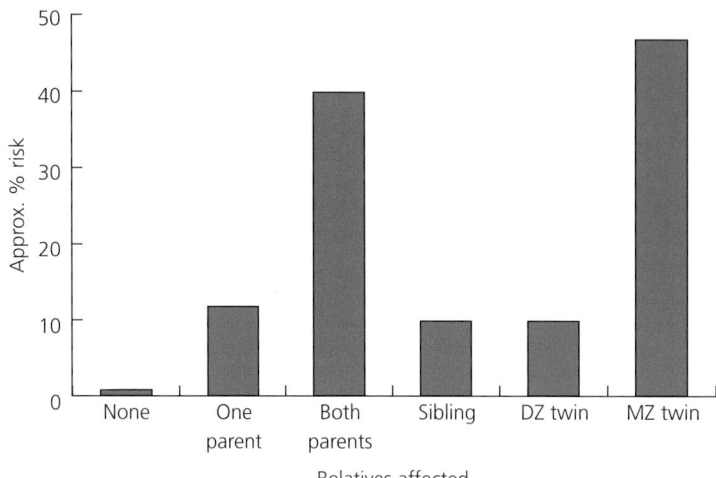

Figure 4.4 Lifetime risks of schizophrenia according to relative(s) affected.

Family studies

The lifetime risks of schizophrenia according to relative(s) affected are illustrated in Figure 4.4.

Adoption studies

Biological offspring of schizophrenic parents adopted by non-schizophrenic parents maintained their increased risk, but biological offspring of non-schizophrenic parents adopted by schizophrenic parents did not have an increased risk at all.

Neurochemical abnormalities

The dopamine hypothesis of schizophrenia states that schizophrenia results from increased levels of dopamine in the brain.

Snyder formulated the dopamine hypothesis of schizophrenia in 1976 based on four sets of findings:

- Amphetamines increase dopamine release and in high doses can induce a schizophrenia-like psychosis ('amphetamine psychosis')
- Amphetamines and other dopaminergic agents exacerbate the symptoms of schizophrenia
- Dopamine antagonists, specifically phenothiazines such as chlorpromazine and butyrophenones such as haloperidol, are effective in the treatment of schizophrenia

- The clinical potency of these typical antipsychotics is correlated to their affinity for dopamine (D_2) receptors. In addition:
- Amphetamine psychosis responds to antipsychotics
- Antipsychotics used in the treatment of schizophrenia can result in parkinsonian side-effects
- L-dopa used in the treatment of Parkinson's disease can result in schizophrenia-like symptoms
- Post-mortem studies suggest that there are increased levels of dopamine and dopamine receptors in the brains of schizophrenia sufferers (although this finding may have resulted from antipsychotic treatment and not from the disease process itself).

Unfortunately, not all findings support the dopamine hypothesis of schizophrenia. In particular:

- Schizophrenia is a relapsing and remitting disorder that presents in a variety of clinical pictures. Such a complex disorder is unlikely to be accounted for by the dopamine hypothesis
- The clinical effects of antipsychotics are only apparent several days after starting treatment, and then only in about 70–85% of schizophrenia sufferers
- Studies of brain tissue, cerebrospinal fluid, and plasma levels of dopamine and its metabolites (homovanillic acid, HVA) do not uniformly support an increase in dopamine levels. In some cases, levels of HVA in the cerebrospinal fluid have even been found to be *decreased*
- Increased levels of dopamine can transiently improve the negative symptoms of schizophrenia.

In light of this conflicting evidence, Davis and colleagues revised the dopamine hypothesis by theorising that the positive symptoms of schizophrenia resulted from dopamine overactivity (hyperdopaminergia) in the **mesolimbic system**, as previously thought, but that the negative symptoms of schizophrenia resulted from dopamine *underactivity* (hypodopaminergia) in the **mesocortical system** (Figure 4.5).

One of the strengths of this revised dopamine hypothesis is its ability to account for the effects of antipsychotic treatment. Typical antipsychotics such as chlorpromazine are unselective in their blocking effect at the dopamine D_2 receptor, and thus decrease the positive symptoms and increase the negative symptoms of schizophrenia (thus making patients 'indifferent'). Atypical antipsychotics such as clozapine, on the other hand, are less likely to increase the negative symptoms of schizophrenia or cause extrapyramidal side-effects because they are selective for the D_2 receptor subtype in the mesolimbic system or because they act primarily on serotoninergic receptors.

Indeed, other neurotransmitters such as serotonin (5-HT), glutamate, noradrenaline, and gamma aminobutyric acid (GABA) also seem to play a role in the aetiology of schizophrenia.

- Findings in support of a role for serotonin:
  - LSD (lysergic acid diethylamide), a 5-HT receptor agonist, can induce a schizophrenia-like psychosis
  - Clozapine, a combined dopaminergic and serotonergic antagonist, is more effective than any other antipsychotic in treatment-resistant schizophrenia.
- Findings in support of a role for glutamate:
  - NMDA antagonists such as phencyclidine hydrochloride (PCP, 'angel dust') and ketamine can induce a schizophrenia-like psychosis
  - Certain studies have reported increased levels of glutamate receptors in the brains of schizophrenia sufferers.

It is probable that altered levels of dopamine and other neurotransmitters such as serotonin and glutamate are interrelated, once more raising the age-old problem of the chicken and the egg.

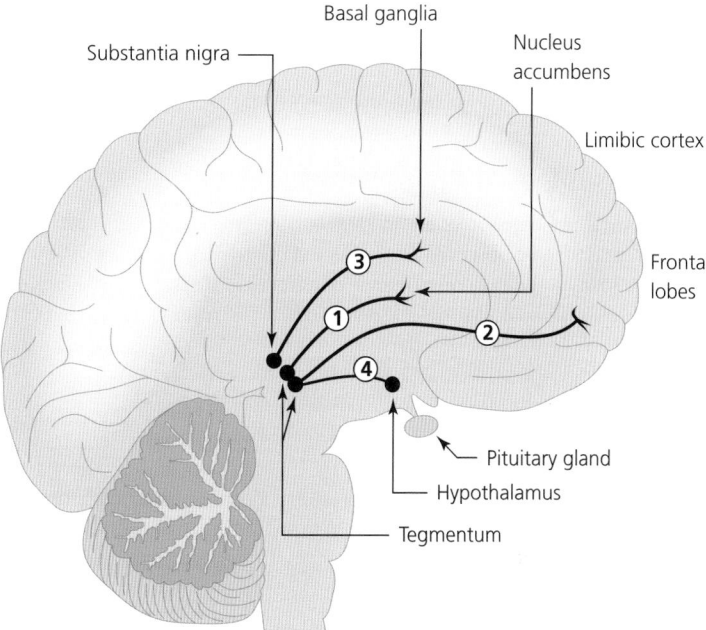

Figure 4.5 Dopamine projections in the brain.

① Mesolimbic tract – positive symptoms of schizophrenia

② Mesocorticol tract – negative symptoms of schizophrenia

③ Nigrostriatal tract – extrapyramidal side-effects of antipsychotic medication

④ Tuberoinfundibular tract – endocrine side-effects of antipsychotic medication

4

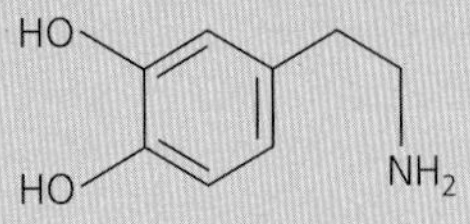

Figure 4.6 Chemical structure of dopamine.

Tyrosine

↓   *Tyrosine hydroxylase*

DOPA

↓   *Dopa decarboxylase*

Dopamine

↓   *Dopamine beta-hydroxylase*

Noradrenaline

Figure 4.7 Synthesis.

Inactivation is through reuptake through the dopamine transporter and either repackaging into vesicles or enzymatic degradation by monoamine oxidase (MAO, in the presynaptic terminal) or catechol-O-methyltransferase (COMT, in synapses).

Receptors
There are five types of dopamine receptor, all of them G-coupled metabotropic receptors. They are divided into the D1-like family (D1 and D5) and the D2-like family (D2, D3, and D4). Activation of D1-like receptors results in increases in cAMP and is typically excitatory. In contrast, activation of D2-like receptors results in decreases in cAMP and is typically inhibitory. D1-like receptors are principally postsynaptic, whereas D2-like receptors are both pre- and post-synaptic.

Functions
Arousal, motivation, desire, pleasure, sociability (mesolimbic and mesocortical tracts), motor control (nigrostriatal tract), release of prolactin from the anterior pituitary (tuberoinfundibular tract), and vomiting (chemoreceptor trigger zone).

Other neurological abnormalities

As structural abnormalities are evident at first presentation and may also be observed in unaffected relatives, they are more likely to be the consequence of a developmental anomaly than that of chronic illness or of its treatment. Structural abnormalities include:
- Reduction in brain mass and size by about 3%, principally affecting the frontal and temporal lobes and medial temporal lobe structures such as the hippocampus, parahippocampus, and amygdala. Reduction in brain mass and size seems to result from a decrease in neuronal size rather than from a neurodegenerative process
- Ventricular enlargement of about 25%, although the distribution of ventricular volumes in schizophrenia sufferers overlaps with that of normal control subjects
- Cytoarchitectural abnormalities.
  Functional abnormalities include:
- 'Hypofrontality', that is, poor performance on tests of frontal lobe function

- Soft neurological signs such as abnormalities of stereognosis and proprioception
- Abnormal eye-tracking performance
- Electroencephalograph (EEG) changes, e.g. increased theta activity, fast activity, and paroxysmal activity, and decreased alpha activity.

Developmental factors

The cytoarchitectural abnormalities and lack of gliosis in the brains of schizophrenia sufferers point to a neurodevelopmental rather than a neurodegenerative pathological process. Studies of the children of schizophrenic parents and of pre-schizophrenic children have suggested subtle manifestations of the schizophrenic genotype characterised by cognitive, motor, and social impairments, and quasi-psychotic symptoms (the so-called premorbid phase).

Further support for a neurodevelopmental pathological process comes from the 'season of birth effect' (see previously). Some studies have suggested that this effect may result from prenatal exposure to the influenza virus or to other viruses. In this respect, it is interesting to note that a season of birth effect has also been reported for autism, depression, and bipolar affective disorder.

Obstetric complications, childhood head injury, and childhood encephalitis have also been suggested as aetiological factors in schizophrenia.

Life events and background stressors

Studies have found that schizophrenia sufferers experience more adverse life events in the month prior to the onset of acute symptoms of the illness. Although this finding suggests that schizophrenia is precipitated by adverse life events, the opposite might also be true. It is also important to remember that most of the stress that a person experiences on a daily basis does not come from life events, but from seemingly smaller 'background' stressors such as tense relationships, painful memories (especially memories of physical or sexual abuse), isolation, discrimination, poor housing, and unpaid bills.

Expressed emotion

Expressed emotion can be thought of as a specific type of stress. It refers to the amount of critical, hostile, or emotionally over-involved attitudes directed to the schizophrenia sufferer by his or her relatives and carers. Such attitudes often originate in a misunderstanding that the schizophrenia sufferer is actually in control of his or her illness and 'choosing' to be ill. Alternatively, over-involvement can result from an unjustified sense of guilt about the schizophrenia sufferer's illness, and a desire on the part of the relative or carer to 'share out' the burden of the illness. A number of studies have demonstrated that high expressed emotion is an important risk factor for relapse in schizophrenia, and that it can increase the risk of relapse by up to four times. As with the relationship between life events and schizophrenia, the relationship between high expressed emotion and schizophrenia is far from being a simple one: in some cases, high expressed emotion may reflect legitimate feelings of anxiety and distress at the illness of a loved one.

Cannabis and other drugs of abuse

Research has found that people who smoke cannabis are up to six times more likely to develop schizophrenia, and that people with schizophrenia who smoke cannabis have more frequent and severe relapses in the illness. Other drugs that have been associated with schizophrenia include stimulant drugs such as amphetamines, ecstasy, and cocaine.

Clinical features

F20 Schizophrenia

The schizophrenic disorders are characterized in general by fundamental and characteristic distortions of thinking and perception, and by inappropriate or blunted affect. Clear consciousness and intellectual capacity are usually maintained, although certain cognitive deficits may evolve in the course of time. The disturbance involves the most basic functions that give the normal person a feeling of individuality, uniqueness, and self-direction. The most intimate thoughts, feelings and acts are often felt to be known to or shared by others, and explanatory delusions may develop, to the effect that natural or supernatural forces are at work to influence the afflicted individual's thoughts and actions in ways that are often bizarre. The individual may see himself or herself as the pivot of all that happens. Hallucinations, especially auditory, are common and may comment on the individual's behaviour or thoughts. Perception is frequently disturbed in other ways: colours or sounds may seem unduly vivid or altered in quality, and irrelevant features of ordinary things may appear more important than the whole object or situation. Perplexity is also common early on and frequently leads to a belief that everyday situations possess a special, usually sinister, meaning intended uniquely for the individual. In the characteristic schizophrenic disturbance of thinking, peripheral and irrelevant features of a total concept, which are inhibited in normal directed mental activity, are brought to the fore and utilized in place of those that are relevant and appropriate to the situation. Thus thinking becomes vague, elliptical, and obscure, and its expression in speech sometimes incomprehensible. Breaks and interpolations in the train of thought are frequent, and thoughts may seem to be withdrawn by some outside agency. Mood is characteristically shallow, capricious, or incongruous. Ambivalence and disturbance of volition may appear as inertia, negativism, or stupor. Catatonia may be present …

ICD-10

4

The onset of schizophrenia is often preceded by an insidious prodromal phase. This prodromal phase can last several years and consists of subtle and non-specific problems in language, cognitive ability, and behaviour that result in a **loss of function**. (Compare this with schizotypal disorder below.)

The symptoms of schizophrenia have traditionally been divided into positive symptoms and negative symptoms, but more recently factor analytical studies have identified a third cluster or dimension of symptoms referred to as 'disorganised symptoms' (Table 4.2). Positive symptoms consist of delusions and hallucinations ('psychotic symptoms'), and are usually most prominent in the acute phase of schizophrenia. Disorganised symptoms involve various cognitive difficulties and are sometimes referred to as 'thought disorder'. They are often detectable in the prodromal phase before the onset of positive symptoms and, although less evident than positive symptoms, they can be just as distressing and disabling. Whereas positive symptoms can be thought of as an excess or distortion of normal functions, negative symptoms can be thought of as a diminution or loss of normal functions. Compared to positive symptoms, negative symptoms tend to be more subtle and less noticeable, but also more persistent. Indeed, they can remain even through periods of remission, long after the positive symptoms have burnt out or faded into the background. During such periods of remission, the severity of any residual negative symptoms is an important determinant of the schizophrenia sufferer's quality of life and ability to function. Unfortunately, negative symptoms are often misconstrued by the general public – and sometimes also by relatives and carers – as laziness or obstreperousness. They can also be difficult to differentiate from symptoms of depression, which are common in schizophrenia sufferers, and from the motor side-effects of antipsychotic medication (see later).

Schizophrenia and creativity

Some highly creative people have suffered from schizophrenia, including Syd Barrett (1946–2006), the early driving force behind the rock band Pink Floyd; John Nash (born 1928), the father of 'game theory'; and Vaclav Nijinsky (1889–1950), the legendary choreographer and dancer. The cases of Barrett, Nash, and Nijinsky are exceptional, and most people with schizophrenia are intensely disabled by the disorder. Even highly creative people with schizophrenia such as Barrett, Nash, and Nijinsky tend to be at their most creative not during active phases of the disorder, but before its onset and during later phases of remission.

Many more highly creative people, whilst not suffering from schizophrenia themselves, have close relatives who do. This was, for example, the case for the physicist Albert Einstein (his son had schizophrenia), the philosopher Bertrand Russell (also his son), and the novelist James Joyce (his daughter). This is unlikely to be simple coincidence, and a number of studies have suggested that the relatives of people with schizophrenia do indeed have above average creative intelligence. According to one theory, both people with schizophrenia and their non-schizophrenic relatives lack lateralisation of function in the brain. Whilst this tends to be a disadvantage for the former, it tends to be an advantage for the latter who gain in creativity from increased use of the right hemisphere and thus from increased communication between right and left hemispheres. This increased communication between right and left hemispheres also occurs in people with schizophrenia, but their thought and language processes tend to be too disorganised for them to make creative use of it.

Table 4.2 Symptoms of schizophrenia.

Positive symptoms	Disorganised symptoms	Negative symptoms
Hallucinations	Disorganised thinking/speech	Affective flattening
Delusions	Disorganised behaviour	Apathy
	Inappropriate affect	Avolition
		Anergy
		Anhedonia
		Alogia
		Asociality
		Attentional impairment

Diagnosis and types

ICD-10 diagnostic criteria for schizophrenia

A minimum of one very clear symptom (and usually two or more if symptoms are less clear-cut) from groups (a) to (d), or symptoms from at least two of the groups (e) to (h).

These symptoms should have been present for most of the time during a period of **one month** *or more. If present for less than one month, a diagnosis of* **acute** *schizophrenia-like* **psychotic disorder** *should be made.*

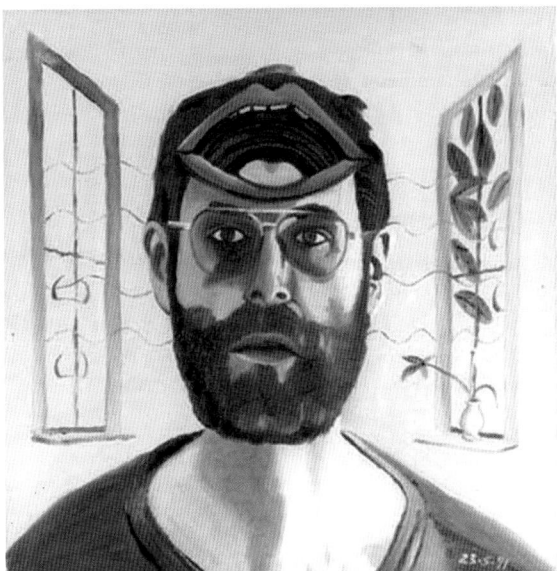

Figure 4.8 Self-portrait of a schizophrenia sufferer with thought broadcasting, which is a symptom of the first rank. Courtesy of SANE/Bryan Charnley.

(a) *Thought echo, thought insertion or withdrawal, thought broadcasting.*

(b) *Delusions of control, influence, passivity; delusional perception.*

(c) *Hallucinatory voices of running commentary, third-person discussion, or other types of voices coming from some part of the body.*

(d) *Persistent delusions of other kinds that are culturally inappropriate and completely impossible.*

(e) *Persistent hallucinations in any modality if accompanied by fleeting or half-formed delusions that are not affective delusions, or by persistent over-valued ideas, or if occurring every day for months on end.*

(f) *Breaks in the train of thought resulting in incoherence, irrelevant speech, or neologisms.*

(g) *Catatonic behaviour such as excitement, posturing, waxy flexibility, negativism, mutism, and stupor.*

(h) *'Negative symptoms' such as apathy, paucity of speech, blunting or incongruity of emotional responses, social withdrawal not due to depression or neuroleptic medication.*

(i) *Significant and consistent change in overall quality of some aspects of personal behaviour, manifest as loss of interest, aimlessness, idleness, a self-absorbed attitude, and social withdrawal.*

ICD-10 types of schizophrenia

F20.0	Paranoid schizophrenia	**F20.4**	Postschizophrenic depression
F20.1	Hebephrenic schizophrenia	**F20.5**	Residual schizophrenia
F20.2	Catatonic schizophrenia	**F20.6**	Simple schizophrenia
F20.3	Undifferentiated schizophrenia	**F20.8**	Other schizophrenia
		F20.9	Schizophrenia, unspecified

Paranoid schizophrenia

Paranoid schizophrenia is the commonest type of schizophrenia. In paranoid schizophrenia, the clinical picture is dominated by relatively stable, often paranoid, delusions, usually accompanied by hallucinations and perceptual disturbances. Disturbances of affect, volition, and speech and catatonic symptoms are *not* prominent. Onset tends to be later than for hebephrenic or catatonic schizophrenia, and the course may be either episodic or chronic.

Hebephrenic schizophrenia

Hebephrenic schizophrenia is marked by prominent affective changes. Mood is inappropriate and often accompanied by giggling or self-satisfied, self-absorbed smiling, or by a lofty manner, grimaces, mannerisms, pranks, hypochrondriacal complaints, and reiterated phrases. Thought is disorganised and speech rambling and incoherent. Behaviour is characteristically aimless and empty of purpose. Compared to paranoid schizophrenia, delusions and hallucinations are fleeting and fragmentary. Hebephrenic schizophrenia is normally diagnosed for the first time only in adolescents or young adults, and has a poor prognosis due to the rapid development of negative symptoms.

Catatonic schizophrenia

Catatonic schizophrenia or catatonia is diagnosed in the presence of prominent psychomotor disturbances that may alternate between extremes such as hyperkinesis and stupor, and automatic obedience and negativism (see Chapter 2 for a full description of catatonia). Catatonia has become rare in occidental and occidentalised societies, perhaps as a result of antipsychotic treatment, or perhaps because the clinical profile of schizophrenia is culturally determined and therefore mutable.

Undifferentiated schizophrenia

Undifferentiated schizophrenia is a diagnosis reserved for conditions meeting the general diagnostic criteria for schizophrenia but not conforming to any of the above subtypes, or exhibiting the features of more than one of them without a clear predominance of a particular set of diagnostic characteristics.

Postschizophrenic depression

A diagnosis of postschizophrenic depression can only be made if the patient has had a schizophrenic illness in the past 12 months, and if some schizophrenic symptoms are still present although no longer dominating the clinical picture. The depressive symptoms must independently fulfil the diagnostic criteria for a depressive episode.

Residual schizophrenia

For a diagnosis of residual schizophrenia to be made, there must have been a clear progression from an early stage (comprising one or more episodes with psychotic symptoms that meet the general criteria for schizophrenia) to a later stage characterised by long-term, although not necessarily irreversible, negative symptoms. For a confident diagnosis of residual schizophrenia to be made, this later stage should already have lasted for at least one year and conditions such as dementia, chronic depression, or institutionalisation should have been excluded.

Simple schizophrenia

Simple schizophrenia is characterised by the insidious but progressive development of oddities of conduct, an inability to meet the demands of society, and a decline in total performance. The characteristic negative symptoms of residual schizophrenia develop without having been preceded by any overt positive or psychotic symptoms. The diagnosis is difficult to make and unreliable.

NB: At this point it is interesting to note that, whilst the biological validity of all these types is questionable, paranoid schizophrenia tends to be dominated by positive symptoms, hebephrenic schizophrenia by disorganised symptoms, and simple schizophrenia by negative symptoms (see Table 4.2).

DSM-IV diagnostic criteria for schizophrenia

A. *Characteristic symptoms: two or more of the following, each present for a significant portion of time during a 1-month period (or less if successfully treated):*
   - *Delusions*
   - *Hallucinations*
   - *Disorganised speech*
   - *Grossly disorganised or catatonic behaviour*
   - *Negative symptoms, i.e. affective flattening, alogia, or avolition.*
   NB: Only one Criterion A symptom is required if delusions are bizarre or hallucinations consist of a voice keeping up a running commentary on the person's behaviour or thoughts, or if there are two or more voices conversing.

B. *Social/occupational dysfunction: for a significant portion of time since the onset of the disturbance, one or more major areas of functioning such as work, interpersonal relations, or self-care are markedly below the level achieved prior to the onset (or when the onset is in childhood or adolescence, failure to achieve expected level of interpersonal, academic, or occupational achievement).*

C. *Duration: continuous signs of the disturbance persist for at least six months. This six-month period must include at least one month of symptoms (or less if successfully treated) that meet Criterion A (i.e. active-phase symptoms) and may include periods of prodromal or residual symptoms. During these periods of prodromal or residual symptoms, the signs of the disturbance may be manifested by only negative symptoms or by two or more symptoms listed in Criterion A present in an attenuated form, e.g. odd beliefs, unusual perceptual experiences. (NB: ICD-10 differs from DSM-IV principally in that it does not specify a six-month period of continuous signs of the disturbance, and in that it does not require criterion B on social/occupational dysfunction.)*

D. **Schizoaffective and mood disorder exclusion:** *schizoaffective disorder and mood disorder with psychotic features have been ruled out because either (1) no major depressive episode, manic episode, or mixed episode have occurred concurrently with the active-phase symptoms; or (2) if mood episodes have occurred during active-phase symptoms, their total duration has been brief relative to the duration of the active and residual periods.*

E. **Substance/general medical condition exclusion:** *the disturbance is not due to the direct physiological effects of a substance or a general medical condition.*

F. **Relationship to a pervasive developmental disorder:** *if there is a history of autistic disorder or another pervasive developmental disorder, the additional diagnosis of schizophrenia is made only if prominent delusions or hallucinations are also present for at least one month (or less if successfully treated).*

DSM-IV types of schizophrenia		
295.10	Disorganised type	Disorganised speech or behaviour; flat or inappropriate affect
295.20	Catatonic type	Catalepsy, excessive motor behaviour, rigid posture, mutism, posturing, grimacing, echolalia, or echopraxia
295.30	Paranoid type	Preoccupation with delusions or auditory hallucinations
295.60	Residual type	Absence of prominent positive symptoms but continuing evidence of disturbance
295.90	Undifferentiated type	Non-specific; used when criteria are not met for paranoid, disorganised, or catatonic types

4

The difficulty with diagnosing schizophrenia

The majority of medical conditions are defined by their cause ('aetiology') or by the damage to the body that they result from ('pathology'), and so are relatively easy to diagnose. For example, if a person is suspected of having malaria, a blood sample can be taken and examined under a microscope for malarial parasites of the genus *Plasmodium*. If a person is suspected of having had a cerebral infarction ('stroke'), a brain scan can be taken to look for evidence of obstruction of an artery in the brain. In contrast, mental disorders are concepts that so far can only be defined by their (supposed) predominant symptoms. For this reason, they are more difficult to describe and diagnose, and more open to misunderstanding and misuse. If a person is suspected of having schizophrenia, there are no laboratory or physical tests that can objectively confirm the diagnosis. Instead the psychiatrist must base his or her diagnosis solely on the symptoms manifested by the patient, without the help of any tests. If the symptoms tally with the diagnostic criteria for schizophrenia listed above, then the psychiatrist is able to make a diagnosis of schizophrenia.

The problem here is that the definition of schizophrenia is circular: the concept of schizophrenia is defined according to the symptoms of schizophrenia, and the symptoms of schizophrenia are defined according to the concept of schizophrenia. Thus, it is impossible to be certain that either schizophrenia or its symptoms map onto any real or distinct disease entity. Given the 'menu of symptoms' approach to diagnosing schizophrenia, it is even possible to have two people with completely different symptoms, but one diagnosis of 'schizophrenia'. Perhaps for this reason, a diagnosis of schizophrenia is a poor predictor of either the severity of the disorder or its likely outcome or prognosis. It has also been argued that psychotic symptoms such as delusions or hallucinations of voices are a poor basis for making a diagnosis of schizophrenia, since psychotic symptoms occur in a number of mental disorders and are therefore a relatively non-specific indicator of mental disorder. Furthermore, most of the disability in schizophrenia is caused by cognitive and negative symptoms rather than by positive symptoms. For these reasons, making a diagnosis of schizophrenia based on psychotic symptoms may be akin to making a diagnosis of pneumonia or appendicitis on the basis of little more than a fever.

4

Clinical skills/OSCE: Enquiring about delusions

Begin with an introductory statement and general questions, such as,

I would like to ask you some questions that might seem a little bit strange. These are questions that we ask to everyone who comes to see us. Is that all right with you? Do you have any ideas or opinions that your friends and family do not share?

Then ask specifically about common delusions (make sure you tailor your questions to the individual patient you are speaking to, e.g. you don't need to ask a manic patient about nihilistic delusions):

- Delusions of control and passivity experiences:
  Is someone or something controlling you?
  Is someone forcing you to think/say/do certain things?
- Delusions of thought control:
  Are you able to think clearly?
  Are your thoughts being interfered with?
  Are thoughts which are not your own being put into your head? (thought insertion)
  Are your own thoughts being removed from your head? (thought withdrawal)
  Are your thoughts being heard or otherwise accessed by other people? (thought broadcasting)
- Delusional perception:
  Do things happening around you have a special meaning to you?
- Delusions of persecution:
  How are you getting on with other people?
  Is anyone deliberately trying to harm you or to make your life miserable?
- Delusions of reference:
  Do people talk about you behind your back?
  Do people drop hints about you/say things that have a special meaning for you?

- Delusions of misidentification:
  Do you feel that people are not who they seem to be? For example, do you feel that they been replaced by imposters (Capgras delusion) or disguised to look like other people? (Fregoli delusion)
- Delusions of grandeur:
  How do you see yourself relative to other people?
  Do you feel you have a special mission?
  Do you feel that you have any special abilities or powers?
- Religious delusions:
  Are you a very religious person?
  Are you especially close to God?
- Delusions of guilt:
  Do you have any regrets?
  Do you feel as though you have committed a crime/sinned greatly/deserve punishment?
- Nihilistic delusions:
  Do you feel that something terrible has happened or is about to happen?
  Do you feel that a part of your body has stopped functioning/been removed?
  Do you feel as though you have died?
- Somatic delusions:
  Are you concerned that you might have a serious illness?
- Delusions of jealousy
  How are you getting on with your partner? Does he or she reciprocate your loyalty?

Explore any delusions and ask in particular about their onset, their effect on the patient's life, and the patient's explanation for them (degree of insight).

Clinical skills/OSCE: Enquiring about auditory hallucinations (voices)

Begin with an introductory statement and general questions, such as,

I gather that you have been under quite some pressure recently. When people are under pressure they sometimes find that their imagination plays tricks on them. Have you had any such experiences? Have you heard things which are unusual? Have you heard things which other people cannot hear?

Then ask more closed questions to determine:

- Content: whose voices are they, where are they coming from, and what are they saying? In particular, are they commanding the patient to do anything dangerous (command hallucination)?

- Type: do the voices speak directly to the patient (second person), speak about him (third person), comment on his every thought and action (running commentary), or repeat his thoughts (thought echo)? Differentiate between true hallucinations and pseudohallucinations. Exclude hypnogogic and hypnopompic hallucinations (see Table 2.7)
- Frequency and duration
- Onset and precipitating factors
- Effect on the patient's life
- The patient's explanation for them (degree of insight and, especially important, likelihood to act on any command hallucinations).

Differential diagnosis

Psychiatric disorders

- Drug-induced psychotic disorder (e.g. amphetamines, cocaine, cannabis, alcohol, LSD, phencyclidine, glucocorticoids, and L-dopa). This differential diagnosis is an important one, as drug-induced psychotic disorders are very common
- Schizoaffective disorder (see p. 73)
- Psychotic depression (see Chapter 5)
- Manic psychosis (see Chapter 5)
- Other psychotic disorder such as schizotypal disorder, brief psychotic disorder, persistent delusional disorder, or induced delusional disorder (see later)
- Puerperal psychosis (see p. 96)
- Personality disorder

Organic disorders

- Delirium
- Dementia
- Stroke
- Temporal lobe epilepsy
- Central nervous system infections such as AIDS, neurosyphilis, herpes encephalitis
- Other neurological conditions such as head trauma, brain tumour, Huntington's disease, Wilson's disease
- Endocrine disorders, in particular Cushing's syndrome

- Metabolic disorders, in particular vitamin B12 deficiency and porphyria
- Autoimmune disorders, in particular systemic lupus erythematosus (SLE)

! Chronic or residual schizophrenia must be differentiated from the symptoms of depression and from the motor side-effects of antipsychotic medication (see later). Depressive symptoms are common in schizophrenia, and about a quarter of patients become depressed once their psychotic symptoms have resolved.

Investigations

Investigations for a first episode of psychosis should include full physical (including neurological) examination, a serum and/or urine drug screen, liver, renal and thyroid function tests, full blood count, fasting blood glucose (or HbA1c), and lipids. The aims of these investigations are principally to uncover possible organic causes of psychosis and to establish baselines for the administration of antipsychotic medication. Other, more specific investigations should be considered on a case-by-case basis, and might for example include brain imaging if there is a suggestion of a space-occupying lesion.

Management

Management is discussed under three principal headings:
- Antipsychotic drugs
- Other drugs and electroconvulsive therapy
- Psychosocial treatments.

Antipsychotic drugs

The following are guidelines to treatment.
- Patients are more likely to respond if treatment is started early, so it is usually best to start treatment soon after the diagnosis is established. Antipsychotic drugs are effective against positive symptoms in about 70–85% of patients, but it can be several days before they take effect and a benzodiazepine such as lorazepam may need to be prescribed in the interim if the patient is agitated or difficult to manage.
- Current treatment guidelines recommend using one of the atypical antipsychotics other than clozapine as a first line of treatment. Choice should be guided primarily by side-effect profile and patient choice (see Tables 4.4 and 4.5).
- If the patient has previously been on treatment, the choice of drug should also be guided by the patient's response to treatment and susceptibility to side-effects.
- The starting dose should be small to minimise side-effects and then increased according to clinical response to the **minimum effective dose**.
- If the patient fails to respond to the chosen antipsychotic or cannot tolerate its side-effects, an alternative antipsychotic from a different class should be tried.
- If the patient fails to respond to two or more antipsychotics after an adequate trial of each (6–8 weeks), clozapine should be considered. Clozapine is effective in about 50% of treatment-resistant patients – 'treatment-resistance' in this case being defined as failure to respond to an adequate trial of at least two antipsychotics.
- If a patient has improved on a particular drug, he or she should continue taking the same drug at the same dose for *at least* the next six months, **and preferably for the next 12–24 months**. Long-term antipsychotic treatment has been demonstrated to reduce rates of relapse and rehospitalisation in a substantial number of patients. Patients with chronic schizophrenia may remain on antipsychotic treatment for many years even though antipsychotics are not effective in the treatment of persistent negative symptoms.
- Depot preparations can be used to improve long-term compliance, but only one atypical antipsychotic (ris-peridone) is available in depot form. The principal advantages and disadvantages of oral versus depot preparations are listed in Table 4.3. Upon converting a patient to a depot antipsychotic, it is usual to first administer a small test dose. The first treatment dose can be administered after about seven days if the patient does not suffer from any unacceptable adverse reactions during this time. The treatment dose can then be increased at regular intervals, as the oral antipsychotic is tapered off and stopped.

Typical antipsychotics (previously referred to as neuroleptics or major tranquillizers) used to be the first line of treatment for schizophrenia. They include chlorpromazine, fluphenazine, flupenthixol, zuclopenthixol, and haloperidol. The clinical antipsychotic efficacy of typical antipsychotics is related to their antagonism of the dopamine D_2 receptor. Their common side-effects are listed in Table 4.4. Extrapyramidal side-effects (EPSEs) are particularly common and can occur in up to 70% of patients. They include acute dystonias, akathisia, Parkinson-like symptoms, and tardive dyskinesia (see Table 4.5). Typical antipsychotics are effective once they reach a certain threshold of D_2 receptor occupancy, thought to be around 60%. Beyond a threshold occupancy of 80% there is little additional clinical efficacy and a significantly increased risk of EPSEs.

Table 4.3 Principal advantages and disadvantages of oral versus depot preparations.

	Advantages	Disadvantages
Oral medication	Short duration of action Flexibility	Variable absorption/ first-pass effect Potential for poor compliance Potential for misuse and overdose
Depot medication	Improved bioavailability Less potential for poor compliance	Potential damage to therapeutic alliance Needle injections: pain, potential local complications, e.g. abscess formation
	Less potential for abuse and overdose	Potential delayed side-effects
	Regular contact with CPN	Potential prolonged side-effects

CPN, Community Psychiatric Nurse.

Table 4.4 Side-effects of antipsychotic drugs according to receptor action.

Receptor action	Potential therapeutic effect	Potential side-effects
Antidopaminergic	Improvement in positive symptoms	Extrapyramidal symptoms (see Table 4.5), Hyperprolactinaemia* Neuroleptic malignant syndrome Weight gain
Serotonergic	Improvement in affective symptoms Improvement in negative symptoms	Anxiety Insomnia Change in appetite leading to weight gain Hypercholesterolaemia Diabetes§
Antihistaminergic	Unknown	Sedation (can be a benefit) Weight gain
Antiadrenergic	Unknown	Postural hypotension Tachycardia Ejaculatory failure
Anticholinergic	Unknown	Dry mouth Blurred vision Constipation Urinary retention

* Symptoms of hyperprolactinaemia include loss of libido, amenorrhoea, erectile dysfunction, galactorrhoea, gynaecomastia, and reduced bone density.
§ The prevalence of type II diabetes is increased in schizophrenia sufferers, their relatives, and those on antipsychotic medication (most evidence for clozapine and olanzapine). This may be a result of weight gain or insulin resistance.
NB: Other side-effects of antipsychotics may include neuroleptic malignant syndrome (NMS – see box, p. 69), hypo- or hyper-thermia, convulsions, cardiotoxic side-effects (increased QTc, myocarditis, cardiomyopathy), hepatotoxicity, blood dyscrasias, photosensitivity, and allergic reactions.

> ❗ Although drugs may be used to treat EPSEs, in the first instance it is often preferable to reduce the dose of the antipsychotic or change the antipsychotic to another (usually atypical) antipsychotic. The prophylactic use of anticholinergics to prevent certain EPSEs is a common practice which is best avoided.

Table 4.5 Extrapyramidal side-effects of antipsychotics.

1. Acute dystonias

Often painful spastic contraction of certain muscles or muscle groups most commonly affecting the neck, eyes, and trunk; for example, tongue protrusion, grimacing, torticollis. Acute dystonias may respond to anticholinergics

2. Akathisia (Greek, *not to sit*)

Distressing feeling of inner restlessness manifested by fidgety leg movements, shuffling of feet, pacing, and so on. Akathisia may respond to anticholinergics, propanolol, the antihistamine cyproheptadine, benzodiazepines, or clonidine

3. Parkinson-like symptoms

Triad of parkinsonian tremor, muscular rigidity, and bradykinesia. Parkinson-like symptoms may respond to anticholinergics

4. Tardive dyskinesia (TD)

Involuntary, repetitive, purposeless movements of the tongue, lips, face, trunk, and extremities that may be generalised or affect only certain muscle groups, typically orofacial muscle groups ('rabbit syndrome'). TD occurs after several months or years of antipsychotic treatment and is often irreversible. Risk factors for TD in patients receiving antipsychotic treatment are length and dose of antipsychotic treatment, increased age, female sex, prominent negative symptoms, head injury/brain damage, and organic brain disease. There is no consistently beneficial treatment and the condition may be *exacerbated* by anticholinergics. Although TD is typically thought of as an antipsychotic-related EPSE, it may also occur in untreated schizophrenia and in healthy elderly people

EPSE, extrapyramidal side-effects.

Strictly speaking, the definition of an atypical antipsy-chotic is **a drug which does not produce catalepsy in rats despite having an antipsychotic profile in behavioural tests**, that is, a drug which, unlike typical antipsychotics, has a high therapeutic index in relation to EPSEs. The reason postulated for this is that in contrast to typical anti-psychotics, atypicals undergo 'fast dissociation' at the dopamine D_2 receptor. The group of atypical antipsychot-ics is considered to include clozapine, risperidone, olanzapine, quetiapine, amisulpride, sertindole, ziprasidone, zotepine, and paliperidone. Atypicals are at least as effective as typical antipsychotics and treat positive symptoms, and, it has been argued, also affective symptoms and negative symptoms. As aforementioned, current treatment guidelines recommend using one of the atypical antipsychotics other than clozapine as a first line of treatment for schizophrenia. Clozapine causes agranulocytosis in about 1% of patients and for this reason patients on the drug must have their differential leucocyte counts monitored. Despite this inconvenience, clozapine is the drug of choice in treatment-resistant schizophrenia, in schizophrenia accompanied by marked suicidality, and in the management of disabling tardive dyskinesia.

Aripiprazole is a novel, third-generation antipsychotic that has been described as a **dopamine-serotonin system stabiliser**. The drug has partial agonist activity at D_2 and $5HT_{1A}$ receptors and antagonist activity at $5HT_{2A}$ receptors. It is purported to have good efficacy in treating positive symptoms, negative symptoms, and affective symptoms, and to be better tolerated than other antipsychotics. Principal side-effects include headache, anxiety, insomnia, nausea, vomiting, and light-headedness, but *not* EPSEs, weight gain, or hyperprolactinaemia.

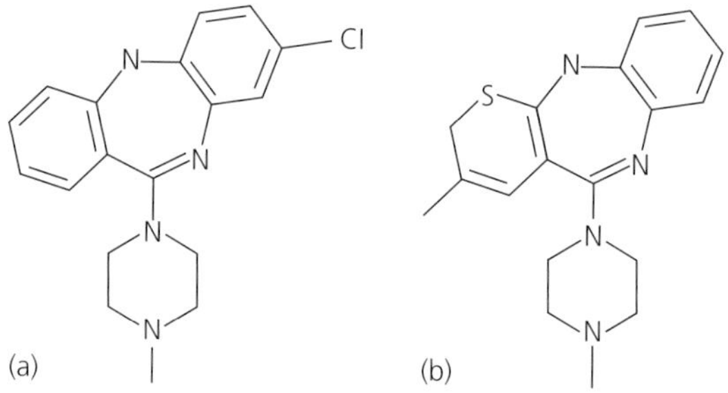

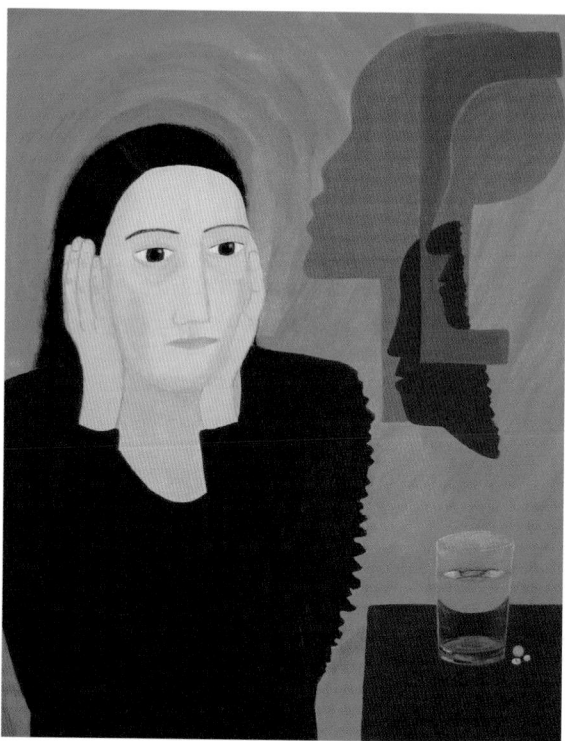

Figure 4.10 'Medication' by Philippa King. Philippa King explains, 'The side-effects I was experiencing on antipsychotic medication were tremors in my arms and hands (illustrated by the wavy line of the sleeve), a dry mouth (another reason for including a glass of water in the picture), and weight gain'.

Figure 4.9 Chemical structures of the aytpical antipsychotics clozapine (left; a dibenzodiazepine) and olanzapine (right; a thienobenzodiazepine). Compare to the structure of chlorpromazine (a phenothiazine) (Figure 4.2).

Table 4.6 Comparison of the side-effect profiles of four commonly prescribed atypical antipsychotics (note that clozapine in particular is also associated with sialorrhoea (hypersalivation), tachycardia, myocarditis, cardiomyopathy, insulin resistance, increased risk of convulsions at higher doses, and agranulocytosis).

Atypical antipsychotic	EPSE	Hyperprolactinaemia	Sedation	Weight gain	Orthostatic hypotension	Anticholinergic side-effects
Risperidone	+	++	+	+	++	0/+
Olanzapine	0/+	+	++	+++	+	+/++
Quetiapine	0/+	0/+	++	++	++	0/+
Clozapine	0	0	+++	+++	+++	+++

EPSE, extrapyramidal side-effects.

! Neuroleptic malignant syndrome

Neuroleptic malignant syndrome (NMS) is a rare but underdiagnosed and potentially fatal idiosyncratic reaction to antipsychotic medication. NMS results from blockade of dopaminergic hypothalamospinal tracts that normally tonically inhibit preganglionic sympathetic neurons. It is characterised by a square of **hyperthermia, muscle rigidity, autonomic instability**, and **altered mental status**. Rhabdomyolysis, as reflected by a high creatinine phosphokinase (CPK) blood level, may lead to renal failure. Other complications include respiratory failure, cardiovascular collapse, seizures, arrhythmias, and disseminated intravascular coagulopathy (DIC). The mainstay of treatment involves stopping the drug and supportive measures such as oxygen, IV fluids, and cooling blankets, although drugs such as dantrolene and lorazepam may also be used to decrease muscle rigidity. **If left untreated, mortality is as high as 20–30%.** Differential diagnosis includes infection, catatonia, parkinsonism, and malignant hyperthermia. Note that atypical antipsychotics, antiparkinsonian drugs, antidepressants, and drugs of abuse such as cocaine or ecstasy can also cause NMS.

Other drugs and electroconvulsive therapy

There may a number of reasons why a patient has not responded to an 'adequate trial' of antipsychotic medication, including ongoing stressors, non-compliance, substance misuse, or an overlooked organic aetiology. If such factors have been excluded or addressed, a **benzodiazepine, lithium**, or **carbamazepine** may be added to the antipsychotic medication. These so-called adjunctive or augmentative treatments are *not* as effective as **clozapine** and should therefore only be used after an adequate trial of clozapine. Clozapine itself is sometimes augmented with **sulpiride** or **risperidone**, but never with carbamazepine which is also linked to agranulocytosis. Nonpharmacological strategies for distressing chronic hallucinations include an IP3 player, subvocal counting or singing, and a pair of earplugs. These strategies should be considered in all treatment-resistant cases, as they are cheap, simple, and empowering, and lacking in side-effects.

Benzodiazepines can also be used in the treatment of ancillary symptom complexes such as anxiety and agitation, and in the emergency treatment of acute psychosis ('rapid transquillisation'). A typical regimen for rapid tranquillisation is lorazepam 1 mg as required, up to 4 mg per 24 hours, delivered either orally or intramuscularly. The atypical antipsychotic haloperidol is also sometimes used for rapid tranquillisation, often in combination with lorazepam. However, this practice is best avoided, as it exposes the patient to a broader range of potential side-effects than lorazepam alone.

Antidepressants and **electroconvulsive therapy** can be used to treat depressive symptoms.

Treatment trials of EPA, an n3 fatty acid contained in fish oil, have so far proven inconclusive.

Clinical skills: Coffee and a cigarette

The vast majority of schizophrenia-sufferers smoke, and typically smoke more heavily than smokers in the general population. This could be because nicotine functions as a neuroprotective agent, or because it stimulates dopamine release in the prefrontal cortex and so alleviates symptoms and improves cognitive performance. Aside from the long-term effects of smoking, nicotine induces the hepatic microsomal enzyme CYP1A2. As clozapine and olanzapine are metabolised by CYP1A2, the levels of these antipsychotics are reduced in smokers. Caffeine is also metabolised by CYP1A2, for which reason smokers tend to drink more coffee than non-smokers. However, caffeine competes with clozapine and olanzapine for CYP1A2, and thereby *increases* the levels of these antipsychotics. Work it out: you probably need an aspirin by now.

Psychosocial treatments

The management of a patient is usually planned at one or several Care Programme Approach (CPA) meetings (see Chapter 3). These meetings are useful to establish the context of the patient's disorder, evaluate his or her current personal circumstances, assess his or her needs, and formulate a detailed care plan to ensure that medical, psychological, and social needs are met. Apart from ensuring that the patient takes his or her medication and that he or she is regularly seen by a member of the mental healthcare team, the care plan should involve a number of psychosocial measures, possibly including supportive therapy, patient self-help groups, family education/therapy, cognitive-behavioural therapy (CBT), and rehabilitation (social skills training and sheltered employment programmes). **Although under-utilised, psychosocial**

Table 4.7 Summary of commonly used atypical, typical, and depot antipsychotics.

Antipsychotic	Trade name	Licensed daily dose range in adults under the age of 65
Atypical antipsychotics		
Risperidone	Risperdal	2–16 mg (rarely exceed 10 mg)
Olanzapine	Zyprexa	5–20 mg
Quetiapine	Seroquel	50–750 mg in two doses, up to 800 mg in mania (usual dose range 300–450 mg)
Amisulpride	Solian	400–1200 mg in two doses
Clozapine	Clozaril/Denzapine	25–900 mg (usual dose range 200–450 mg)
Aripiprazole	Abilify	10–30 mg
Typical antipsychotics		
Phenothiazines		
Chlorpromazine	Largactil	75–1000 mg
Fluphenazine	Modecate/Moditen	2–20 mg
Butyrophenones		
Haloperidol	Haldol/Dozic/Serenace	3–30 mg (18 mg if administered IM/IV)
Diphenylbutylpiperidines		
Pimozide	Orap	2–20 mg (ECG monitoring required)
Thioxanthenes		
Flupenthixol	Depixol	3–18 mg
Zuclopenthixol	Clopixol	20–150 mg
Substituted benzamides		
Sulpiride	Dolmatil/Sulpitil/Sulpor	400–2400 mg
Depot antipsychotics		
Risperidone	Risperdal Consta	Max 50 mg fortnightly
Fluphenazine decanoate	Modecate	Test dose 12.5 mg Max 100 mg fortnightly
Flupenthixol decanoate	Depixol	Test dose 20 mg Max 400 mg/week
Zuclopenthixol decanoate	Clopixol	Test dose 100 mg Max 600 mg/week
Pipiotazine palmitate	Piportil depot	Test dose 25 mg Max 200 mg/4 weeks

NB: Prior to starting an antipsychotic, it is good practice to obtain at the very least: urea and electrolytes, liver function tests, fasting plasma glucose, blood lipids, and prolactin, as well as recordings of blood pressure and weight. Clozapine additionally requires registration with a monitoring service, baseline full blood count and ECG, and weekly full blood counts for the first 18 weeks. It also requires close monitoring of pulse rate, blood pressure, and temperature during the titration period.

measures are often cost-effective and their importance in the treatment of schizophrenia should not be underestimated.

Supportive therapy should be offered to the patient and his or her relatives by one or several members of the Community Mental Health Team. The patient and his or her relatives can additionally be referred to charitable organisations which offer information and support, and which organise patient self-help groups. These enable patients to meet other schizophrenia sufferers, share their experiences, and thereby normalise and destigmatise them. Family education/therapy is useful as relatives invariably need explanation and support, and need to be involved in the patient's management plan. This can help to reduce high expressed emotion and improve compliance with medication, amongst others. CBT can be useful if the patient continues to suffer from residual symptoms such as drug-resistant delusions, or from negative or depressive symptoms. CBT for drug-resistant delusions typically involves exploring the subjective nature of the delusions, challenging the evidence for them, and subjecting them to reality testing. CBT can also be useful to improve a patient's insight, and so his or her compliance with medication.

Some patients, especially those suffering from prominent negative symptoms, may need a period of rehabilitation. Areas that are considered during rehabilitation are accommodation, activities of daily living, occupational activities, leisure activities, and social skills. Several members of the multidisciplinary team, such as the Community Psychiatric Nurse, Occupational Therapist, and Clinical Psychologist, may be co-opted into the patient's care. Sheltered employment programmes use the place-and-train vocational model and significantly increase the patient's likelihood of re-entering competitive employment. Social skills training involves dividing complex social activities, such as making conversation and participating in recreational activities, into simpler steps that can then be learned and practised through role play. Despite a period of rehabilitation, some patients may remain unable to live independently, and may therefore require long-term supported accommodation. Such supported accommodation is often found in a sheltered home or group home – a house shared by several schizophrenia sufferers and supported by a group homes organisation.

Hospitalisation

Schizophrenia is increasingly managed in the community, but hospitalisation may sometimes be required. The possible functions of hospitalisation are listed in Table 4.8. In many cases, attendance at a day hospital or management by the crisis team (in the short-term) or assertive outreach team (in the longer-term) can prevent a hospital admission or decrease time spent in hospital.

Course and prognosis

The course of schizophrenia can vary considerably from one person to another, but it is often marked by a number of distinct phases. In the acute phase, positive symptoms come to the fore, while any cognitive and negative symptoms that may already be present appear to sink into the background. The patient typically reaches a crisis point, at

Table 4.8 Possible functions of hospitalisation.

- Establishment of a diagnosis
- Stabilisation of medication
- Management of acute exacerbations, e.g. severe psychotic symptoms, non-cooperation, lack of insight
- Management of comorbid conditions
- Safety of the patient and of the community
- Carer respite
- Substitute to community care if patient is lacking a social structure

which time contact with mental health services is made. Antipsychotic medication is started and the acute phase resolves, even though residual positive symptoms may still remain in the background for some time. As the acute phase resolves, the cognitive and negative symptoms may appear to return to the fore and dominate the clinical picture. This chronic phase, if it occurs, may last for a period of months or, in some cases, several years. In some cases it may be interrupted by relapses to the acute phase, particularly if the patient is not taking any antipsychotic medication. Common causes of relapse to the acute phase include reduction or discontinuation of antipsychotic medication, non-compliance with antipsychotic medication, substance misuse, high expressed emotion, life events, and child birth.

The prognosis of schizophrenia can be summarised by the 'rule of thirds' according to which, after an acute psychotic episode:

- About one-third of patients recover and lead normal or almost normal lives
- About one-third of patients improve but continue to experience significant symptoms
- About one-third of patients do not improve significantly and require frequent hospitalisation.

The suicide rate in schizophrenia is estimated to be 5%, but the rate of attempted suicide is significantly higher. Risk factors for suicide include being young, being male, being early in the course of the illness, having good insight into the illness, coming from a high socioeconomic family background, having high intelligence, having high expectations, being unmarried, lacking social support, and being recently discharged from hospital (Table 4.9). Other important causes of death in schizophrenia include accidents and cardiovascular disease. Overall, life expectancy is decreased by about 8 years.

Interestingly, the prognosis of schizophrenia is better in traditional societies than in industrialised ones. This may

Schizophrenia and the abuse of psychiatry

Whilst a lack of scientific validity and reliability is a problem for all psychiatric disorders that are defined and diagnosed according to their clinical manifestations and symptoms, it is a particular problem for schizophrenia, which has a history of being abused for political motives. Beginning in the early 1970s, reports began appearing that political and religious dissidents in the Soviet Union were being incarcerated in maximum-security psychiatric hospitals. In 1989 the Soviet government authorised a delegation of psychiatrists from the United States to make site visits to selected hospitals and to conduct extensive interviews of 27 suspected victims of abuse, of whom 24 had at one time or another received a diagnosis of schizophrenia. This investigation provided unequivocal proof that psychiatry had been abused to imprison people who were not mentally disordered and whose only transgression had been the expression of political or religious dissent. In as many as 14 of the 27 cases, there was no evidence of mental disorder of any kind, let alone mental disorder of a nature and degree requiring hospital treatment. The living conditions in the psychiatric hospitals were found to be primitive and highly restrictive, with 'patients' unable even to keep books or writing materials. Physical restraints were used and high doses of antipsychotic and other drugs were administered by injection. In a paper that dates back to 2002 (R. Bonnie, Political abuse of psychiatry in the Soviet Union and China: complexities and controversies. *Journal of American Academic Psychiatry and the Law* (2002), 30, 136–44), Richard Bonnie writes,

In some cases, abuse was undoubtedly attributable to intentional misdiagnosis and to knowing complicity by individual psychiatrists in an officially directed effort to repress dissident behaviour. In other cases, the elastic conception of mental disorder used in Soviet psychiatry was probably bent to political purposes, with individual psychiatrists closing their eyes to whatever doubts they may have had about the consequences of their actions.

In this respect, it is interesting to note that the prevailing diagnostic system in the Soviet Union accommodated a very broad concept of schizophrenia which included mild ('latent' or 'sluggish') and moderate forms supposedly characterised by 'personality changes'. Such blatant abuses of psychiatry are sadly not confined to the Soviet Union. China, for example, has established a system of maximum-security psychiatric hospitals ('Ankang') similar to that in the Soviet Union, in part for confining political offenders and Falun Gong practitioners who are deemed to be a 'social danger'.

Recommended reading

The Meaning of Madness (2009) Neel Burton. Acheron Press.

The Divided Self: An Existential Study in Sanity and Madness (1990) R. D. Laing. Penguin Books Ltd.

Madness Explained: Psychosis and Human Nature (2004) Richard P. Bentall. Penguin Books Ltd.

The Dialectics of Schizophrenia (1997) Philip Thomas. Free Association Books Ltd.

The Quiet Room: Journey Out of the Torment of Madness (1996) Lori Schiller and Amanda Bennett. Little, Brown & Co.

Summary

Epidemiology
- Prevalence of schizophrenia is around 1%, with males and females more or less equally affected.
- Onset can occur at any age but is typically in early adulthood and earlier in males than in females.

Aetiology
- Genetic factors and environmental factors are both involved in the aetiology of schizophrenia.
- The dopamine hypothesis states that positive symptoms of schizophrenia result from overactivity in the mesolimbic system, and negative symptoms from underactivity in the mesocortical system.

Clinical features
- The onset of schizophrenia is often preceded by an insidious prodromal phase that may last for several years and that consists of subtle and non-specific problems in language, cognitive ability, and behaviour that result in a loss of function.
- The symptoms of schizophrenia can be divided into positive symptoms, disorganised symptoms, and negative symptoms. Acute schizophrenia tends to be dominated by positive symptoms and chronic schizophrenia by negative symptoms. It can sometimes be difficult to differentiate chronic schizophrenia from depressive symptoms and from the motor side-effects of antipsychotic medication.
- Schneider's first rank symptoms are supposed to be specific to, and therefore pathognomonic of, schizophrenia. However, they are neither. They largely consist of florid psychotic symptoms held together by a common theme of loss of control over thoughts, feelings, and the body.

Differential diagnosis
- The differential diagnosis of schizophrenia is from other psychiatric disorders (including drug-induced psychotic disorder) and from medical/neurological disorders.

Management
- Antipsychotic drugs are effective against positive symptoms in about 70–80% of patients.
- Current treatment guidelines recommend using one of the atypical antipsychotics other than clozapine as a first line of treatment.
- Atypical antipsychotics such as risperidone, olanzapine, quetiapine, and clozapine are at least as effective as typical antipsychotics and treat the positive and, it has been argued, the affective and negative symptoms of schizophrenia. They are better tolerated than typical psychotics, principally because they cause considerably fewer extrapyramidal side-effects.
- Clozapine causes agranulocytosis in about 1% of patients and for this reason patients on the drug must have their blood counts monitored. Despite this, clozapine is the drug of choice in treatment-resistant schizophrenia.
- Psychosocial measures in the treatment of schizophrenia include family education, psychotherapy, cognitive-behavioural therapy, self-help groups, and rehabilitation.

Prognosis
- Although complete recovery is possible, schizophrenia tends to be progressive and punctuated by episodes of relapse and remission.
- Good prognostic factors include acute onset, late onset, precipitating factors, florid symptoms or associated mood disorder, female sex, no family history, no substance misuse, good premorbid occupational/social adjustment, good social support, early treatment, and good response to treatment.
- Common causes of relapse to the acute phase include reduction or discontinuation of antipsychotic medication, non-compliance with antipsychotic medication, substance misuse, high expressed emotion, life events, and child birth.

4

Self-assessment

Simply answer with true or false. Answers on p. 217.

1. Kraepelin's description of schizophrenia put more emphasis on thought disorder and on negative symptoms than on positive symptoms.
2. Schizophrenia tends to present earlier in women, and also tends to affect women more severely.
3. The season of birth effect is not mirrored in the southern hemisphere.
4. The lifetime risk of schizophrenia if one parent has been affected is about 12%.
5. According to the revised dopamine hypothesis, the negative symptoms of schizophrenia result from dopamine overactivity in the mesocortical system.
6. The subtle and non-specific problems in language, cognitive ability, and behaviour that form part of the prodromal phase of schizophrenia do not result in a loss of function.
7. Strong religious beliefs can be classified as delusions.
8. Pseudo-hallucinations tend to point towards a diagnosis of personality disorder rather than of schizophrenia.
9. Pseudo-hallucinations typically differ from true hallucinations in that they are perceived to arise from the mind rather than from the sense organs, and in that they are less vivid or less distressing.
10. Second person auditory hallucinations are one of Schneider's first rank symptoms.
11. Third person auditory hallucinations are one of Schneider's first rank symptoms.
12. ICD-10 criteria for the diagnosis of schizophrenia are based on Schneider's first rank symptoms.
13. According to ICD-10, for a diagnosis of schizophrenia to be made, symptoms should have been present for most of the time for a period of one month or more.
14. The main differences between the ICD-10 and DSM-IV criteria for schizophrenia is that ICD-10 specifies a six-month period of continuous signs of disturbance, and has an additional criterion specifying social/occupational dysfunction.
15. About 10% of schizophrenia patients become depressed once their psychotic symptoms have resolved.
16. 'Deficit syndrome' refers to prominent and enduring negative symptoms of schizophrenia.
17. Oculogyric crisis and akathisia are side-effects of both typical and atypical antipsychotics.
18. Tardive dyskinesia can occur in up to 10% of patients on typical antipsychotics.
19. The antiadrenergic side-effects of atypical antipsychotics include postural hypotension and tachycardia, but not ejaculatory failure.
20. Olanzapine typically causes more hyperprolactinaemia than either risperidone or quetiapine.
21. Risperidone typically causes more weight gain than either olanzapine or quetiapine.
22. Patients on clozapine must have their blood counts monitored because they are at risk of thrombocytosis.
23. Symptoms of neuroleptic malignant syndrome include hyperthermia, tremor, autonomic instability, and altered mental status.
24. Anticholinergics are used to treat tardive dyskinesia.
25. Psychotic experiences are common in the general population and, for the most part, do not constitute mental disorder.
26. In DSM-IV schizotypal disorder is classified under personality disorders.
27. Brief psychotic disorder has a short course of less than one week.
28. Brief psychotic disorder is often precipitated by acute stress.
29. *Folie à famille* describes a delusional disorder that is shared by several members of the same family.
30. In *folie imposée*, B maintains his or her delusions even if he or she is separated from A.
31. Schizophreniform disorder is a condition characterised by the development of a single delusion or set of related delusions. The delusions are of a fixed, elaborate, and systematised kind, and can often be related to the patient's life situation.
32. The prognosis for schizoaffective disorders is better than that for schizophrenia.
33. If a patient has improved on a particular drug, he or she should continue taking that same drug at the same dose for at least the next three months.
34. Acute onset is a poor prognostic factor in schizophrenia.
35. Florid positive symptoms and associated mood disorder are good prognostic factors in schizophrenia.
36. Suicide is the most common cause of death in schizophrenia.
37. Having good insight into the illness is a protective factor against suicide in schizophrenia.
38. Having high intelligence is a protective factor against suicide in schizophrenia.

Affective (mood) disorders

5

5

Key learning objectives

- Epidemiological factors in mood disorders
- Aetiological factors in mood disorders, including monoamine hypothesis of depression
- Clinical features of depression, mania, and hypomania
- Differential diagnosis of depression, including organic causes
- Be able to assess a patient with low mood
- Be able to talk to a patient about starting an antidepressant or mood stabiliser
- Be able to talk to a patient about electroconvulsive therapy (ECT)

Testimony of a bipolar sufferer

I have been high several times over the years, but low only once.

When I was high, I became very enthusiastic about some project or another and would work on it with determination and success. During such highs I wrote the bulk of two books and stood for parliament as an independent. I went to bed very late, if at all, and woke up very early. I didn't feel tired at all. There were times when I lost touch with reality and got carried away. At such times, I would jump from project to project without completing any, and did many things which I later regretted. Once I thought that I was Jesus and that I had a mission to save the world. It was an extremely alarming thought.

When I was low I was an entirely different person. I felt as though life was pointless and that there was nothing worth living for. Although I would not have tried to end my life, I would not have regretted death. I did not have the wish or the energy to do even the simplest of tasks. Instead I withered away my days sleeping or lying awake in bed, worrying about the financial problems that I had created for myself during my highs. I also had a feeling of unreality, that people were conspiring to make life seem normal when in actual fact it was unreal. Several times I asked the doctor and the nurses to show me their ID because I just couldn't bring myself to believe that they were real.

Psychiatry, 2e. By Neel Burton. Published 2010 by
Blackwell Publishing.

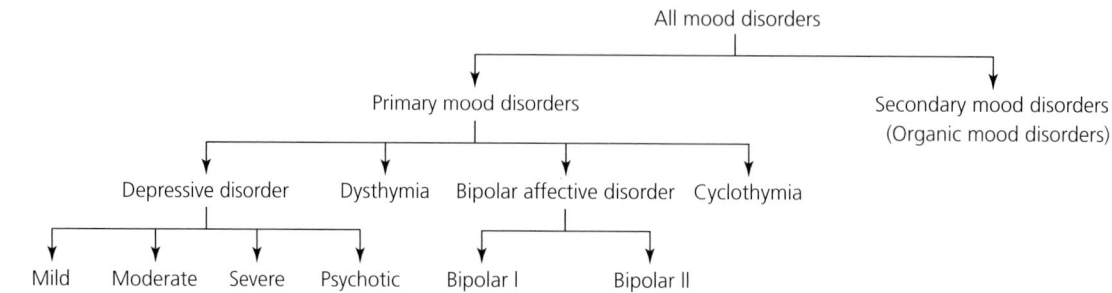

Figure 5.1 Types of mood disorder.

Classification

Primary versus secondary mood disorder

A **primary mood disorder** is one that does not result from another medical or psychiatric condition. A **secondary mood disorder**, on the other hand, is one that results from another medical or psychiatric condition, such as anaemia, hypothyroidism, or substance misuse.

> **!** Once a diagnosis of mood disorder has been made, it is important to consider the possibility that it is a secondary mood disorder. This is not only because a secondary mood disorder is most effectively treated by treating the primary condition that led to it, but also because the primary condition may require medical attention *per se*.

Unipolar depression versus bipolar affective disorder

Broadly speaking, a primary mood disorder is either unipolar (depressive disorder, dysthymia) or bipolar (bipolar affective disorder, cyclothymia) (Figure 5.1). **To meet the criteria for a bipolar mood disorder, the patient must have had one or more episodes of mania or hypomania.** The unipolar–bipolar distinction is an important one to make, as the course and treatment of bipolar affective disorder differ significantly from that of unipolar depression.

Unipolar mood disorders

In ICD-10, depressive disorders are classified according to their severity into **mild, moderate, severe**, and **psychotic** depressive disorder (Figure 5.1). If a patient has had more

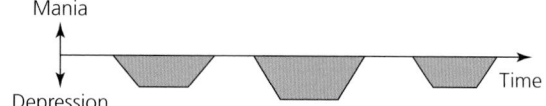

Figure 5.2 Recurrent depressive disorder.

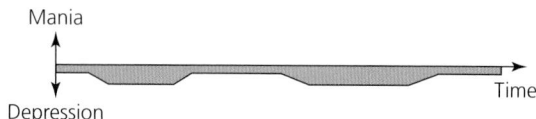

Figure 5.3 Dysthymia.

than one episode of depressive disorder, the term **recurrent depressive disorder** is used, and the current episode is classified as for a single episode, e.g. 'recurrent depressive disorder, current episode moderate' (Figure 5.2). In DSM-IV the term 'major depression' is used instead of depressive disorder, and major depression is simply subclassified as 'single episode' or 'recurrent'.

Not all people suffering from depressive symptoms have a depressive disorder. **Dysthymia** can be described as a mild chronic depression and as such is characterised by depressive symptoms that are not sufficiently severe to meet a diagnosis of depressive disorder (Figure 5.3).

Bipolar mood disorders

According to ICD-10, bipolar affective disorder consists of repeated (2+) episodes of depression and mania or hypomania (Figure 5.4).

In the absence of episodes of mania or hypomania, the diagnosis is one of recurrent depressive disorder.

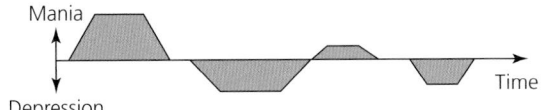

Figure 5.4 Bipolar affective disorder (DSM-IV Bipolar I).

In the absence of episodes of depression, the diagnosis is either one of bipolar affective disorder or of hypomania, **i.e. recurrent episodes of mania are diagnosed as bipolar affective disorder**. This is not only because sooner or later a depressive episode is almost certain to supervene, but also because recurrent episodes of mania resemble bipolar affective disorder in their course and prognosis.

According to DSM-IV, 'bipolar disorder' can be diagnosed after even a single episode of mania, whereas in ICD-10 a single episode of mania (without a history of depressive episodes) is simply diagnosed as 'manic episode'. The separation of bipolar disorder into bipolar I and bipolar II in DSM-IV may have implications for treatment response. **Bipolar I** consists of episodes of major depression and mania (Figure 5.4), and **bipolar II** of episodes of major depression and *hypomania*.

Cyclothymia can be described as mild chronic bipolar affective disorder and is characterised by recurrent episodes of mild elation and mild depressive symptoms that are not sufficiently severe or prolonged to meet the criteria for bipolar affective disorder or recurrent depressive disorder (Figure 5.5).

5

ICD-10 classification of affective disorders

F30 Manic episode
    F30.0 Hypomania
    F30.1 Mania without psychotic symptoms
    F30.2 Mania with psychotic symptoms
    F30.8 Other manic episodes
    F30.8 Manic episode, unspecified

F31 Bipolar affective disorder (BAD)
    F31.0 BAD, current episode hypomanic
    F31.1 BAD, current episode manic without psychotic symptoms
    F31.2 BAD, current episode manic with psychotic symptoms
    F31.3 BAD, current episode mild or moderate depression
    F31.4 BAD, current episode severe depression without psychotic symptoms
    F31.5 BAD, current episode severe depression with psychotic symptoms
    F31.6 BAD, current episode mixed
    F31.7 BAD, current episode in remission
    F31.8 Other bipolar affective disorders
    F31.9 Bipolar affective disorder, unspecified

F32 Depressive episode
    F32.0 Mild depressive episode
    F32.1 Moderate depressive episode
    F32.2 Severe depressive episode without psychotic symptoms
    F32.3 Severe depressive episode with psychotic symptoms
    F32.8 Other depressive episodes
    F32.9 Depressive episode, unspecified

F33 Recurrent depressive disorder
    F33.0 Recurrent depressive disorder, current episode mild

    F33.1 Recurrent depressive disorder, current episode moderate
    F33.2 Recurrent depressive disorder, current episode severe without psychotic symptoms
    F33.3 Recurrent depressive disorder, current episode severe with psychotic symptoms
    F33.4 Recurrent depressive disorder, currently in remission
    F33.8 Other recurrent depressive disorders
    F33.9 Recurrent depressive disorder, unspecified

F34 Persistent mood disorders
    F34.0 Cyclothymia
    F34.1 Dysthymia
    F34.8 Other persistent mood disorder
    F34.9 Persistent mood disorder, unspecified

F38 Other mood disorders
    F38.0 Other single mood disorders
    F38.1 Other recurrent mood disorders
    F38.8 Other specified mood disorders

F39 Unspecified mood disorders

DSM-IV classification of affective disorders
Depressive disorders
  Major depressive disorder
    Single episode
    Recurrent
  Dysthymic disorder
Bipolar disorders
  Bipolar disorder I
  Bipolar disorder II
  Cyclothymic disorder
Mood disorder due to a general medical condition
Substance-induced mood disorder

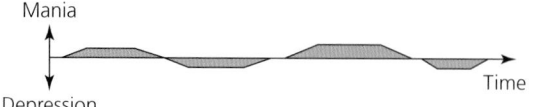

Figure 5.5 Cyclothymia.

Depressive disorders

(…) I have of late – but
wherefore I know not – lost all my mirth, forgone all
custom of exercises; and indeed it goes so heavily
with my disposition that this goodly frame, the
earth, seems to me a sterile promontory, this most
excellent canopy, the air, look you, this brave
o'erhanging firmament, this majestical roof fretted
with golden fire, why, it appears no other thing to
me than a foul and pestilent congregation of vapours.
What a piece of work is a man! how noble in reason!
how infinite in faculty! in form and moving how
express and admirable! in action how like an angel!
in apprehension how like a god! the beauty of the
world! the paragon of animals! And yet, to me,
what is this quintessence of dust? man delights not
me: no, nor woman neither, though by your smiling
you seem to say so.

Shakespeare, *Hamlet*, Act II, Scene 2

Epidemiology

Depression is so common that the costs of treating it
exceed the costs of treating hypertension and diabetes
combined. Figures for the lifetime incidence or lifetime
risk of depressive disorders depend on the criteria used
to define 'depressive disorders'. Using the criteria for
major depressive disorder (DSM-IV), the **lifetime risk
of depressive disorders is about 15%**. The prevalence
of depressive disorders at any one time or **point prevalence is about 5%**. This figure masks an uneven gender distribution, as **females are more affected than males
by a ratio of about 2:1**. The reasons for this uneven
gender distribution are unclear but are thought to be

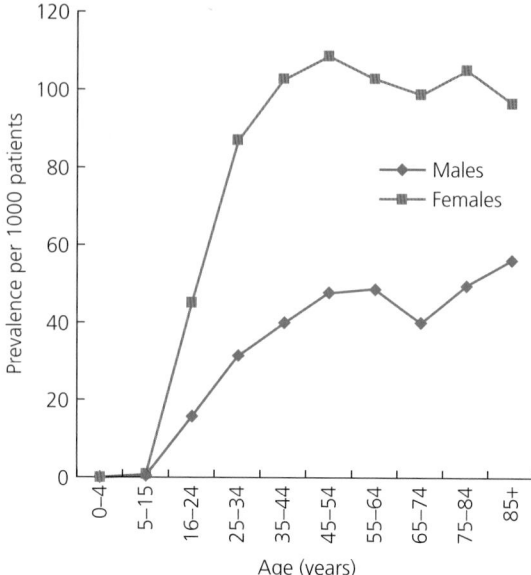

Figure 5.6 Prevalence of 'treated depression' according to age
and sex. Note prevalences and peaks. (Adapted from *Key Health
Statistics from General Practice* 1998.)

partly biological (genetic predisposition, hormonal
influences), and partly sociocultural (social pressures,
readiness to admit to depressive symptoms, diagnostic
bias in clinicians). Although depressive disorders can
occur at any age, their peak prevalence in males is in
old age, and in females it is in middle age (Figure 5.6).
They are relatively uncommon in children, or present
differently (see Chapter 13). Interestingly, the overall
prevalence of depressive disorders appears to be rising.

There are important geographical variations in the
prevalence rates of depressive disorders, and these
can at least in part be accounted for by sociocultural factors. For example, somatic presentations of
depression are particularly common in Asian and
African cultures and may therefore be difficult to recognise as depression. **As a clinician it is important
to remember that sociocultural factors can affect
the presentation not only of depression but also of
other psychiatric and non-psychiatric conditions** (see
Table 7.3).

Aetiology

Genetics

The prevalence rate for major depression in first-degree relatives is about 15%, compared to about 5% in the general population. Although first-degree relatives of a depressed patient are at increased risk of depressive disorders, they are *not* at increased risk of bipolar affective disorder or schizoaffective disorder. **The concordance rate for major depression in monozygotic twins is 46%, compared to 20% in dizygotic twins.** There is thus an important genetic component to the aetiology of depressive disorders. The inheritance pattern is no doubt polygenic, but more research is needed to identify the genes involved.

Neurochemical abnormalities

The monoamine hypothesis of depression suggests that depression results from the depletion of the monoamine neurotransmitters noradrenaline, serotonin, and dopamine. In its revised version the monoamine hypothesis of depression recognises that depression may actually result not from a depletion of the monoamine neurotransmitters, but from a change in their receptors' function.

Support for the original monoamine hypothesis of depression comes from several findings, notably:

- Antidepressants increase the levels of the monoamine neurotransmitters:
  - Monoamine oxidase inhibitors (MAOIs) inhibit the degradation of monoamines presynaptically;
  - Tricyclic antidepressants (TCAs) inhibit the reuptake of noradrenaline from the synaptic cleft;
  - Selective serotonin reuptake inhibitors (SSRIs) inhibit the reuptake of serotonin from the synaptic cleft
- Amphetamines and cocaine increase the levels of monoamines in the synaptic cleft and can elevate mood
- Reserpine decreases the levels of monoamines presynaptically and can depress mood
- CSF levels of 5-hydroxyindoleacetic acid (5-HIAA), a serotonin metabolite, are decreased in depression sufferers.

Psychopharmacology: Serotonin in the brain

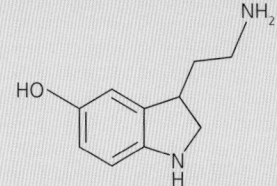

Figure 5.7 Chemical structure of serotonin.

Tryptophan

$\downarrow$ *Tryptophan hydroxylase*

5-hydroxy tryptophan
(5-HTP)

$\downarrow$ *5-HTP decarboxylase*

Serotonin

Figure 5.8 Synthesis.

Inactivation is by reuptake from the synapse into the presynaptic neuron through the 5-HT reuptake transporter, which can be inhibited by serotonin-selective reuptake inhibitors, tricyclic antidepressants, cocaine, and ecstasy. Degradation is by monoamine oxidase (MAO), which converts serotonin to 5-hydroxyindole acetaldehyde, which is then to converted 5-hydoxyindole acetic acid, the major excreted metabolite of serotonin.

Receptors
The raphe nuclei are the principal source of serotonin in the brain: they are grouped in pairs and distributed along the entire length of the brainstem. There are at least seven families of serotonin receptors. They are all G-coupled metabotropic receptors except for the 5-HT$_3$ receptor, which is a ligand-gated ion channel.

Functions
Mood, anxiety, sleep, appetite, sexuality, vomiting, regulation of body temperature.

Other neurological abnormalities

Computed tomographic and magnetic resonance imaging findings in major depression include enlarged lateral ventricles and loss of volume in the frontal and temporal lobes, hippocampus, and basal ganglia, but these findings are inconsistent.

Endocrine abnormalities and immune function

The fact that depression occurs in a variety of endocrine disorders (Cushing's syndrome, Addison's disease, hypothyroidism, hyperparathyroidism) suggests that endocrine abnormalities play a role in the aetiology of depressive disorders. It has been found that plasma cortisol levels are increased in about 50% of depression sufferers and that about 50% of depression sufferers fail to respond to the dexamethasone suppression test. These endocrine abnormalities may have their origins in disturbances of the hypothalamic–pituitary–adrenal axis, which may at least in some cases result from changes in immune regulation.

Organic causes

The organic causes of depression are listed in Table 5.1.

Personality traits

Personality disorders and certain personality traits such as neuroticism and obsessionality predispose to depression. Personality disorders are covered in Chapter 8.

Table 5.1 Organic causes of depression.
(NB: This list is non-exhaustive.)

Neurological	Stroke, Alzheimer's disease/dementia, Parkinson's disease, Huntington's disease, multiple sclerosis, epilepsy, intracranial tumours
Endocrine	Cushing's syndrome, Addison's disease, hypothyroidism, hyperparathyroidism
Metabolic	Iron deficiency, B_{12}/folate deficiency, hypercalcaemia, hypomagnesaemia
Infective	Influenza, infectious mononucleosis, hepatitis, HIV/AIDS
Neoplastic	Non-metastatic effects of carcinoma
Drugs	L-dopa, steroids, beta-blockers, digoxin, cocaine, amphetamines, opioids, alcohol

Environmental factors

Early adverse life events such as loss of a parent, neglect, or sexual abuse may predispose to depression in later life, and an 'excess of life events' has been found to occur in the months preceding the onset of a depressive episode. A depressive episode that appeared to result from life events and lacked somatic symptoms (see p. 83) used to be called a *reactive* depression and contrasted with an *endogenous* depression, but both epithets and their cognates have been abandoned in favour of the realisation that all depressive episodes ultimately result from a combination of both genetic and environmental factors. Interestingly, the so-called 'kindling hypothesis' suggests that, over the course of several years, successive depressive episodes become less and less attributable to life events.

> ### Historical study: The Brown and Harris study
>
> In 1978, Brown and Harris studied working class women in inner London boroughs and found that certain circumstances acted as so-called 'vulnerability factors' for depression. These included:
>
> - Loss of mother by death or separation before the age of 11
> - Excess of life events or major difficulties prior to onset of depression
> - Lack of a supportive relationship
> - Three or more children under the age of 14 at home
> - Not working outside the home.

Seasonal affective disorder

Seasonal affective disorder (SAD) is a depressive disorder that recurs every year at the same time of year and may be marked by increased sleep and carbohydrate craving. The condition is thought to result from changes in the seasons, particularly in the length of daylight, and may respond to bright artificial lights given at 2500 lux in the morning and late evening. There is usually complete summer remission and, occasionally, summer hypomania or mania which, along with Shakespeare, may be at the origin of the expression, 'This is very midsummer madness'.

Psychological theories

Three of the most influential psychological theories of depression are considered in Tables 5.2 and 5.3.

Table 5.2 Psychological theories of depression.

According to	Depression results from
Bowlby's attachment theory	Maternal deprivation
Freud's psychoanalytical theory	Loss of the loved object and mixed feelings of love and hatred, so-called *ambivalence*
Beck's cognitive theory	Beck's triad (negative appraisal of the self, of the present, and of the future) and Beck's cognitive distortions (see Table 5.3).

Table 5.3 Beck's cognitive distortions or thinking errors in depression.

Arbitrary inference	Drawing a conclusion in the absence of evidence, e.g. *The whole world hates me*
Overgeneralisation	Drawing a conclusion on the basis of a single incident, e.g. *My nephew did not come to visit me – the whole world hates me*
Selective abstraction	Focussing on a single event to the detriment of others, e.g. *She gave me an annoyed look three days ago. (But never mind that she spent an hour talking to me this morning)*
Personalisation	Relating independent events to oneself, e.g. *The nurse went on holiday because she was fed up looking after me*
Dichotomous thinking	'All-or-nothing' thinking, e.g. *If he doesn't come to see me today then he doesn't love me*
Magnification/ minimisation	Over- or under-estimating the importance of an event, e.g. *Now that my cat is dead, I'll never have anything to look forward to*
Catastrophic thinking	Exaggerating the consequences of an event or situation, e.g. *The pain in my knee is getting worse. I'm probably going to end up in a wheelchair. Then I won't be able to go to work and pay the mortgage, so I'll lose my house and end up living in the street*

'Learned helplessness' and depression

In 1975 Seligman demonstrated that dogs that had learnt that they could not escape from an electric shock did not try to escape from it even once the situation permitted them to do so. In other terms, once the dogs had learnt that they could not exert control over their environment, they permanently gave up the will to do so. Extended to human behaviour, this so-called 'learned helplessness' has provided an influential cognitive-behavioural model of depression.

Man's Search for Meaning

We who lived in concentration camps can remember the men who walked through the huts comforting others, giving away their last piece of bread. They may have been few in number, but they offer sufficient proof that everything can be taken from a man but one thing: the last of human freedoms – to choose one's attitude in any given set of circumstances – to choose one's own way.

Victor Frankl (1905–1997), psychiatrist, neurologist, holocaust survivor, author of *Man's Search for Meaning*, and founder of logotherapy and existential psychotherapy

Frankl observed that those who survived longest in the concentration camps were not those who were physically the strongest, but those who succeeded in retaining a sense of individual purpose and control over their lives.

Table 5.4 Symptoms of depression.

Core symptoms	Low mood
	Loss of interest and enjoyment
	Fatigability
Psychological symptoms	Poor concentration
	Poor self-esteem
	Guilt
	Pessimism
Somatic symptoms	Sleep disturbance
	Early morning waking
	Morning depression
	Loss of appetite and weight loss
	Loss of libido
	Anhedonia
	Agitation or retardation

Clinical features

The symptoms of depression can be divided into core symptoms, psychological symptoms, and physical or somatic symptoms (Table 5.4). 'Anhedonia' refers to the loss of the capacity to experience pleasure from previously pleasurable activities.

Although the most common symptom of depression is depressed mood, many patients never complain of this and instead present with cognitive, behavioural, or somatic symptoms. For example, they may present because they are feeling tired all the time, because they cannot concentrate on their job, or because they can no longer partake in their marital or social roles.

Mild depression is the commonest form of depression and tends to present, if at all, to GPs. The patient often complains of feeling depressed and tired all the time, and sometimes also of feeling stressed or anxious (so-called 'mixed anxiety–depression'). There are none of the somatic features of depression and, although suicidal thoughts can occur, self-harm is uncommon.

Moderate depression is the classic textbook description of depression that is often treated in primary care but

that can be severe enough to be referred to a psychiatrist. **Many if not most of the clinical features of depression are present to such an intense degree that the patient finds it difficult to fulfil his or her social obligations.** Somatic features are present and anhedonia is characteristic. Suicidal ideation is common and may be acted upon.

Severe depression is an exaggerated form of moderate depression. It is characterised by intense negative feelings and psychomotor agitation or retardation. Depressive stupor may supervene upon psychomotor retardation, and in such cases urgent ECT treatment may be required (see p. 91). **Psychotic symptoms** may present in 10–25% and are usually mood-congruent, e.g. nihilistic delusions, delusions of guilt, delusions of poverty (see Chapter 2). Suicidal risk is high and, in the retarded patient, may paradoxically be even more so once treatment is initiated and the patient develops sufficient motivation and energy to act on his or her suicidal thoughts.

The subjective experience of depression

In depression this faith in deliverance, in ultimate restoration, is absent. The pain is unrelenting, and what makes the condition intolerable is the foreknowledge that no remedy will come – not in a day, an hour, a month, or a minute. If there is mild relief, one knows that it is only temporary; more pain will follow. It is hopelessness even more than pain that crushes the soul. So the decision-making of daily life involves not, as in normal affairs, shifting from one annoying situation to another less annoying – or from discomfort to relative comfort, or from boredom to activity – but moving from pain to pain. One does not abandon, even briefly, one's bed of nails, but is attached to it wherever one goes.

William Styron (1925–2006), *Darkness Visible: A Memoir of Madness*

Styron is also the author of *Sophie's Choice* and other novels.

When the shadow of the sash appeared on the curtains it was between seven and eight o'clock and then I was in time again, hearing the watch. It was Grandfather's and when Father gave it to me he said I give you the mausoleum of all hope and desire; it's rather excruciatingly apt that you will use it to gain the reducto absurdum of all human experience which can fit your individual needs no better than it fitted his or his father's. I give it to you not that you may remember time, but that you might forget it now and then for a moment and not spend all your breath trying to conquer it. Because no battle is ever won he said. They are not even fought. The field only reveals to man his own folly and despair, and victory is an illusion of philosophers and fools.

William Faulkner (1897–1962), *The Sound and the Fury*

Clinical skills: The omega sign and Veraguth's fold

The omega sign is a fold that looks like the Greek letter 'Ω' in the forehead just above the root of the nose. It is sometimes produced in depression through the action of the corrugator muscle, which is the muscle of grief and suffering.

Another clinical sign that is sometimes produced in depression is Veraguth's fold, which is an oblique skin fold in the upper eyelid that runs medially and superiorly.

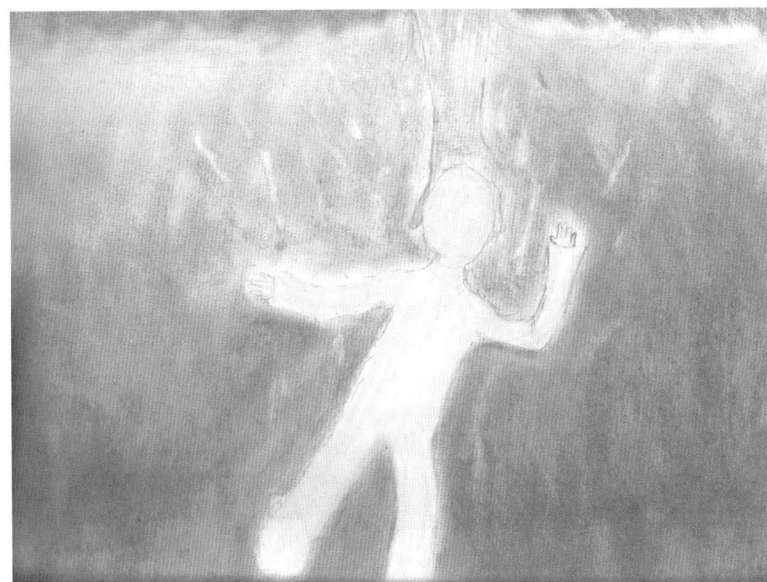

Figure 5.9 A drawing by an inpatient suffering from severe depression. She is drowning, and each time she struggles up near the surface, she is pushed back down.

5

Dysthymia

Dysthymia is characterised by mild chronic depressive symptoms that are not sufficiently severe to meet the criteria for mild depressive disorder. Although dysthymia has sometimes been regarded as a 'depressive personality', genetic studies suggest that it is in fact a chronic, mild form of depressive disorder. If it develops into a depressive disorder, it is then referred to as 'double depression' (Figure 5.10). Its lifetime prevalence is about 3% and, as it is a very chronic condition, its point prevalence is not significantly different. Dysthymia may respond to drug treatment and to psychological treatments, although there is no firm evidence base for the latter.

Diagnosis

ICD-10 criteria for depressive episode

In typical depressive episodes of all three varieties described in ICD-10 (mild, moderate, and severe), the individual usually suffers from depressed mood, loss of interest and enjoyment, and reduced energy leading to increased fatiguability and diminished activity. Marked tiredness after only slight effort is common. Other common symptoms are:

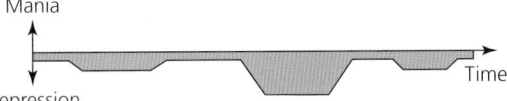

Figure 5.10 Dysthymia and double depression.

- *Reduced concentration and attention*
- *Reduced self-esteem and self-confidence*
- *Ideas of guilt*
- *Pessimism*
- *Ideas of self-harm or suicide*
- *Disturbed sleep*
- *Poor appetite.*

*Mood varies little from day to day and is often unresponsive to circumstances. In some cases, anxiety, distress, and motor agitation may be more prominent than depressed mood. For depressive episodes of all three grades of severity a duration of at least **two weeks** is usually required for diagnosis, **but shorter periods may be reasonable if symptoms are unusually severe and of rapid onset**. The categories of mild, moderate, and severe depressive episodes should only be used for a single (first) depressive episode, and further episodes should be classified under one of the subdivisions of recurrent depressive disorder.*

ICD-10 criteria for mild depressive episode

At least two of depressed mood, loss of interest and enjoyment, and increased fatiguability should be present, plus at least two of the other symptoms described above, for a minimum period of two weeks. None of the symptoms should be present to an intense degree.

ICD-10 criteria for moderate depressive episode

At least two of the three most typical symptoms noted for mild depressive episode should be present, plus at least three (and preferably four) of the other symptoms for a minimum of two weeks. Several symptoms are likely to be present to an intense degree.

An individual with a moderately severe depressive episode will usually have considerable difficulty in continuing with social, work, or domestic activities.

ICD-10 criteria for severe depressive episode

There is considerable distress or agitation, unless retardation is a marked feature. Loss of self-esteem and feelings of uselessness or guilt are likely to be prominent, and suicide is a distinct danger in particularly severe cases. Psychotic symptoms may be present and are usually mood-congruent.

DSM-IV criteria for major depressive episode

A. *Five or more of the following symptoms have been present for the same **two-week** period and represent a change from previous functioning; at least one of the symptoms is either depressed mood, or loss of interest or pleasure:*
  A. *Depressed mood most of the day, nearly every day*
  B. *Markedly diminished interest or pleasure in all, or almost all, activities most of the day, nearly every day*
  C. *Significant weight loss or weight gain or decrease or increase in appetite*
  D. *Insomnia or hypersomnia*
  E. *Psychomotor agitation or retardation*
  F. *Fatigue or loss of energy*
  G. *Feelings of worthlessness or excessive or inappropriate guilt*
  H. *Diminished ability to think or concentrate*
  I. *Recurrent thoughts of death, recurrent suicidal ideation, or suicide attempt*
B. *Symptoms do not meet criteria for a mixed episode*
C. *Symptoms cause significant distress or impairment on social, occupational, or other important areas of functioning*
D. *The symptoms are not due to the direct physiological effects of a substance or a general medical condition*
E. *The symptoms are not better accounted for by bereavement*

DSM-IV criteria for major depressive disorder, single episode

A. *Presence of a single major depressive episode*
B. *The major depressive episode is not better accounted for by schizoaffective disorder and is not superimposed on schizophrenia, schizophreniform disorders, delusional disorder, or psychotic disorder not otherwise specified*
C. *There has never been a manic episode, a mixed episode, or a hypomanic episode*

NB: Does not apply if these episodes are substance- or treatment-induced or the direct physiological effects of a general medical condition.

DSM-IV criteria for major depressive disorder, recurrent

A. *Presence of two or more major depressive episodes*
B. *The major depressive episodes are not better accounted for by schizoaffective disorder and are not superimposed on schizophrenia, schizophreniform disorders, delusional disorder, or psychotic disorder not otherwise specified*
C. *There has never been a manic episode, a mixed episode, or a hypomanic episode*

NB: Does not apply if these episodes are substance- or treatment-induced or the direct physiological effects of a general medical condition.

> ! Note that neither ICD-10 nor DSM-IV requires the presence of depressed mood for a diagnosis of depressive disorder to be made.

Differential diagnosis

- Normal reaction to life event or situation, or to fresh insight

Depressive realism

And I gave my heart to know wisdom, and to know madness and folly: I perceived that this also is vexation of spirit.
For in much wisdom is much grief: and he that increaseth knowledge increaseth sorrow.

Ecclesiastes 1:17–18 (KJV)

Whilst people with depression can suffer from cognitive distortions about everyday events, the scientific literature suggests that they can also have more accurate judgement about the outcome of so-called contingent events (events which may or may not occur) and a more realistic perception of their role, abilities and limitations. This so-called 'depressive realism' may enable a person with depression to shed the Pollyanna-ish optimism and rose-tinted spectacles that shield us from reality, to see life more accurately, and to judge it accordingly.

Psychiatric disorders

- Adjustment disorder (see Chapter 7)
- Bereavement (see Chapter 7)
- Seasonal affective disorder (SAD)
- Dysthymia
- Cyclothymia
- Bipolar disorder
- Mixed affective states (during transition from mania to depression or *vice versa*)
- Schizoaffective disorder
- Schizophrenia, including:
  - Depression superimposed upon schizophrenia
  - Negative symptoms of schizophrenia
  - Extrapyramidal side-effects of antipsychotic drugs
- Schizophreniform disorder
- Delusional disorder
- Generalised anxiety disorder
- Obsessive–compulsive disorder
- Post-traumatic stress disorder
- Eating disorder

Medical or organic disorders

The organic causes of depression are listed in Table 5.1. In all cases, it is important to consider the possibility that a depressive disorder is secondary to a primary, organic condition. This is not only because a secondary mood disorder is most effectively treated by treating the primary condition that led to it, but also because the primary condition may require medical attention *per se*.

5

Clinical skills/OSCE: Assess a patient with low mood

- First ask open questions about his or her current mood and feelings, listening attentively and gently encouraging him or her to open up.
- Aim to cover:
  The core symptoms of depression:
  - Depressed mood
  - Loss of interest
  - Fatiguability.
  The psychological symptoms of depression:
  - Poor concentration
  - Poor self-esteem and self-confidence
  - Guilt
  - Pessimism.
  The somatic symptoms of depression:
  - Sleep disturbance
  - Early morning waking
  - Morning depression
  - Loss of appetite and/or weight loss
  - Loss of libido

  - Anhedonia
  - Agitation and/or retardation.
- Ask about anxiety, obsessions, hallucinations, delusions, and mania, to exclude other possible psychiatric diagnoses.
- Ask about the onset of illness, and about its possible triggers and causes.
- Assess the severity of the illness and the effect that it is having on everyday life.
- **Ask about suicidal intent. If the patient so much as hints that he or she is actively suicidal, you must carry out a full risk assessment (see Chapter 6).**
- Take brief psychiatric, medical, drug, and family histories.
- Ask him or her if there is anything else he or she might add that you have forgotten to ask about.
- Thank him or her and, if appropriate, offer a further course of action (see p. 88).

Adapted from *Clinical Skills for OSCEs*, 3e (2009), by Neel Burton, Scion Publishing

Management

Clinical skills: Investigations in depression

Laboratory investigations should be ordered on a case-by-case basis to exclude potential medical or organic causes of depression (see above), to exclude complications of illness such as malnutrition or dehydration, and as a baseline for starting drug treatment. Laboratory investigations to consider include FBC, U&E, LFTs, TFTs, ESR, vitamin B$_{12}$ and folate, toxicology screen, antinuclear antibody, HIV test, and dexamethasone suppression test. A CT or MRI scan of the brain should also be considered if clinically indicated.

Methods of treatment include:
- Antidepressants:
  - Serotonin-selective reuptake inhibitors (SSRIs)
  - Tricyclic antidepressants (TCAs)
  - Monoamine oxidase inhibitors (MAOIs)
  - Other antidepressants
- Other drugs
- Electroconvulsive therapy
- Psychological and social treatments

Antidepressants

History of antidepressants

The first MAOI, iproniazid, was originally developed in the 1950s as a treatment for tuberculosis. Although it revolutionised the treatment of depression, patients had to adhere to a strict diet to avoid its most dangerous side-effect, the tyramine reaction (see p. 90).

The first TCA, imipramine, was originally developed in the late 1950s as a treatment for schizophrenia. Although patients no longer had to adhere to a strict diet, they continued to suffer from a number of other troublesome and potentially dangerous side-effects.

It took another 30 years for the next class of antidepressants to be developed, and the first SSRI, fluoxetine, only gained regulatory approval in 1987. Since then other classes of dual action and selective antidepressants have been developed, such as venlafaxine, mirtazepine, and reboxetine, but their exact role in the treatment of depression remains to be established.

Table 5.5 Factors involved in choosing an antidepressant.

Factor	Explanation or example
Patient preference	Patients should be explained the common and potentially dangerous side-effects of the main alternatives and given a reasonable degree of choice
Previous treatment	If a patient has had a previous positive response to an antidepressant, that same antidepressant should be re-started
Type and severity of symptoms	Prefer an SSRI for mixed anxiety–depression; prefer a sedative antidepressant if there is insomnia
Suicidality	Avoid TCAs and MAOIs as they are more toxic in overdose (and prescribe any drug in smaller amounts)
Past history of elevated mood	All antidepressants may promote 'manic switch' in bipolar depression, but this is particularly true of TCAs. If a patient has a history of elevated mood, ask for a psychiatric opinion before starting an antidepressant
Age and physical health	Prefer an SSRI in elderly and physically ill patients
Pregnancy	Prefer the SSRI fluoxetine and the TCAs nortriptyline, amitriptyline, and imipramine in pregnancy, and the SSRIs paroxetine or sertraline in breastfeeding.

MAOI, monoamine oxidase inhibitor; SSRI, serotonin selective reuptake inhibitor; TCA, tricyclic antidepressant.

! Explanation and reassurance are an important part of treatment in all depressions, and in the acute milder depressions may be the only form of treatment that is either necessary or appropriate.

If it is decided to start an antidepressant, several factors need to be considered in choosing it (Table 5.5).

The chosen antidepressant should be prescribed at its therapeutic dose and trialled for an adequate period of time (at least one month), unless intolerable side-effects develop. After recovery the antidepressant should be continued **at the same dose** for at least six months before being tapered off. Patients should be educated about antidepressants, not least because this significantly improves compliance. In particular, they should be told that:

- Although it is true that antidepressants are not a solution to life's problems, they can lift your mood and give you a better chance of addressing them
- Antidepressants are effective in over 60% of patients but it can be 10–20 days before you start noticing an effect. Better sleep is often the first sign of improvement
- Antidepressants may have troublesome side-effects, but these do tend to resolve in the first month of treatment. (List the common and potentially dangerous side-effects of the main alternatives)
- Antidepressants should not be stopped suddenly once treatment is established.

If a patient fails to respond to an adequate trial of an antidepressant (i.e. the antidepressant has been prescribed at its therapeutic dose for a period of at least one month), check compliance. If the patient has been compliant, the diagnosis is not in doubt, and there are no significant perpetuating factors (e.g. hypothyroidism, alcoholism, social factors), increase the dose to the recommended maximum or tolerated dose. If the patient still fails to respond, try another drug from the same class or from a different class. If the patient still fails to respond, this is referred to as 'treatment-resistant depression'. A third antidepressant can be tried, although it is important to remember that antidepressants are not the only form of treatment for depression (see later).

Serotonin-selective reuptake inhibitors

Serotonin-selective reuptake inhibitors (SSRIs) such as fluoxetine, fluvoxamine, paroxetine, sertraline, citalopram, and escitalopram (the pharmacologically active S-enantiomer of citalopram) selectively inhibit the reuptake of serotonin. SSRIs have replaced TCAs as the first line of treatment, notably because of their lesser need for dose titration and their safety in overdose. They are particularly useful in the elderly and the physically ill, in mixed anxiety–depression, and in suicidal patients. The response rate to SSRIs is 55–70%, but improvement in mood may be delayed for 10–20 days. Side-effects include dry mouth, nausea, vomiting, diarrhoea, dizziness, sedation, sexual dysfunction, agitation, akathisia, parkinsonism (rare), and convulsions (rare). As fluoxetine, fluvoxamine, and paroxetine in particular are potent inhibitors of the cytochrome P450 isoenzymes, they can also cause important pharmacokinetic drug interactions.

The **SSRI discontinuation syndrome** consists of headache, dizziness, shock-like sensations, paraesthesia, gastrointestinal symptoms, lethargy, insomnia, and changes in mood (depression, anxiety/agitation), and occurs most frequently after the abrupt discontinuation of paroxetine, which has a comparatively short half-life. Note that the fact that a discontinuation syndrome has been described does not mean that SSRIs are 'addictive' in the sense that people do not experience a 'high' from them, and do not seek or crave them as they might a drug of abuse such as cocaine or heroin.

! The serotonin syndrome

The **serotonin syndrome** is a rare but potentially fatal acute syndrome resulting from increased serotonin (5-HT) activity. It is most often caused by SSRIs but can be caused by other drugs too, e.g. TCAs or lithium.

Symptoms include:
- Psychological symptoms: agitation, confusion
- Neurological symptoms: nystagmus, myoclonus, tremor, seizures
- Other symptoms: hyperpyrexia, autonomic instability.

The principal differential of serotonin syndrome is from neuroleptic malignant syndrome. Management involves the discontinuation of the drug and institution of supportive measures.

Recent doubts about the efficacy of SSRIs

Doctors often tell people starting on an SSRI that they have a 55–70% chance of responding to their medication. However, a recent paper (E. H. Turner et al, Selective publication of antidepressant trials and its influence on apparent efficacy. New England Journal of Medicine (2008), 358(3), 252–260) suggested that the effectiveness of SSRIs is greatly exaggerated as a result of a bias in the publication of research studies. Of 74 studies registered with the United States Food and Drug Administration (FDA), 37 of 38 studies with positive results were published in academic journals. In contrast, only 14 of 36 studies with negative results were published in academic journals, and 11 of these were published in such a way that they conveyed a positive outcome. Thus, whilst 94% of published studies conveyed a positive outcome, only 51% of all studies actually demonstrated one.

Continued...

Another recent paper (I. Kirsch I et al, Initial severity and antidepressant benefits: A meta-analysis of data submitted to the Food and Drug Administration. *Public Library of Science Medicine* (2008)) combined 35 studies submitted to the FDA before the licensing of four antidepressants, including the SSRIs fluoxetine and paroxetine. The authors of the study found that, whilst the antidepressants performed better than a placebo, the effect size was very small for all but very severe cases of depression. Furthermore, the authors attributed this increased effect size in very severe cases of depression not to an increase in the effect of the antidepressants, but to a decrease in their placebo effect.

If, as these studies suggest, the efficacy of SSRIs has been greatly exaggerated, their cost–benefit urgently needs to be re-evaluated. In any case, there can be little doubt that at least some of the benefit of an antidepressant is attributable to its placebo effect.

Table 5.6 Principal side-effects of TCAs.

Anticholinergic	Dry mouth, blurred vision, glaucoma, constipation, urinary retention
Antihistaminergic	Sedation, weight gain
α-Noradrenergic blockade	Sedation, postural hypotension
5-HT$_2$ blockade	Weight gain, sexual dysfunction
Cardiotoxic	Arrhythmias*, myocardial depression
Neurotoxic	Delirium, movement disorders, convulsions

* ECG changes indicative of cardiotoxicity include prolonged PR and QT intervals, and ST segment and T wave changes.

Tricyclic antidepressants

Tricyclic antidepressants (TCAs) inhibit the reuptake of noradrenaline and serotonin and also have antagonist activities at a variety of neurotransmitter receptors. As their name suggests, they have a three-ringed structure with an attached side-chain (Figure 5.11). Tertiary amines such as amitriptyline, imipramine, and clomipramine are more sedating and cause more anticholinergic side-effects than secondary amines such as nortriptyline, dothiepin, and lofepramine. See Table 5.6 for other common side-effects. Plasma monitoring may be required in certain circumstances, e.g. lack of a therapeutic response, coexisting medical disorder, or possibility of drug interaction. Although TCAs may be more effective than SSRIs for severe depression in in-patients, they must be used cautiously in the elderly and the physically ill, and should be avoided in suicidal patients. Principal contraindications are cardiovascular disease (TCAs delay ventricular conduction time), severe liver disease, glaucoma, and prostatic hypertrophy. Important drug inter-

actions include dental anaesthetics containing lignocaine ('lidocaine') and MAOIs. The response rate to TCAs is 55–70% but improvement in mood may be delayed for 10–20 days. Better sleep is usually the first sign of improvement.

Monoamine oxidase inhibitors (MAOIs)

Patients on the older or irreversible MAOIs (phenelzine, isocarboxacid, and tranylcypromine) must adhere to strict dietary restrictions to avoid the so-called tyramine (or 'cheese and chianti') reaction – a hypertensive crisis that can result in subarachnoid haemorrhage. For this reason MAOIs are seldom used, and then only in treatment-resistant depression or atypical depression (depression with increased sleep, increased appetite, and phobic anxiety).

> **!** Substances that can provoke the tyramine reaction include:
> - Tyramine containing foods such as cheese (except cottage cheese and ricotta), game, yeast extracts, broad bean pods, pickled herring, beef or chicken liver, and some alcoholic drinks
> - Sympathomimetic drugs, including non-prescription cold remedies.

MAOIs inactivate monoamine oxidase enzymes that oxidise the monoamine neurotransmitters dopamine, noradrenaline, serotonin (5-HT), and tyramine. There are two isoforms of monoamine oxidase enzymes, MAO-A and MAO-B. Moclobemide is a more recent, reversible MAOI that binds selectively to MAO-A, leaving MAO-B

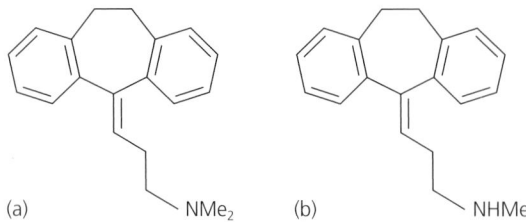

(a)　　　　　　NMe$_2$　　(b)　　　　　　NHMe

Figure 5.11 Chemical structures of (a) amitriptyline and (b) nortriptyline.

free to metabolise tyramine and eliminating the need for dietary restrictions.

Other side-effects of MAOIs include anticholinergic side-effects, weight gain, insomnia, postural hypotension, tremor, paraesthesia of the limbs, and peripheral oedema.

> **!** A TCA or SSRI should not be started until two weeks after stopping a MAOI (three weeks in the case of clomipramine and imipramine). Conversely, a MAOI should not be started until at least 7–14 days after stopping a TCA or SSRI (three weeks in the case of clomipramine and imipramine, and as many as five weeks in the case of fluoxetine). Other drugs that interact with MAOIs include insulin, pethidine, and barbiturates.

Other antidepressants

Table 5.7 lists some of the other antidepressants available.

Other drugs

Lithium, tryptophan, tri-iodothyronine, buspirone (a 5-HT1$_A$ partial agonist), or pindolol (a beta-blocker and 5-HT1$_A$ antagonist) can be used to augment antidepressant treatment.

Antipsychotics can be used in addition to antidepressants if there are psychotic symptoms.

Electroconvulsive therapy

> ### History of electroconvulsive therapy
>
> In pre-modern times it had been observed that convulsions induced by camphor could improve schizophrenia and depression. In 1933 the German psychiatrist Sakel began the practice of using insulin injections to induce convulsions, but a period of panic and impending doom prior to convulsing
>
> Continued...

5

Table 5.7 Other antidepressants.

Antidepressant	Class	Notes
Venlafaxine	Serotonin and noradrenaline reuptake inhibitor (SNRI)	Usually used in treatment-resistant depression Arguably has a more rapid onset of action and greater efficacy than SSRIs, especially in severe depressive disorder Similar side-effect profile to SSRIs and may cause hypertension and heart disease Should not be used in patients with heart disease, uncontrolled hypertension, or electrolyte imbalance. An ECG and a blood pressure measurement should be undertaken prior to starting treatment and blood pressure measurements should be undertaken at regular intervals thereafter Relatively safe in overdose
Reboxetine	Noradrenaline reuptake inhibitor (NARI)	Highly specific noradrenaline reuptake inhibitor Usually used as a second- or third-line treatment for depression Arguably more effective than SSRIs in severe depression Less likely than SSRIs to trigger mania in bipolar depression or convulsions in epilepsy Common side-effects include dry mouth, constipation, and insomnia Safe in overdose
Mirtazapine	Noradrenaline and serotonin-specific antidepressant (NaSSa)	Enhances noradrenergic and serotonergic neurotransmission but has no significant effect on the reuptake of monoamines Usually used as a second or third line treatment for depression Commoner side-effects are weight gain, sedation, and dry mouth. Mirtazapine becomes *less* sedative as the dose is increased Less sexual side effects than other antidepressants Safe in overdose
Trazodone	Phenylpiperazine	Weak serotonin reuptake inhibitor Commonly used in the elderly Mildly sedating, can cause priapism in 0.1% Safe in overdose

made the treatment very difficult to tolerate. The Hungarian psychiatrist Meduna replaced insulin by metrazol, but similar problems remained. Then in 1938 the Italian neuropsychiatrist Cerletti began the practice of using electric shocks. Cerletti's method, first tested on a vagrant that he found at *Roma Termini* (the main train station in Rome), soon superseded Sakel's insulin injections and Meduna's metrazol injections as the least unpopular method of inducing convulsions. The advent of suitable short-acting anaesthetics and muscle relaxants in the 1950s made the electric shocks much safer by reducing complications such as muscle pains and bone fractures. Since then many drugs have been invented, but electroconvulsive therapy (ECT) is still occasionally used as an alternative form of treatment. Its mechanism of action is unclear, although it is known to decrease $5\text{-}HT_1$ and increase $5\text{-}HT_2$ receptors in the brain.

Indications

Table 5.8 lists the main indications for ECT.

Contraindications

As ECT is a potentially life-saving treatment, it has no absolute contraindications. Relative contraindications include:
- Cardiovascular disease
- Raised intracranial pressure
- Dementing illnesses
- Epilepsy and other neurological disorders
- Cervical spine disease.

Note that old age and pregnancy are not contraindications to ECT.

Method

The patient is given a standard anaesthetic such as propofol and a muscle relaxant such as suxamethonium, and the seizure duration is monitored using an electroencephalograph (EEG) recording (Figure 5.12). The modern approach is to deliver constant current, brief-pulse ECT that is at a voltage above the patient's individual seizure threshold. The choice of bilateral or unilateral (usually right-sided) ECT should be made on a case-by-case basis: although bilateral ECT is more effective than unilateral ECT, unilateral ECT has less cognitive side-effects (see below). Most patients respond to a course of four to eight ECT treatments, delivered over the course of two to four weeks. Prior to starting a course of ECT treatments, a patient should have a physical examination, an

Table 5.8 Indications for ECT.

Depression	Severe depression is by far the most common indication for ECT. The treatment is especially indicated in treatment resistance or in the presence of psychotic features, pronounced psychomotor retardation, or high suicidal risk. Its efficacy is *at least equal* to that of antidepressants, and its speed of action is faster – an important factor in life-threatening situations
Mania	The use of ECT in mania is uncommon and restricted to acute mania that is refractory to drug treatment or if drug treatment is contraindicated
Schizophrenia	The use of ECT in schizophrenia is uncommon and restricted to acute episodes of schizophrenia in the presence of marked catatonia or affective symptoms

electrocardiograph (ECG), and blood tests including FBC and U&Es – and should be 'nil by mouth' from the previous midnight. Informed consent is needed except if being treated under the provision of the Mental Health Act. The Mental Health Act 2007 introduces new safeguards for the use of ECT. In short, ECT may not be given to a person with the capacity to refuse consent, and it may only be given to a person without the capacity to refuse consent if this does not conflict with any advance directive, decision of a donee or deputy, or decision of the Court of Protection.

Common side-effects

- Side-effects of anaesthesia
- Headache
- Muscle aches
- Nausea
- Confusion
- Temporary anterograde memory impairment

Note that mortality is similar to that of any minor surgical procedure and mostly results from cardiovascular complications such as arrhythmias. Although memory impairment is a recognised side-effect of ECT, most patients actually feel their memory improving as their depression lifts. Interestingly, emerging evidence suggests that the use of repetitive transcranial magnetic stimulation (rTMS) could in some cases provide a safer and less off-putting alternative to ECT in depression and other psychiatric disorders.

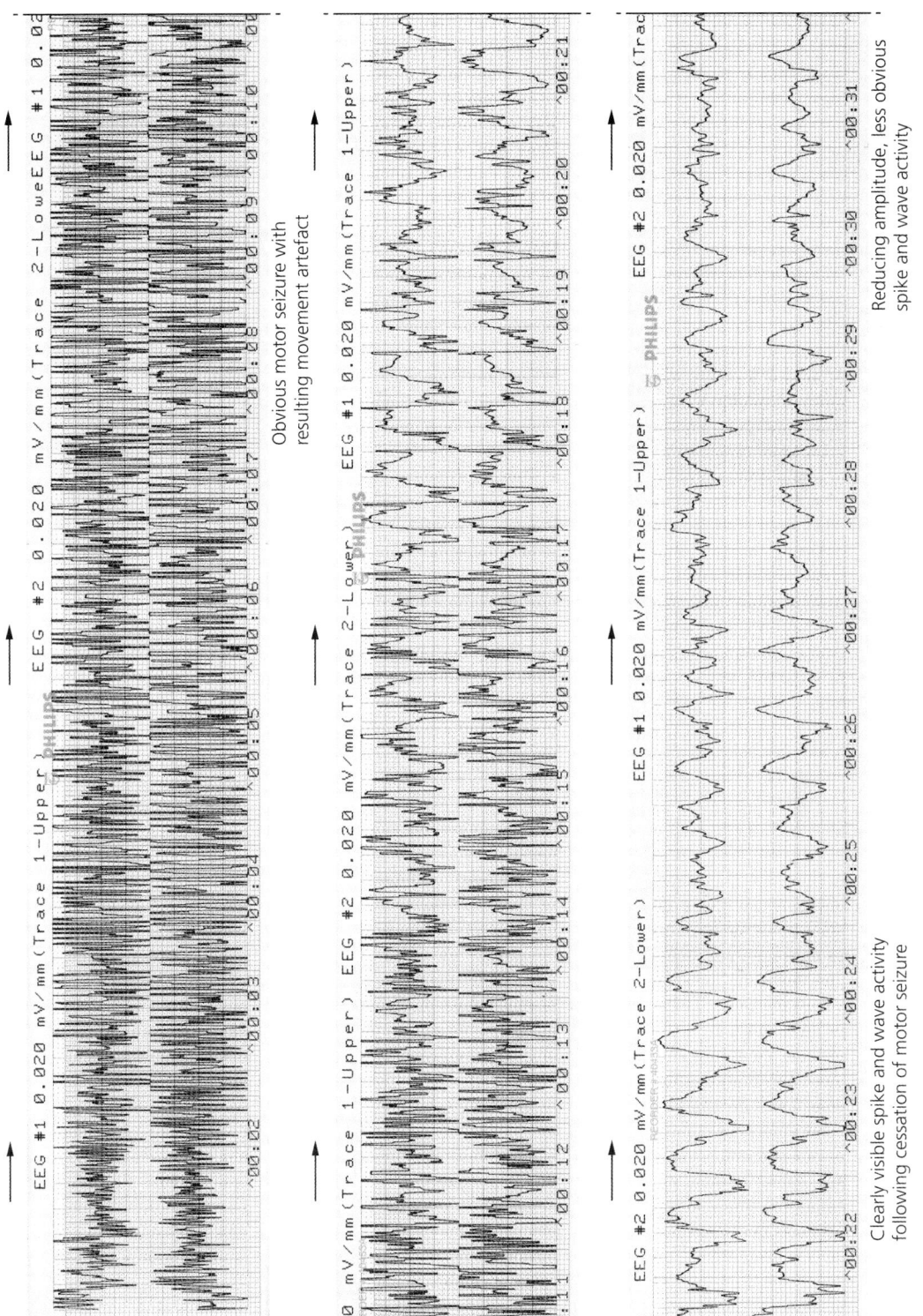

Obvious motor seizure with resulting movement artefact

Clearly visible spike and wave activity following cessation of motor seizure

Reducing amplitude, less obvious spike and wave activity

Figure 5.12 EEG activity following the delivery of bilateral constant current, brief-pulse ECT at a voltage above the patient's seizure threshold.

5

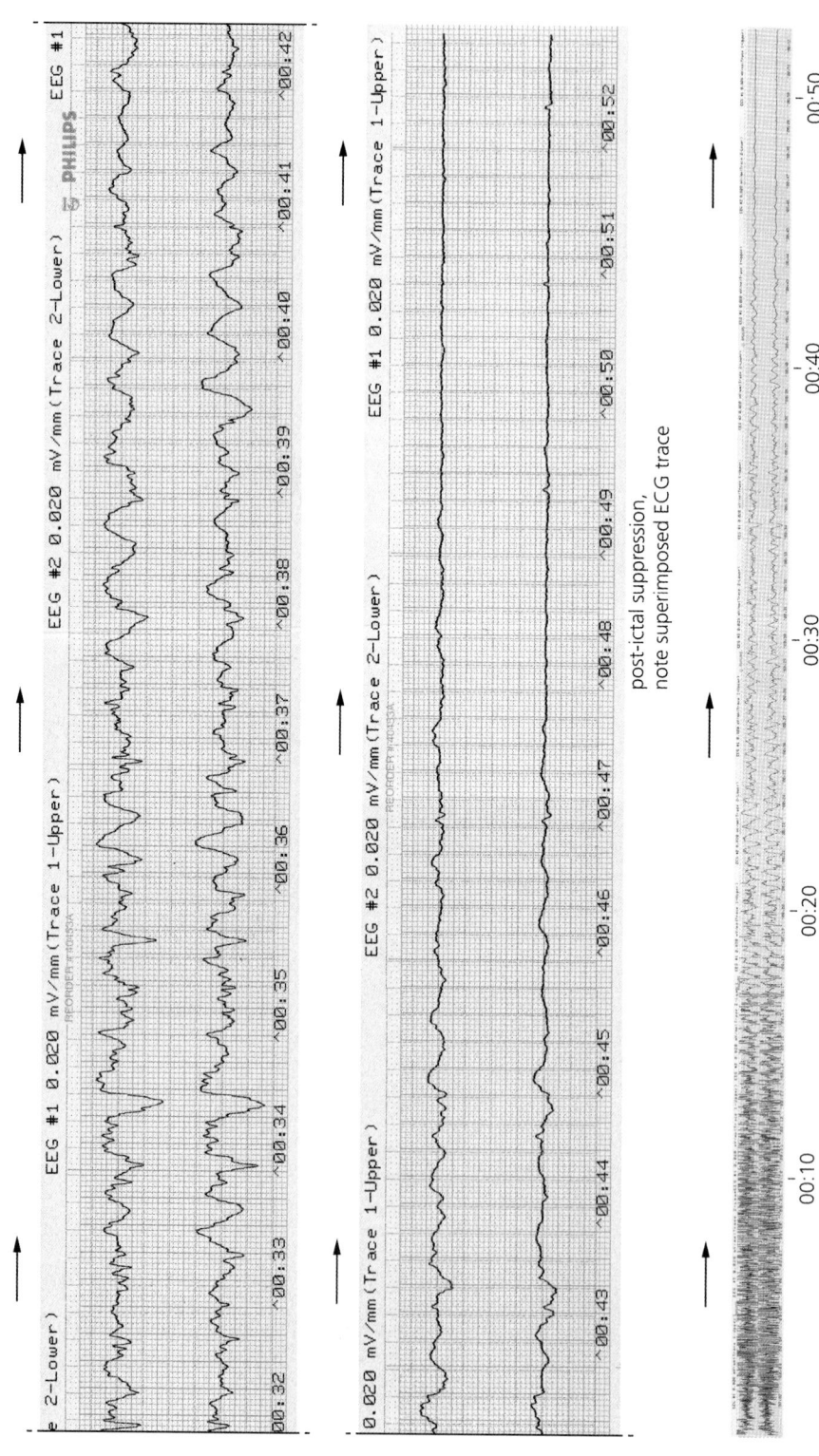

Figure 5.12   Continued

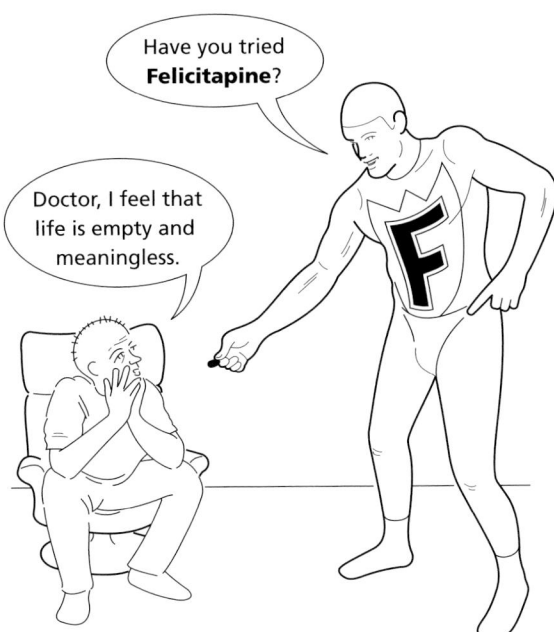

Figure 5.13 Drugs are not the only answer.

Psychological and social treatments

Although drug treatments are the most readily available treatment option, psychological and social interventions can in many cases be more effective. They are often preferred by patients because they are (correctly) seen to address underlying problems rather than simply treating symptoms. The types of psychological treatment that are

---

Peter Tchaikovsky (1840–1893)

Born in 1840, the composer Tchaikovsky suffered from depression throughout most of his short life. He began suffering from depression after his mother died in 1854 and never completely recovered. During his depressive episodes, Tchaikovsky experienced not only a pervasive melancholy, but also insomnia, lack of appetite, and other classical symptoms of depression. Although he suffered greatly from these symptoms, there is no doubt that he used his mental state as a source of inspiration. Tchaikovsky died only nine days after the première of his sixth symphony, the aptly named *Symphonie Pathétique*, a piece of inconsolable anguish and grief. Some say that he died from cholera but others, by suicide.

Table 5.9 Psychological treatments used in depression.

Counselling	Identification and resolution of current life difficulties
	Explanation, reassurance, and support
Cognitive-behavioural therapy	Identification of cognitive distortions and associated behaviours
	Cognitive restructuring and behavioural modifications
Interpersonal psychotherapy	A systematic and standardised treatment approach to personal relationships and life problems
Individual dynamic psychotherapy	Effecting change through a higher level of self-understanding
Family therapy	Effecting change by addressing the dysfunctional aspects of family relationships that contributed to the depressive episode

most appropriate for depression are listed in Table 5.9. The type of psychological treatment that is chosen depends not only on the individual clinical case, but also, deplorably, on the financial and human resources that are locally available. Although there is no substantial evidence for a marked benefit from combining psychological and drug treatments, this should be considered in treatment-resistant cases.

Course and prognosis

The average length of a depressive episode is about six months, although depressive episodes lasting for more than one year are not uncommon. After a first depressive episode, about 80% of patients have further depressive episodes. These episodes tend to become progressively longer and the inter-episode intervals progressively shorter. About 10% of patients develop a chronic unremitting disorder, and about 10% of patients eventually have a manic episode and so 'convert' to bipolar affective disorder.

! The overall lifetime suicide rate for major depression is about 7% in males and 1% in females, but the figures for severe depression requiring inpatient treatment are significantly higher.

5

Puerperal disorders

The puerperium is characterised by unique hormonal and psychological stresses that lead to a number of clinically distinct psychiatric disorders (Table 5.10).

Table 5.10 Comparison of puerperal disorders.

Puerperal disorder	Incidence (%)	Time of onset postpartum
Maternity blues	50	3–4 days
Postnatal depression	10–15	<1 month
Puerperal psychosis	0.2	7–14 days

Maternity blues

Maternity blues (also called 'baby blues') is a minor mood disturbance occurring in about 50% of mothers on the third or fourth day postpartum. The condition is more common in primiparous mothers and is thought to result from a precipitous decline in sex steroids and from the psychological stresses of childbirth and mothering. Clinical features include tearfulness, irritability, and – characteristically – lability of affect. No specific treatment other than explanation and reassurance is required, and the condition usually resolves spontaneously in a matter of days.

Postnatal depression

Postnatal depression occurs in about 10–15% of mothers in the first month postpartum. The condition is thought to result from the stresses of mothering, and from feelings of anxiety and guilt about caring for the baby. It is more common if the mother has a past psychiatric history or lacks social support. Tiredness, irritability, and anxiety are often more prominent than depressed mood, and the baby may be at short-term risk of neglect and harm. Treatment involves explanation and reassurance and, in some cases, antidepressants or psychological treatments. If hospital admission is required, it should be to a mother-and-baby unit so that the mother–baby relationship is maintained and bonding is not compromised.

Puerperal psychosis

Puerperal psychosis affects about 0.2% of mothers, and is more common if the mother is primiparous or has a psychiatric history or family history of psychiatric illness. Onset is about 7–14 days postpartum. Puerperal psychosis can present in one of three clinical pictures: delirious, affective (bipolar disorder and schizoaffective disorder), and schizophreniform. The delirious picture results from puerperal sepsis and is in effect an organic psychosis; it has become relatively rare since the advent of antibiotics. In puerperal psychosis the mother may be deluded about the baby and may for example believe that it is abnormal or evil. This may put the baby at high risk of neglect and harm. Hospital admission is likely and treatment often involves antidepressants and antipsychotics. ECT usually leads to a dramatic recovery and may, depending on the clinical features and severity, be the treatment of choice. Although recovery is the norm, the long-term relapse rate is in the order of 25%.

Mania and bipolar affective disorder

Nessun maggior dolore
Che ricordarsi del tempo felice
Nella miseria.

[There is no greater pain
Than to recall happy times
In times of misery.]

Dante, *Inferno* V

! Important reminder on classification and diagnosis

According to ICD-10, bipolar affective disorder consists of repeated (2+) episodes of depression and mania or hypomania.

In the absence of episodes of mania or hypomania, the diagnosis is one of recurrent depressive disorder.

In the absence of episodes of depression, the diagnosis is either one of bipolar affective disorder or of hypomania, i.e. **recurrent episodes of mania are diagnosed as bipolar affective disorder**. In DSM-IV a single episode of mania is sufficient to diagnose bipolar disorder.

Epidemiology

The lifetime risk for bipolar affective disorder (BAD) ranges from 0.3% to 1.5% and because it is a chronic disorder, the prevalence rate is fairly similar. All races and both sexes are equally affected, although a recent study found that the incidence rates of BAD in ethnic minority groups in London, Bristol, and Nottingham are several times higher than those in comparison Caucasian groups (T. Lloyd *et al*, Incidence of bipolar affective disorder in three UK cities: results from the AESOP study. *British Journal of Psychiatry* (2005), 186, 126–131). The mean age of onset is 21 years and, although the age of onset is variable, a first episode of mania after the age of 50 should lead to an investigation for a primary cause such as organic brain disease or an endocrine or metabolic disorder. Interestingly, the prevalence rate of BAD is higher in higher socioeconomic groups. This may be because genetic susceptibility to BAD tends to favour unaffected relatives and sometimes even bipolar sufferers themselves, such that they are more creative, and hence more successful, than average. In *Touched by Fire: Manic Depressive Illness and the Artistic Temperament*, Professor Kay Redfield Jamison estimates that the prevalence of BAD is 10–40 times higher amongst artists than amongst the general public. Artists who suffered (or are thought to have suffered) from bipolar disorder include the authors Hans Christian Andersen, Honoré de Balzac, F. Scott Fitzgerald, Ernest Hemingway, Victor Hugo, Edgar Allan Poe, Mary Shelley, Mark Twain, and Virginia Woolf; the poets William Blake, Emily Dickinson, T. S. Eliot, John Keats, Robert Lowell, Sylvia Plath, Alfred Lord Tennyson, and Walt Whitman; and the composers Ludwig van Beethoven, Hector Berlioz, George Frederic Handel, Gustav Mahler, Sergei Rachmaninoff, Robert Schumann, and Peter Tchaikovsky.

Aetiology

Genetics

First-degree relatives of a bipolar sufferer have a 10% lifetime risk of BAD, and also have increased risks of unipolar depression and schizoaffective disorder. The concordance rate for BAD in monozygotic twins is 79% – higher than in either depressive disorders or schizophrenia – as compared to only 19% in dizygotic twins. Furthermore, children of bipolar sufferers remain at increased risk of affective disorders even after adoption by unaffected foster parents. There is thus a strong genetic component to the aetiology of BAD, stronger, in fact, than in any other psychiatric disorder. The inheritance pattern is most likely to be polygenic, but more research is needed to identify the genes involved.

Neurochemical abnormalities

The monoamine hypothesis of depression suggests that mania results from increased levels of noradrenaline, serotonin, and dopamine, and it has been observed that stimulant drugs such as cocaine and amphetamines can exacerbate mania. Unfortunately, neurochemical abnormalities in mania have not been as extensively studied as in depression.

5

That fine madness

I am come of a race noted for vigor of fancy and ardour of passion. Men have called me mad; but the question is not yet settled, whether madness is or is not the loftiest intelligence – whether much that is glorious – whether all that is profound – does not spring from disease of thought – from moods of mind exalted at the expense of the general intellect. They who dream by day are cognizant of many things which escape those who dream only by night. In their grey visions they obtain glimpses of eternity… They penetrate, however ruderless or compassless, into the vast ocean of the 'light ineffable'.

Edgar Allan Poe, *Eleonora*

But if a man comes to the door of poetry untouched by the madness of the Muses, believing that technique alone will make him a good poet, he and his sane companions never reach perfection, but are utterly eclipsed by the performances of the inspired madman.

Plato, *Phaedrus*

Other neurological abnormalities

Findings of neuroimaging studies suggest ventricular enlargement and structural abnormalities in the prefrontal cortex, striatum and amygdala, but these findings are inconsistent.

Life events/environmental factors

Life events, severe stresses, and disruptions in daily routines and circadian rhythms (e.g. missing a night's sleep or flying from London to Tokyo) may provoke the onset of a first manic or hypomanic episode. There is an excess of manic episodes in late spring and summer, and also in the postpartum period.

Clinical features of mania

As previously noted, BAD consists of repeated (two or more) episodes of depression and mania or hypomania. Manic episodes usually begin abruptly and last for a median duration of about four months. Depressive episodes last for a median duration of about six months and rarely for more than one year, except in the elderly. The frequency and severity of episodes is very variable, as is the proportion of manic to depressive episodes. **Rapid cycling** is more common in females and refers to four or more episodes of mania, hypomania, and/or depression in a period of one year (DSM-IV).

People with mania are often dressed in colourful clothing or in unusual, haphazard combinations of clothing which they complement with inappropriate accessories, such as hats and sunglasses, and excessive make-up, jewellery, or body art. Their behaviour is typically hyperactive, and may appear to others as entertaining, charming, flirtatious, vigilant, assertive, or aggressive, and sometimes all of these in turn. Whilst people with mania are typically euphoric, optimistic, self-confident, and grandiose, they may also be irritable or tearful, with rapid and unexpected shifts from one extreme to another. Their thoughts race through their mind at high speed and as a result their speech is pressured and voluble and difficult to interrupt. The author, artist, and art critic John Ruskin (1819–1900) described the experience thus, 'I roll on like a ball, with this exception, that contrary to the usual laws of motion I have no friction to contend with in my mind, and of course have some difficulty in stopping myself when there is nothing else to stop me … I am almost sick and giddy with the quantity of things in my head – trains of thought beginning and branching to infinity, crossing each other, and all tempting and wanting to be worked out'. Sometimes their speech is so rambling or disorganised that they are unable to stick to one topic or to make a point; they may ignore the strictures of grammar, step outside the confines of an English dictionary, and even talk in rhyme and puns. An example of talking in rhymes and puns is, 'They thought I was in the pantry at home … Peekaboo … there's a magic box. Poor darling Catherine, you know, Catherine the Great, the fire grate, I'm always up the chimney. I want to scream with joy … Hallelujah!' (Andrew Sims, *Symptoms in the Mind: An Introduction to Descriptive Psychopathology* (1988)). All this can make it very difficult for anyone else to be heard, let alone understood, by the person with mania.

People with mania are typically full of grandiose and unrealistic plans that they begin to act upon but soon abandon. They often engage in impulsive, pleasure-seeking, and disinhibited behaviour that may, for example, involve driving recklessly, taking illegal drugs, spending vast amounts of money with careless abandon, or engaging in sexual activity with near-strangers. As a result, they may end up harming themselves or others, getting into trouble with the police and authorities, or being exploited by those lacking in scruples. People with mania may also experience psychotic symptoms such as hallucinations or delusions that make their behaviour seem all the more bizarre and out of character. Delusional themes are usually congruent or in keeping with the elevated mood, and often involve delusions of grandeur, that is, delusions of exaggerated self-importance – of special status, special purpose, or special abilities. For example, a person with mania may believe that he or she is a brilliant scientist on the verge of finding a cure for AIDS, or that he or she is an exceptionally talented entrepreneur engaged by the Queen to rid the country of poverty. People with mania generally have very poor insight into their mental state, and typically find it very difficult to accept that they are ill. As a result, they are likely to delay getting the help that they need and, in the meantime, cause tremendous damage to their relationships, careers, finances, and health. A typical case of mania is that of Mrs S.

Hypomania

Hypomania is a lesser degree of mania and as such its clinical features are very similar to those seen in mania. **The mood is elevated, expansive, or irritable but, in con-**

The story of Mrs S

Ten months ago Mrs S, a Community Psychiatric Nurse, started feeling happier and more energetic. She took on many extra hours and extra roles, but to her surprise one of her colleagues reported her as unsafe. She promptly resigned, claiming that she needed more time to devote to her many plans and projects. By then she couldn't stop her thoughts from racing and was sleeping only three or four hours a night. She rented a launderette and set out to transform it into a multipurpose centre. Then she bought three houses to rent out to the poor.

She became very outgoing and acted completely out of character, dressing garishly, smoking marijuana, and getting herself arrested for being 'drunk and disorderly'. Four months ago her mood began dropping and she felt dreadful and ashamed. Today she is feeling better but has had to sell her house to pay off her debts. Her psychiatrist suggested that she start on a mood stabiliser, but she is reluctant to take his advice.

When you're high it's tremendous. The ideas and feelings are fast and frequent like shooting stars and you follow them until you find better and brighter ones. Shyness goes, the right words and gestures are suddenly there, the power to captivate others a felt certainty. There are interests found in uninteresting people. Sensuality is pervasive and desire to seduce and be seduced is irresistible … But, somewhere this changes … Everything previously moving with the grain is now against – you are irritable, angry, frightened, uncontrollable, and emerged totally in the blackest caves of the mind.

Kay Redfield Jamison, *An Unquiet Mind*

Clinical skills/OSCE: Mental state examination in mania

Appearance	Flamboyant clothing, unusual combinations of clothing, heavy makeup and jewellery
Behaviour	Hyperactive, entertaining, flirtatious, hypervigilant, assertive, aggressive
Speech	Pressured speech, neologisms, clang associations
Mood/affect	Euphoric, irritable, labile
Thought	Optimistic, self-confident, grandiose, pressure of thought, flight of ideas, loosening of associations, circumstantiality, tangentiality, mood-congruent delusions or less commonly mood-incongruent delusions
Perception	Hallucinations
Cognition	Poor concentration but intact memory and abstract thinking
Insight	Very poor insight

trast to mania, there are no psychotic features and no *marked* impairment of social functioning. The differential diagnosis of hypomania includes mania, cyclothymia, agitated depression, substance misuse, hyperthyroidism, and anorexia. Hypomania may herald mania, and in such cases the diagnosis is simply one of mania.

Cyclothymia

Cyclothymia can be described as mild chronic BAD and is characterised by numerous episodes of mild elation and mild depressive symptoms that are not sufficiently severe or prolonged to meet the criteria for BAD or recurrent depressive disorder. Cyclothymia usually develops in early adult life and is more common in the relatives of bipolar sufferers and no doubt also in medical students. Unless it progresses to BAD (15–50% of cases), it rarely comes to medical attention.

Diagnosis

ICD-10 criteria for manic episode

ICD-10 specifies three degrees of severity for manic episode: **hypomania, mania without psychotic symptoms,** and **mania with psychotic symptoms.**

ICD-10 criteria for hypomania

A lesser degree of mania in which abnormalities of mood and behaviour are too persistent and marked to be included under cyclothymia but are not accompanied by hallucinations or delusions. There is a persistent mild elevation of mood (for at least several days on end), increased energy and activity, and usually marked feelings of well-being and both physical and mental efficiency. Increased sociability, talkativeness, overfamiliarity, increased sexual energy, and a decreased need for sleep are often present but not to the extent that they lead to severe disruption of work or result in social rejection. Irritability, conceit, and boorish behaviour may take the place of the more usual euphoric sociability.

ICD-10 criteria for mania without psychotic symptoms

Mood is elevated out of keeping with the individual's circumstances and may vary from carefree joviality to almost uncontrollable excitement. Elation is accompanied by increased energy, resulting in overactivity, pressure of speech, and a decreased need for sleep. Normal social inhibitions are lost, attention cannot be sustained, and there is often marked distractibility. Self-esteem is inflated, and grandiose or over-optimistic ideas are freely expressed.

Perceptual disorders may occur, such as the appreciation of colours as especially vivid (and unusually beautiful), a preoccupation with fine details of surfaces or textures, and subjective hyperacusis. The individual may embark on extravagant and impractical schemes, spend money recklessly, or become aggressive, amorous, or facetious in inappropriate circumstances. In some manic episodes the mood is irritable and suspicious rather than elated.

The episode should last for at least one week and should be severe enough to disrupt ordinary work and social activities more or less completely.

DSM-IV criteria for hypomanic episode

*A distinct period of persistently elevated, expansive, or irritable mood, **lasting throughout at least 4 days**, that is clearly different from the usual non-depressed mood.*

A. *During the period of mood disturbance, three (or more) of the following symptoms have persisted (four if the mood is only irritable) and have been present to a significant degree:*
  1. *Inflated self-esteem or grandiosity*
  2. *Decreased need for sleep*
  3. *More talkative than usual or pressure to keep talking*
  4. *Flight of ideas or subjective experience that thoughts are racing*
  5. *Distractibility*
  6. *Increase in goal-directed activity or psychomotor agitation*
  7. *Involvement in pleasurable activities that can have painful consequences.*

NB: *These symptoms are exactly the same as those listed under manic episode (see below).*

B. *The episode is associated with an unequivocal change in functioning that is uncharacteristic of the person when not symptomatic.*
C. *The disturbance in mood and the change in function are observable by others.*
D. ***The episode is not severe enough to cause marked impairment in social or occupational functioning, or to require hospitalisation, and there are no psychotic features.***
E. *The symptoms are not due to a substance or general medical condition.*

DSM-IV criteria for manic episode

A. *A distinct period of abnormally and persistently elevated, expansive, or irritable mood, **lasting at least one week** (or any duration if hospitalisation is necessary).*
B. *During the period of mood disturbance, three (or more) of the following symptoms have persisted (four if the mood is only irritable) and have been present to a significant degree:*
  1. *Inflated self-esteem or grandiosity*
  2. *Decreased need for sleep*
  3. *More talkative than usual or pressure to keep talking*
  4. *Flight of ideas or subjective experience that thoughts are racing*
  5. *Distractibility*
  6. *Increase in goal-directed activity or psychomotor agitation*
  7. *Involvement in pleasurable activities that can have painful consequences.*
C. *The symptoms do not meet criteria for a mixed episode.*
D. ***The mood disturbance is sufficiently severe to cause marked impairment in occupational functioning or in usual social activities or relationships with***

others, or to require hospitalisation to prevent harm to self or others, or there are psychotic features.

E. *The symptoms are not due to a substance or a general medical condition.*

DSM-IV criteria for mixed episode

A. **The criteria are met both for a manic episode and for a major depressive episode (except for duration) nearly every day during at least a one-week period.**

B. *The mood disturbance is sufficiently severe to cause marked impairment in occupational functioning or in usual social activities or relationships with others, or to require hospitalisation to prevent harm to self or others, or there are psychotic features.*

C. *The symptoms are not due to a substance or a general medical condition.*

Differential diagnosis

Psychiatric disorders

- Mixed affective states (simultaneous manic and depressive symptoms)
- Schizoaffective disorder
- Schizophrenia
- Cyclothymic disorder
- Attention-deficit hyperactivity disorder
- Drugs such as alcohol, amphetamines, cocaine, hallucinogens, antidepressants, L-dopa, steroids

Medical/neurological disorders

- Organic brain disease of the frontal lobes such as cerebrovascular accident, multiple sclerosis, intracranial tumours, epilepsy, AIDS, neurosyphilis
- Endocrine disorders, e.g. hyperthyroidism, Cushing's syndrome
- Systemic lupus erythematosus
- Sleep deprivation

Management

Clinical skills: Investigations in mania

Laboratory investigations should include a serum and/or urine drug screen, liver, renal and thyroid function tests, full blood count, ESR, and a urine test (including pregnancy test). The aim of these investigations is to rule out drug abuse, establish baselines for the administration of mood-stabilising medication, and uncover possible medical causes for the patient's symptoms. Other, more specific, investigations such as antinuclear antibody and urine copper level should be considered on a case-by-case basis. A pretreatment ECG is important prior to starting lithium and some other drugs. If the patient is already on lithium, a lithium level should be taken.

Treatment

Methods of treatment for mania and BAD include:
- Mood stabilising and other drugs
- Electroconvulsive therapy (rarely used)
- Psychosocial treatments.

The choice of medication in BAD is largely determined by current symptoms. In a manic episode, the treatment most often prescribed is antipsychotic medication. In a depressive episode, the treatment most often prescribed is antidepressant medication, often in conjunction with a mood stabiliser to avoid 'manic switch', that is, overtreatment into mania. In rare instances, a depressive episode may be so severe or unresponsive to medication that ECT might be indicated. ECT might also be indicated for mania that cannot be treated by medication, either because it is unresponsive to medication or because medication is contraindicated. Finally, in the long term the patient should be prescribed a mood stabiliser to prevent further relapses into mania and depression. Although medication plays a central role in the management of BAD, there are a number of psychological and social interventions that can play a major role not only in improving outcome, but also in improving quality of life.

5

Antipsychotic medication

If a person with mania is not already on a long-term mood stabiliser, the most common practice is to start an antipsychotic and to wait for the person to recover before a long-term mood stabiliser is started. Often, a person with mania is already on a long-term mood stabiliser, in which case it is common to continue the mood stabiliser and increase the dose and/or add an antipsychotic. Antipsychotics are fast-acting and effective in the treatment of mania, but relatively high doses are required and, unlike mood stabilisers, they do not protect against further depressive episodes. For these reasons some psychiatrists prefer to start a mood stabiliser rather than an antipsychotic, or to start both simultaneously. The disadvantage of starting a mood stabiliser during a manic episode is that the patient cannot participate in the decision to start the mood stabiliser. This compromises his or her long-term compliance, which is crucial in ensuring the effectiveness of the mood stabiliser. Once started, the antipsychotic should be continued until full remission has been achieved. In some cases, the antipsychotic can be continued in the long term instead of or in addition to a mood stabiliser, particularly if the illness is characterised by prominent psychotic symptoms, mixed states, rapid cycling, or treatment resistance. For full coverage of antipsychotic medication, see Chapter 4.

Other drugs used in mania

In the initial stages of treatment of mania, the patient may be highly agitated and difficult to manage, and a very fast-acting sedative such as lorazepam may be given in addition to an antipsychotic or mood stabiliser. If the patient is sleep-deprived, as he or she is most likely to be, a sleeping tablet such as temazepam or zopiclone may also be given. A sleeping tablet can be especially useful in the early hypomanic stages, when it might succeed in aborting a full-scale manic episode. In contrast, any antidepressant medication should be rapidly tapered off and stopped.

Mood stabilisers: lithium

The Australian John Cade described the antimanic properties of lithium in 1949, but the drug took another 20 years to enter mainstream practice. Today lithium is commonly used in the treatment of acute manic episodes and in the long-term prophylaxis of BAD and recurrent depressive disorder. It has a response rate of 75% in the treatment of acute manic episodes, but takes several days to have an effect. In the prophylaxis of BAD, it reduces the rate of relapse by about one-third, but is more effective against mania than against depression. Despite its popularity and many side-effects, its mode of action is unclear. It is understood to have a range of effects in the CNS, including effects on cation transport, intracellular second messenger systems, and certain neurotransmitters and neurotransmitter receptors.

Lithium should only be started if there is a clear intention to continue it for at least three years, as poor compliance and intermittent treatment may lead to rebound mania. The starting dose of lithium should be cautious, e.g. 400 mg of lithium carbonate at night, and depends on several factors, including the preparation used (i.e. lithium carbonate or lithium citrate). Lithium is eliminated unchanged by the kidney and its half-life is related to renal function. It is therefore important to check renal function before starting the drug. The therapeutic range is **0.5–1.0 mmol/L** (0.8–1.0 mmol/L for the acute treatment of mania), although this can vary slightly from hospital to hospital.

> **! Lithium toxicity**
>
> Lithium toxicity usually occurs beyond 1.5 mmol/L and is characterised by gastrointestinal disturbances such as anorexia, nausea, vomiting and diarrhoea; nystagmus, coarse tremor, dysarthria, ataxia, and, in severe cases, loss of consciousness, seizures, and death.

Serum levels should be taken at 12 hours post-dose (usually in the morning) and monitored at 5–7 day intervals until the patient is stabilised, and at 3–4 monthly intervals thereafter. Renal and thyroid function should also be monitored.

Once started on lithium some patients stop taking it because of its side-effects (Table 5.11). In addition to the side-effects listed in Table 5.11, lithium is teratogenic, and the risk of cardiovascular malformations in the foetus is 0.5–1 per 1000 births. The most common cardiovascular malformation is Epstein anomaly, which describes downward displacement of the tricuspid valve into the right ventricle. As lithium is excreted into breast milk, breast-feeding is not advisable.

If lithium is started but not tolerated or found to be ineffective, it can be stopped abruptly. However, it should

Table 5.11 Side-effects of lithium.

Short-term	Long-term
Fine tremor	Weight gain
Gastrointestinal	Oedema
disturbances	Goitre and hypothyroidism*
Muscle weakness	Hyperparathyroidism
Polyuria	Nephrogenic diabetes insipidus
Polydipsia	Irreversible renal damage**
Stuffy nose, metallic	Cardiotoxicity§
taste in the mouth	Exacerbation of acne and psoriasis
	Raised leucocyte and platelet count

* Check TFTs before starting therapy and monitor every six months.
** Check U&Es before starting therapy and monitor every six months.
§ Perform ECG before starting therapy. During therapy, lithium cardiotoxicity is manifest as T wave flattening.

only be stopped gradually (say, over the course of two or three months) following successful long-term treatment, as stopping it abruptly in these circumstances can precipitate an episode of rebound mania. Patients on lithium should be advised to drink plenty of fluids and to avoid reducing their salt intake, as dehydration and sodium depletion can precipitate lithium toxicity. Common lithium drug interactions are listed in Table 5.12.

Table 5.12 Some lithium drug interactions.

Drug	Explanation
Diuretics, especially thiazides	Sodium depletion increases lithium levels, resulting in lithium toxicity
Carbamazepine	Can result in neurotoxicity, prefer valproate
NSAIDs	Most NSAIDs can increase lithium levels, resulting in lithium toxicity
ACE inhibitors	Lithium toxicity

ACE, acetylcholinesterase inhibitor; NSAIDs, non-steroidal anti-inflammatory drugs.

Mood stabilisers: anticonvulsants

The use of anticonvulsants (principally valproate and, more recently, lamotrigine) in the prophylaxis of BAD is increasing. Anticonvulsants enhance the action of the inhibitory neurotransmitter gamma aminobutyric acid (GABA), but their precise mode of action in the prophylaxis of BAD is as yet unclear.

Valproate, in the form of semisodium valproate (Depakote), is used alone or as an adjunct to lithium or other drugs in the treatment and prophylaxis of BAD, and in the USA has become the most frequently prescribed mood stabiliser. Compared to lithium, it has a similar efficacy but a quicker onset of action, and is of particular benefit in rapid-cycling BAD. Although valproate can have a number of side-effects it is often better tolerated than lithium, particularly if lithium levels need to be

A flight of angels

Despite its proven efficacy, many people with bipolar disorder are reluctant to start on lithium because of the complexities and potential risks involved. This is often especially true of those who value or depend on their creativity, and fear that lithium may dampen it or make them feel lethargic, restless, or 'drugged into a haze'. As the German poet Rainer Maria Rilke (1875–1926) put it, 'If my devils were to leave me, I am afraid my angels will take flight as well.' Yet lithium can be effective in many people, and need not result in side-effects. The psychiatrist Kay Redfield Jamison, who herself suffers from BAD, wrote:

I have often asked myself whether, given the choice, I would choose to have manic–depressive illness. If lithium were not available to me, or didn't work for me, the answer would be a simple no … and it would be an answer laced with terror. But

lithium does work for me, and therefore I can afford to pose the question. Strangely enough, I think I would choose to have it. It's complicated … Depression is awful beyond words or sounds or images … So why would I want anything to do with this illness? Because I honestly believe that as a result of it I have felt more things, more deeply; had more experiences, more intensely; loved more, and have been more loved; laughed more often for having cried more often; appreciated more the springs, for all the winters … Depressed, I have crawled on my hands and knees in order to get across a room and have done it for month after month. But normal or manic I have run faster, thought faster, and loved faster than most I know. And I think much of this is related to my illness – the intensity it gives to things.

Kay Redfield Jamison, *An Unquiet Mind*

maintained above 0.8 mmol/L. Side-effects include nausea, tremor, sedation, weight gain, alopecia, blood dyscrasias, hepatoxicity, and pancreatitis. Valproate can cause neural tube defects and other malformations in the foetus, and for these reasons it should be avoided in women of child-bearing age. It is important to check blood cell counts and liver function before valproate is started, and to continue monitoring these at 6–12 month intervals.

Lamotrigine is more effective against relapses of depression than it is against relapses of mania, and it can be used both in the treatment of relapses of bipolar depression and in the prophylaxis of BAD. Compared with lithium and valproate, lamotrigine has fewer side-effects and does not usually require long-term monitoring with blood tests. Common side-effects include nausea and vomiting, headaches, dizziness, clumsiness, and blurred vision and diplopia. Other side-effects include flu-like symptoms, sedation, insomnia, skin rash, and severe skin reactions.

Carbamazepine is generally used as a second- or third-line drug in the prophylaxis of BAD, and is thought to be of particular value in treatment-resistant cases and in rapid-cycling. Side-effects include nausea, headache, dizziness, sedation, diplopia, ataxia, skin rashes, rare but potentially fatal blood dyscrasias, and hepatotoxicity. Bloods should be monitored regularly for leukopaenia, hyponatraemia, and raised LFTs. Carbamazepine can cause spina bifida if used in pregnancy, but it is not excreted in breast milk and so can be used by breast-feeding mothers. As it is a strong inducer of hepatic microsomal enzymes, it increases the metabolism of a number of other drugs.

Psychosocial treatments

Education about the symptoms, course, and treatment of the disorder, education about the importance of drug compliance, advice about lifestyle (e.g. avoidance of triggers for relapse such as sleep deprivation and substance misuse), and identification of early signs of relapse are an important aspect of the management of all bipolar sufferers. Most cases of bipolar disorder can be managed on an outpatient basis with the support of the Community Mental Health Team or the Crisis Team. However, hospitalisation may be required in severe cases (see Table 4.8).

Course and prognosis

The average length of a manic episode is about four months. After a first manic episode, about 90% of patients experience further manic and depressive episodes, and the inter-episode interval tends to become progressively shorter. The prognosis is therefore quite poor, but is more so in rapid-cycling, and less so in bipolar II. About 10% go on to commit suicide, but the rate of attempted suicide is much higher.

Virginia Woolf (1882–1941)

I married, and then my brains went up like a shower of fireworks. As an experience, madness is terrific I can assure you, and not to be sniffed at; and in its lava I still find most of the things I write about. It shoots out of one everything shaped, final, not in mere driblets as sanity does. And the six months … that I lay in bed taught me a good deal about what is called oneself.

Quoted from a letter to her dear friend Ethel Smyth

She felt very young; at the same time unspeakably aged. She sliced like a knife through everything; at the same time was outside, looking on … far out to sea and alone; she always had the feeling that it was very, very dangerous to live even one day.

Quoted from the novel *Mrs Dalloway*

Virginia Woolf, the novelist and member of the Bloomsbury Group, suffered from BAD from the age of 13. She committed suicide at the age of 59 by walking into the River Ouse with a large rock in her pocket (beautifully portrayed in The Hours, a film loosely based on the novel *Mrs Dalloway* and starring Nicole Kidman as Virginia Woolf). This is her suicide note to her husband.

Dearest, I feel certain I am going mad again. I feel we can't go through another of those terrible times. And I shan't recover this time. I begin to hear voices, and I can't concentrate. So I am doing what seems the best thing to do. You have given me the greatest possible happiness. You have been in every way all that anyone could be. I don't think two people could have been happier till this terrible disease came. I can't fight any longer. I know that I am spoiling your life, that without me you could work. And you will I know. You see I can't even write this properly. I can't read. What I want to say is I owe all the happiness of my life to you. You have been entirely patient with me and incredibly good. I want to say that – everybody knows it. If anybody could have saved me it would have been you. Everything has gone from me but the certainty of your goodness. I can't go on spoiling your life any longer. I don't think two people could have been happier than we have been.

V.

Recommended reading

Darkness Visible: A Memoir of Madness (2001) William Styron. Vintage.

The Noonday Demon (2002) Andrew Solomon. Vintage.

Churchill's Black Dog and other Phenomena of the Human Mind (1997) Anthony Storr. HarperCollins.

An Unquiet Mind (1997) Kay Redfield Jamison. Picador.

Touched with Fire: Manic Depressive Illness and the Artistic Temperament (1996) Kay Redfield Jamison. Simon & Schuster.

Summary

Depressive disorders
Classification
- In ICD-10 depressive disorders are classified according to their severity into mild, moderate, severe, and psychotic depressive disorder. In DSM-IV the term 'major depression' is used instead of depressive disorder. Major depression is simply sub-classified as 'single episode' or 'recurrent'.

Epidemiology
- The lifetime risk of depressive disorders is about 15%. The point prevalence is about 5%.
- Females are more affected than males by a ratio of about 2:1. Peak prevalence in males is in old age, but in females it is in middle age.

Aetiology
- Genetic factors and environmental factors are both involved in the aetiology of depressive disorders.
- The monoamine hypothesis of depression suggests that depression results from underactivity of monoamine projections.
- Organic causes of depression include neurological conditions, endocrine conditions, metabolic abnormalities, infections, and drugs.

Clinical features
- The clinical features of depression can be divided into core features, other common features, and somatic features.
- Dysthymia is characterised by mild chronic depressive symptoms that are not sufficiently severe to meet the criteria for mild depressive disorder.

Differential diagnosis
- The differential diagnosis of depression is from other psychiatric disorders and from secondary depression (depression due to medical or organic causes).

Management
- Methods of treatment include antidepressants, other drugs, electroconvulsive therapy, and psychological and social treatments.

- Psychological and social treatments are often preferred by patients because they are seen to address underlying problems rather than simply treating symptoms.

Prognosis
- The average length of a depressive episode is about six months. After a first depressive episode, about 80% of patients have further depressive episodes.

Disorders of the puerperium
- Maternity blues occurs in about 50% of mothers on the third or fourth day postpartum.
- Postnatal depression occurs in about 10–15% of mothers in the first month postpartum.
- Puerperal psychosis occurs in about 0.2% of mothers at about 7–14 days postpartum.

Mania and bipolar affective disorder
Classification
- In DSM-IV a single episode of mania is sufficient to meet the criteria for bipolar disorder. Bipolar I consists of episodes of mania and major depression, bipolar II of episodes of hypomania and major depression.

Epidemiology
- The lifetime risk for bipolar disorder ranges from 0.3% to 1.5%. Mean age of onset is 21 years. All races and both sexes are equally affected.

Aetiology
- Although genetic factors and environmental factors are both involved in the aetiology of bipolar affective disorder, genetic factors play an especially important role.
- The monoamine hypothesis of depression suggests that mania results from overactivity of monoamine projections.

Clinical features
- The frequency and severity of episodes is very variable, as is the proportion of manic to depressive episodes.

Continued...

5

- In hypomania the mood is elevated, expansive or irritable, but in contrast to mania, there are no psychotic features and no *marked* impairment of social functioning.
- Cyclothymia is characterised by numerous episodes of mild elation and mild depressive symptoms that do not meet the criteria for bipolar depression or recurrent depressive disorder.

Differential diagnosis
- The differential diagnosis of mania and bipolar affective disorder is from other psychiatric disorders, drugs, and medical and neurological conditions.

Management
- Choice of medication in bipolar disease is to a large extent determined by the patient's current symptoms.

  - Antipsychotics, benzodiazepines, and/or mood stabilisers for an acute manic episode
  - Antidepressants and mood stabilisers for an acute depressive episode
  - Mood stabilisers to prevent relapses.
- Psychological treatments include education about the symptoms, course, and treatment of the disorder, education about the importance of drug compliance, advice about lifestyle, and identification of early signs of relapse.

Prognosis
- After a first manic episode, about 90% of patients experience further manic and depressive episodes, and the inter-episode interval tends to become progressively shorter.

5

Self-assessment

Simply answer with true or false. Answers on p. 217.

1. Poor self-esteem is a core symptom of depression.
2. The peak prevalence of depressive disorders in females is in middle age.
3. Somatic presentations of depression are common in Asian cultures.
4. Monoamine neurotransmitters include noradrenaline, serotonin, and GABA.
5. Plasma cortisol levels are increased in all depression sufferers.
6. Alcohol misuse is a common cause of depressive symptoms.
7. Stimulant misuse can lead to both mania and depression.
8. According to the 'kindling hypothesis', successive depressive episodes become more and more attributable to life events.
9. One of the vulnerability factors for depression is loss of a parent by death or separation before the age of 11.
10. According to attachment theory, depression results from loss of the loved object and mixed feelings of love and hatred (ambivalence).
11. Beck's triad involves negative appraisal of the self, of the past, and of the future.
12. Selective abstraction involves drawing a conclusion on the basis of a single incident.
13. Low mood is not strictly required for a diagnosis of depressive disorder to be made.
14. In mild depression the patient finds it difficult to fulfil his or her social obligations.
15. Psychotic symptoms are more common in mania than in bipolar depression, and more common in bipolar depression than in unipolar depression.
16. Double depression refers to a depressive episode on a background of dysthymia.
17. In the treatment of bipolar depression, SSRIs are particularly likely to induce 'manic switch'.
18. Sertraline is a good choice of antidepressant for a breast-feeding woman.
19. In some respects, people with depression may have a more realistic perception of the world.
20. Serotonin syndrome should be managed in a general hospital.

21. The SSRI discontinuation syndrome occurs most frequently upon discontinuing imipramine.
22. Tertiary amines such as amitriptyline, imipramine, and clomipramine are less sedating and cause fewer anticholinergic side-effects than secondary amines such as nortriptyline, dothiepin, and lofepramine.
23. The tyramine reaction is a hypertensive crisis that can result in subarachnoid haemorrhage.
24. Trazodone is a mildly sedating antidepressant that is commonly used in the elderly.
25. Better sleep is often the first sign of improvement after starting antidepressant medication.
26. Pregnancy is a contraindication to ECT.
27. Under the Mental Health Act, ECT may be given to a person with the capacity to refuse to consent to it.
28. Interpersonal psychotherapy involves effecting change through a higher level of self-understanding.
29. If a patient has only recurrent episodes of mania, a diagnosis of bipolar affective disorder can be made.
30. In the DSM-IV classification, bipolar II consists of episodes of major depression and mania.
31. Rapid-cycling refers to four or more episodes of mania in a period of one year.
32. The concordance rate for bipolar disorder in monozygotic twins is higher than in either depressive disorders or schizophrenia.
33. Toxic effects of lithium are usually experienced beyond 1.5 mmol/L.
34. Serum levels of valproate should be taken at 12 hours post-dose and monitored at 5–7 day intervals until the patient is stabilised, and at 3–4 monthly intervals thereafter. Renal and thyroid function should also be monitored.
35. In contrast to lithium, lamotrigine is more effective against relapses of mania than it is against relapses of depression.
36. Side-effects of carbamazepine include nausea, headache, dizziness, sedation, diplopia, ataxia, skin rashes, blood dyscrasias, and hepatotoxicity.
37. The average length of a manic episode is six months.
38. Suicide is more common in bipolar sufferers than in depression sufferers.

5

Suicide and deliberate self-harm

6

Key learning objectives

- The definitions of the terms 'deliberate self-harm', 'parasuicide', 'attempted suicide', and 'suicide'

- Sociodemographic and clinical risk factors for suicide
- Assessment and management of suicidal risk

Introduction

And so it was I entered the broken world
To trace the visionary company of love, its voice
An instant in the wind (I know not whither hurled)
But not for long to hold each desperate choice.
    Hart Crane (1899–1932), quoted from *The Broken Tower*

This poem was written not long before the poet committed suicide by jumping from the steamship SS Orizaba into the Gulf of Mexico.

Suicide is a neologism coined from *sui caedes*, Latin for 'murder of oneself', and has been defined by the sociologist Emile Durkheim as applying to 'all cases of death resulting directly or indirectly from a positive or negative act of the victim himself, which he knows will produce this result'. Suicide can simply be defined as the act of intentionally killing oneself, although sometimes intentionally killing oneself with the primary aim of saving or helping others is seen as self-sacrifice rather than as suicide. Thus suicide might best also be defined as the act of intention-

Psychiatry, 2e. By Neel Burton. Published 2010 by Blackwell Publishing.

ally killing oneself, **with the primary aim of dying**. In some acts of suicide, the primary aim is not entirely clear. For example, in 1941 Virginia Woolf killed herself by walking into the River Ouse with a large rock in her pocket. In her suicide note to her husband she mentions both that her manic depressive illness is deteriorating *and* that she is spoiling her husband's life (see p. 104).

Suicide should also be distinguished from assisted suicide, the making available to a person of the means to end his or her life; and from voluntary euthanasia, the deliberate ending of the life of another person who has requested it and is physically unable to commit suicide. The act of suicide itself should be distinguished from other forms of self-harm, and particularly from attempted suicide and parasuicide. Attempted suicide is the act of intentionally trying to kill oneself but failing to do so, and parasuicide is an act that looks like suicide but that does not result in death. The intention of parasuicide may have been to kill oneself, but this is not necessarily so – it may have been a means of attracting attention, a 'cry for help', an act of revenge, or an expression of despair. Suicide, attempted suicide and parasuicide are all forms of deliberate self-harm, which is the act of intentionally injuring oneself, irrespective of the actual degree of injury sustained.

In summary then:

- **Suicide** is the act of intentionally killing oneself with the primary aim of dying

6

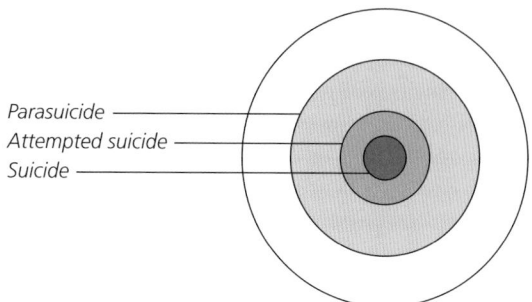

Figure 6.1 Different types of deliberate self-harm.

- **Attempted suicide** is the act of intentionally trying to kill oneself with the primary aim of dying, but failing to do so
- **Parasuicide** is an act that looks like suicide but does not result in death. Parasuicide can be tantamount to attempted suicide, but this is not necessarily so – it can also be a means of attracting attention, a 'cry for help', an act of revenge, or an expression of despair
- **Deliberate self-harm** is the universal set: the act of intentionally injuring oneself, irrespective of the actual degree of injury sustained.

The ethics of suicide

But the life of man is of no greater importance to the universe than that of an oyster (…) I thank providence, both for the good which I have already enjoyed, and for the power with which I am endowed of escaping the ill that threatens me.

David Hume (1711–1776), *Of Suicide*

Deus non sibi potest mortem consciscere si velit, quod homini dedit optimum in tantis vitæ pœnis.
[God cannot commit suicide even if He wishes, but man can do so at any time he chooses.]

Pliny the Elder (23–79), *Natural History*

The Catholic Church has consistently argued that one's life is the property of God and thus that to commit suicide is to deride God's prerogatives. The counterargument, by the empiricist philosopher David Hume (1711–1776) is that, if such is the case, then to save someone's life is also to deride God's prerogatives. Most religions share the Catholic Church's belief in the sanctity of life, although some have come to regard at least some suicides as an hon-

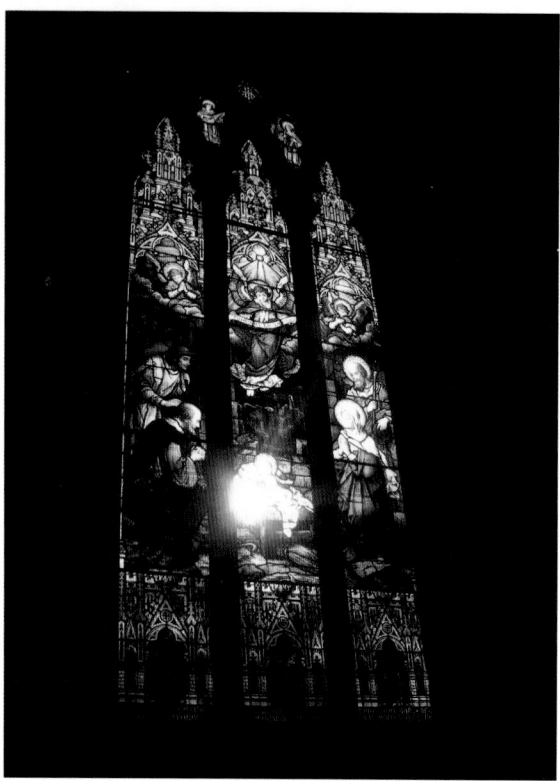

Figure 6.2 The Catholic Church has consistently argued that one's life is the property of God and thus that to commit suicide is to deride God's prerogatives. Photo by Neel Burton.

ourable death. Some Tibetan monks, for example, have committed suicide to protest against the Chinese occupation of Tibet.

Legal systems have historically been informed by religion, such that in many jurisdictions suicide and attempted suicide are still illegal. Some jurisdictions even go so far as punishing attempted suicide by death, although this is usually more in the spirit than in the practice. In the UK the Suicide Act 1961 decriminalised attempted suicide and suicide. Voluntary euthanasia is still a crime, but this may change as the voice of pro-choicers becomes louder than that of pro-lifers. Broadly speaking, pro-choicers argue that a person's life belongs to no one but himself or herself and that a person's decision to commit suicide, especially if justified as a rational solution to real problems (e.g. chronic and disabling pain), should be respected and assisted. Pro-lifers on the other hand believe that a person's life is not his or hers to take, regardless of the circumstances. Some of the stronger arguments in favour of voluntary euthanasia are that people should be free agents, that it preserves dignity and prevents unnecessary suffering, and that it frees up valuable healthcare resources. On the other hand, voluntary euthanasia is difficult to regulate and open to abuse by relatives and doctors. Furthermore, people with a physical or mental disorder may lack the mental capacity to make a rational decision about such an important issue.

Unlike most people, certain philosophers do not think about suicide in terms of ethics. Existentialist philosophers 'turn the tables round' by arguing that life has no meaning and there is therefore no reason *not* to commit suicide. For them, a person must *justify* not committing suicide by giving his or her life a meaning and fulfilling his or her unique potential through this meaning. As Jean-Paul Sartre (1905–1980), the leading exponent of existentialism, once noted, 'One lives one's death, one dies one's life'. Nihilistic (from the Latin *nihil*, 'nothing') philosophers differ from existential philosophers in that they believe that a person cannot justify his or her life even by

giving it an individual meaning. For them nothing can have a meaning, not even suicide itself. Interesting as all this may be, it should be noted that psychiatrists believe that more than 90% of cases of suicide are not the result of a rational decision (the so-called 'rational suicide'), but of a mental disorder.

> Then would I stretch my languid frame
> Beneath the wild wood's gloomiest shade,
> And try to quench the ceaseless flame
> That on my withered vitals preyed;
> Would close mine eyes and dream I were
> On some remote and friendless plain
> And long to leave existence there,
> If with it I might leave the pain
> That with a finger cold and lean
> Wrote madness on my withering mien.
>
> Percy Bysshe Shelley (1792–1822)
> The Retrospect: Cwn Elan (1812), lines 25–34

Thomas Nagel on life and death

In his influential paper of 1970, tersely entitled '*Death*', the American philosopher Thomas Nagel (b. 1937) asks the question, If death is the permanent end of our existence, is it an evil? Either it is an evil because it deprives us of life, or it is a mere blank because there is no subject left to experience the loss. Thus, if death is an evil, this is not in virtue of any positive attributes but in virtue of what it deprives us from, namely, life. For Nagel, the bare experience of life is intrinsically invaluable, regardless of the balance of its good and bad elements.

The longer one is alive, the more one 'accumulates' life. In contrast, death cannot be accumulated – it is not 'an evil of which Shakespeare has so far received a larger portion than Proust'. Most people would not consider the temporary suspension of life as an evil, nor would they regard the long period before they were born as an evil. Therefore, if death is an evil this is not because it involves a period of non-existence, but because it deprives us of life.

Nagel points out three objections to this view, but only so as to later counter them. First, it is doubtful whether anything can be an evil unless it actually causes displeasure. Second, in the case of death there is no subject left on whom to impute an evil. As long as a person exists, he has not yet died; and once he has died, he no longer exists. So there seems to be no time at which the evil of death might occur. Third, if most people would not regard the long period before they were born as

an evil, then why should they regard the period after they are dead any differently?

Nagel counters these three objections by arguing that the good or evil that befalls a man depends on his history and possibilities rather than on his momentary state, such than an evil can befall him even if he is not here to experience it. For example, if an intelligent person receives a head injury that reduces his mental condition to that of a contented infant, this should be considered a serious evil even if the person himself (in his current state) is unable to appreciate this. Thus, if these three objections are invalid, it is essentially because they ignore the direction of time. Even though a person cannot survive his death, he can still suffer evil; and even though a person does not exist during the time before his birth or during the time after his death, the time after his death is time of which he has been deprived, time in which he could have continued to enjoy the good of living.

The question remains as to whether the non-realization of further life is an absolute evil, or whether this depends on what can naturally be hoped for: the death of Keats at 24 is commonly regarded as tragic, but that of Tolstoy at 82 is not. 'The trouble,' says Nagel, 'is that life familiarizes us with the goods of which death deprives us … Death, no matter how inevitable, is an abrupt cancellation of indefinitely extensive goods'.

Epidemiology

In the UK there are around 5500 recorded suicides per year, and suicide is one of the leading causes of death in young adults. Whilst deliberate self-harm is far more common in women, completed suicide is three times more common in men. This may be because men are more likely to use violent and effective means of suicide, or because men with suicidal thoughts find it more difficult to obtain and engage with the help and support that they need. According to the Office for National Statistics, men in the 15–44 age group are at the highest risk of suicide, with a suicide rate of about 18 per 100,000 per year. One major problem with figures such as this is that they reflect the reported rates of suicide, which in turn reflect verdicts reached in Coroners' Courts. Thus, the actual suicide rate may be significantly higher than the statistics suggest.

As methods of reporting suicide vary from one country to another, it is difficult to make robust international comparisons. The global suicide rate has increased from about 10 per 100,000 in 1950 to 16 per 100,000 today, but this may simply be due to better identification and reporting of cases. In Europe, there is a marked tendency for suicide rates to increase the more north and the more east one travels. Thus Russia, Lithuania, and Estonia report suicide rates of about 40 per 100,000; in contrast, Greece, Ireland, and Italy report suicide rates of less than 6 per 100,000. In the USA, the reported suicide rate is about 11 per 100,000, compared to about 8 per 100,000 in the UK.

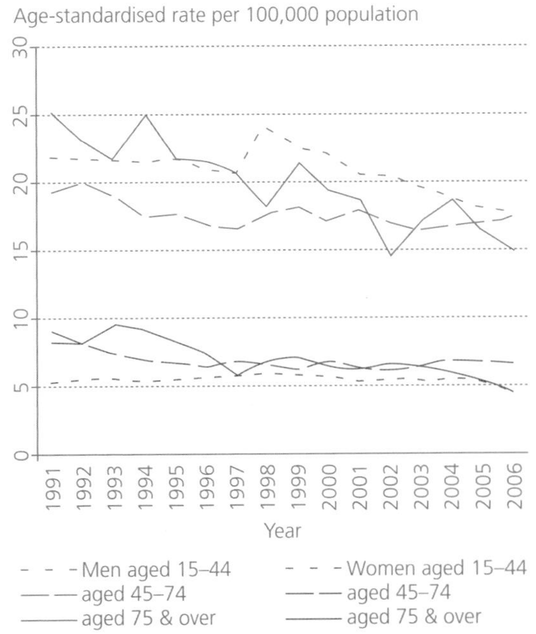

In British men the most common method of suicide is hanging, which accounts for just under half of all completed suicides. This is surprisingly high given that hanging is both violent and likely to fail, but highlights the important influence of culture on chosen methods of suicide. In British women the most common method of suicide is poisoning, which accounts for about half of all completed suicides. The drugs most commonly used are antidepressants, paracetamol, and non-steroidal anti-inflammatory drugs (NSAIDs) such as aspirin and ibuprofen. Compared to countries such as the USA, gunshot is an uncommon method of suicide, highlighting that the choice of the method of suicide is influenced by its availability and accessibility. For example, the proliferation of barbiturates in the early 1960s led to a marked increase in poisoning as a method of suicide. In the UK, about 1% of suicides involve a suicide pact in which two or more people – more often an elderly couple than a pair of star-cross'd lovers – agree to commit suicide at or around the same time.

Several factors can affect the suicide rate, such as the time of year, the state of the economy, and what predominates in media reporting. Contrary to popular belief, the suicide rate peaks in the springtime, not the wintertime. This is probably because the rebirth that occurs in the springtime accentuates feelings of hopelessness in those already contemplating suicide. As expected the suicide rate increases during times of economic depression, but less expected is that it also increases during times of economic prosperity. This is probably because people feel 'left behind' if people around them all seem to be racing ahead. The suicide rate also increases after the depiction or prominent reporting of a suicide in the media. A suicide that is inspired by another suicide, either in the media or in real life, is sometimes referred to as a 'copycat suicide', and the phenomenon itself is sometimes referred to as the 'Werther effect', after Goethe's eponymous fictional character. Sometimes copycat suicides can spread through an entire local community with one copycat suicide inspiring the next, and so on. Such a 'suicide contagion' is most

Figure 6.3 Suicide rates in England and Wales, by sex and age group, 1991–2006. Source: ONS.

likely to occur in vulnerable population groups such as disaffected teenagers and the mentally ill. On the other hand, the suicide rate decreases during times of national cohesion or coming together, such as during a war or its modern substitute, the international football tournament. During such times there is not only a feeling of 'being in it together', but also a sense of anticipation and curiosity as to 'what is going to happen next'.

> **!** It is estimated that about two-thirds of people who commit suicide had told someone of their intentions, and that about half had visited a GP in the month prior to killing themselves. Talking about suicide can be uncomfortable, but it is essential that healthcare professionals feel confident broaching the subject.

Risk factors

Risk factors for suicide can be divided into sociodemographic risk factors (Table 6.1) and clinical risk factors (Table 6.2).

Table 6.1 Sociodemographic risk factors for suicide.

Male sex	Suicide rate is three times higher in males than in females
Age	Suicide rate is highest in males aged 25–44 years
Marital status	Single, widowed, or separated/divorced
Employment status	Unemployed, insecurely employed, or retired
Occupation	Veterinary surgeons, farmers, pharmacists, doctors
Socioeconomic status	Socioeconomic groups IV and V
Poor level of social support	The elderly, prisoners, immigrants, refugees, the bereaved
Other	Recent life crisis, victim of physical or sexual abuse, access to victims, access to means

Table 6.2 Clinical risk factors for suicide.

History of deliberate self-harm	After an act of DSH, the risk of completing suicide in the subsequent year is approximately **100 times** greater than in the general population. Up to half of all completed suicides have a history of DSH, making a history of DSH the strongest risk factor for suicide
Mental disorder	Especially depressive disorders, substance misuse, schizophrenia, and personality disorders – some of these disorders may, and often do, coexist. Treatment resistance and non-compliance further increase risk. Specific factors in the mental state that increase risk are suicidal ideation and expressed intent, anger, hostility, revenge-seeking, suspiciousness, delusions of persecution, delusions of control, delusions of jealousy, delusions of guilt, and second person command hallucinations
Physical illness	Notably cancer, AIDS, epilepsy, multiple sclerosis, cerebrovascular accident, endocrine and metabolic disorders
Family history of DSH	There is strong evidence that suicidal behaviour clusters in families, although this may simply reflect a genetic predisposition to mental disorders

6

Risk assessment

Clinical skills/OSCE: Assess suicidal risk

- Ask about the history of the current episode of self-harm (if any) to determine degree of suicidal intent (higher intent/lower intent – guidelines only):
  - What was the precipitant for the attempt? (Serious precipitant/trivial precipitant)
  - Was it planned? (Planned/unplanned)
  - What was the method of self-harm? (Violent method/non-violent method)
  - Did the patient leave a suicide note? (Suicide note/no suicide note)
  - Was he or she alone? (Alone/not alone)
  - Was he or she intoxicated? (Depends on individual case)

Continued…

- Did he or she take any precautions against discovery? (Precautions/no precautions)
- Did he or she seek help after the attempt? (Did not seek help/sought help)
- How did he or she feel when he was found? (Angry or disappointed/relieved).
- Ask about the risk factors for suicide (these are more easily remembered if subdivided into sociodemographic risk factors and clinical risk factors, as above).
- Examine the mental state, especially current mood.
- Assess the current situation:
  - Ask if the patient is going to be returning to the same situation, i.e. has anything changed?
  - Ask about his outlook on the future.
  - Ask about current suicidal intent. Has he or she made any plans?
  - Ask about homicidal intent.
- Assess suicidal risk. Does the patient have any protective factors?
- Formulate a treatment plan and try to convince the patient to accept it. Based primarily upon suicidal risk, decide upon inpatient, day-patient, or outpatient management. Always discuss your management plan with a senior colleague.

Management

The management plan should depend on your assessment of risk, and should in all cases be discussed with a senior colleague and, preferably, a psychiatrist. In most cases, the patient can be discharged back into the community, particularly if he or she has a strong social support network upon which he or she can rely. In some cases a discharge can be facilitated by the Crisis Team, which can step in to provide the patient with additional support. The patient should also be referred to his or her GP for a follow-up and, in some cases, also to the local Community Mental Health Team. If the patient is already under the care of the local Community Mental Health Team, he or she should be referred to his or her care coordinator as soon as possible, preferably by telephone or answerphone.

Simple advice that you can give to people with suicidal thoughts is:

- Whatever thoughts you are having, and however bad you are feeling, remember that you have not always felt this way, and that you will not always feel this way.

- Many people who have attempted suicide and survived ultimately feel relieved that they did *not* end their lives.
- The risk of someone committing suicide is highest in the combined presence of (1) suicidal thoughts, (2) the means to commit suicide, and (3) the opportunity to commit suicide. If you are prone to suicidal thoughts, ensure that the *means* to commit suicide have been removed. For example, give tablets and sharp objects to someone for safekeeping, or put them in a locked or otherwise inaccessible place.
- At the same time, ensure that the *opportunity* to commit suicide is lacking. The surest way of doing this is by remaining in close contact with one or more relatives or friends, e.g. by inviting them to stay with you. Share your thoughts and feelings with these people, and don't be reluctant to let them help you.
- If no one is available or no one seems suitable, there are a number of emergency telephone lines that you can ring at any time. You can even ring 999 for an ambulance or take yourself to an Accident and Emergency department.
- Do not use alcohol or drugs as these can make your behaviour more impulsive and significantly increase your likelihood of attempting suicide. In particular, do not drink or take drugs alone, or end up alone after drinking or taking drugs.
- Make a list of all the positive things about yourself and a list of all the positive things about your life, including the things that have so far prevented you from committing suicide (you may need to get help with this). Keep the lists on you, and read them to yourself each time you are assailed by suicidal thoughts.
- On a separate sheet of paper, write a safety plan for the times when you feel like acting on your suicidal thoughts. Your safety plan could involve delaying any suicidal attempt by at least 48 hours, and then talking to someone about your thoughts and feelings as soon as possible. Discuss your safety plan with your GP, psychiatrist or key worker, and commit yourself to it.
- Sometimes even a single good night's sleep can significantly alter your outlook, so it is important not to underestimate the importance of sleep. If you are having trouble sleeping, speak to your GP or psychiatrist about this.

Deliberate self-harm

Acts of self-harm are carried out for a variety of reasons, most commonly to express and relieve bottled-up anger or tension, feel more in control of a seemingly desperate life situation, punish oneself for being a 'bad person', or combat feelings of numbness and deadness and feel more 'connected' and alive. Acts of self-harm reflect very deep distress, and are most often used as a desperate and reluctant last resort – a method of surviving rather than of ending one's life, and sometimes also a method of attracting much-needed attention. For some people, the pain inflicted by self-harm is preferable to the numbness and emptiness that it replaces: it is something rather than nothing, and a salutatory reminder that one is still able to feel, that one is still alive. For others, the pain inflicted by self-harm merely replaces a different kind of pain that they can neither understand nor control. Self-harm may be a one-off response to a severe emotional crisis or it may be a more long-term problem. Some people continue to self-harm because they continue to suffer from the same problems, or they may stop self-harming for a period – sometimes even several years – only to return to it at the next major emotional crisis.

> *I slashed my wrist again and again, as deeply as I could. I knew perfectly well that it would not kill me, not like the times before. They have been something quite different. As my writing to you comes to a close, the pain is so unbearable inside me that a force of such strength has driven me to inflict a physical pain on myself in the hope of appeasing the other.*
>
> Sarah Ferguson (1973), *A Guard Within*

The true extent of deliberate self-harm (DSH) is difficult to establish. In the UK each year, approximately 170,000 cases of DSH present to hospitals. This number has been increasing for several years, but now appears to be levelling off. About 80% of acts of DSH involve drug overdoses, and self-cutting accounts for a significant proportion of the remainder. The most frequently used drugs are paracetamol and paracetamol compounds, antidepressants, minor tranquillisers and sedatives, and NSAIDs (cf. suicide). Alcohol is taken as part of the act of DSH in about 30% of cases. The most frequently cited problems at the time of DSH are relationships, alcohol, employment/studies, finances, housing, social isolation,

bereavement, and physical health. About 40% of cases have a major psychiatric disorder excluding personality disorder, alcohol misuse, and substance misuse, and about 25% report high suicidal intent on the Beck Suicide Intent Scale. Finally, about 20–25% of cases repeat DSH in the first year. These statistics are based on data collected in 2006 from the John Radcliffe Hospital in Oxford by the University of Oxford Centre for Suicide Research.

Simple advice that you can give to people with thoughts of self-harm is:

- If you are plagued by thoughts of self-harm, try to take your mind off them by using one of several coping strategies or distraction techniques.
- A useful coping strategy is to find someone you trust such as a friend, relative, or teacher, and to be with them and share your feelings with them. If no one is available or there is no one you feel comfortable with, there are a number of emergency telephone lines that you can ring at any time.
- Engaging in creative activities such as writing, drawing, or playing a musical instrument can also take your mind off thoughts of harming yourself, and additionally help you to express your feelings and understand them better.
- Other coping strategies include reading a good book, listening to classical music, watching a comedy or nature programme, or even just cooking a meal or going out to the shops.
- Relaxation techniques like deep breathing or yoga and meditation can also help.
- However, avoid alcohol and drugs as these can make your behaviour more impulsive, and significantly increase your likelihood of harming yourself.
- In some cases the urge to harm yourself may be so great that all you can do is to minimise the risks involved. Methods for doing this include holding ice cubes in your palm and attempting to crush them, fitting an elastic band around your wrist and flicking it, or plucking the hairs on your arms and legs.
- If you have harmed yourself and are in pain or unable to control the bleeding, or if you have taken an overdose of any kind or size, call 999 immediately, or get a relative or friend to take you to Accident and Emergency as soon as possible. Going to Accident and Emergency not only enables you to get medical treatment, but also gives you an opportunity to spend time with someone and talk to him or her about your feelings.

6

- Once things are more settled, consider getting yourself referred for a talking treatment such as counselling or cognitive-behavioural therapy. This can give you the opportunity to talk through your feelings in a safe and supportive environment, and to better understand why you sometimes feel the way you do. It can also help you to identify solutions to your problems, as well as alternative strategies for coping with them.
- Joining a local support group enables you to meet other people with similar problems to yours, that is, people who are likely to accept you and understand you, and with whom you may feel better able to share your feelings. However, beware of joining unmonitored online forums and chat groups which are open to all and sundry, and which can sometimes leave you feeling even worse than before.

Recommended reading

Existentialism and Humanism (L'Existentialisme est un humanisme) (1974) Jean-Paul Sartre. Methuen Publishing Ltd.

The Stranger (1989) Albert Camus. Vintage Books.

Night Falls Fast: Understanding Suicide (2000) Kay Redfield Jamison. Vintage Books.

The Practical Art of Suicide Assessment: A Guide for Mental Health Professionals and Substance Abuse Counselors (2002) S. C. Shea. John Wiley & Sons.

Choosing to Live: How to Defeat Suicide through Cognitive Therapy (1996) Thomas E. Ellis and Cory F. Newman. New Harbinger Publications.

6

Self-assessment

Simply answer with true or false. Answers on p. 218

1. The making available to a person of the means to end his or her life is called assisted suicide.
2. The deliberate ending of the life of another person who has requested it and is physically unable to commit suicide is called voluntary euthanasia.
3. The term 'parasuicide' is also used to mean 'attempted suicide.'
4. The majority of suicides are so-called 'rational suicides'.
5. The suicide rate is five times higher in males than in females.
6. Since 1976, the suicide rate in young males has been falling.
7. In females poisoning is the most common method of suicide.
8. Careful planning of the suicidal act suggests a high suicidal intent.
9. The suicide rate increases in spring and around Christmas time.
10. Reliable statistics indicate that in Europe suicide rates tend to be highest in northern and eastern countries.
11. The suicide rates amongst immigrants to the UK closely reflect those of their country of origin, highlighting the important aetiological role of cultural factors in suicidal behaviour.
12. Two-thirds of suicides had visited a GP in the month prior to killing themselves.
13. Males aged 15–19 are at the highest risk of deliberate self-harm.
14. Although the extent of deliberate self-harm is difficult to assess, the number of acts of deliberate self-harm presenting to hospitals has been increasing for several years.
15. The majority of acts of deliberate self-harm are drug overdoses.
16. About 20–25% of cases of deliberate self-harm repeat in the first year (10% if they have no previous history of deliberate self-harm).
17. The most important risk factor for deliberate self-harm is a history of self-harm.
18. In some cases, patients who self-harm can be advised to self-harm in less dangerous ways.

Neurotic, stress-related, and somatoform disorders (anxiety disorders)

7

Key learning objectives

- Psychological and physical symptoms of anxiety
- Definition of phobia and the three different types of phobic anxiety disorder: agoraphobia, social phobia, and specific phobias
- Key features differentiating phobic anxiety disorders from panic disorder and generalised anxiety disorder
- Nature of obsessions and compulsions in obsessive-compulsive disorder
- Diagnostic criteria for adjustment reaction and post-traumatic stress disorder
- Relationship of dissociative and somatoform disorders to factitious disorders and malingering

7

Introduction

Anxiety is a normal response to life experiences, but is considered pathological if it becomes so exaggerated, frequent, and chronic as to result in impairment of function. Such anxiety can be found in a number of psychiatric and medical disorders, but in anxiety disorders it is the primary and most prominent feature.

Anxiety can be defined as **a state consisting of psychological and physical symptoms brought about by a sense of apprehension at a perceived threat**. This perceived threat can be external as in agoraphobia, social phobia, and specific phobias; or internal as in panic disorder, generalised anxiety disorder, and obsessive-compulsive disorder. In each of these anxiety disorders the psychological and physical symptoms of anxiety present in different and characteristic patterns.

The evolutionary basis of anxiety

Anxiety is a normal response to life experiences, a protective mechanism that has evolved both to prevent us from entering into potentially dangerous situations and to enable us to escape from them should they befall us regardless. For example, anxiety may prevent us from coming into close contact with disease-carrying or poisonous animals such as rats, snakes, and spiders; from engaging with a much stronger enemy to whom we are sure to lose out; and even from declaring our undying love to someone who is unlikely to spare our feelings. If we do find ourselves in a potentially dangerous situation, the fight-or-flight response brought on by anxiety may help us mount an appropriate response by priming our body for action and increasing our performance and stamina.

Continued...

Psychiatry, 2e. By Neel Burton. Published 2010 by
Blackwell Publishing.

Although some degree of anxiety can improve our performance on a range of tasks, *severe* anxiety can have the opposite effect and hinder our performance. Thus, whereas a confident and talented actor may perform optimally in front of a live audience, a novice may develop stage-fright and freeze. The relationship between anxiety and performance can be expressed graphically by a parabola or inverted 'U'. This is referred to as the 'Yerkes–Dodson' curve, after the psychologists R. M. Yerkes and J. D. Dodson.

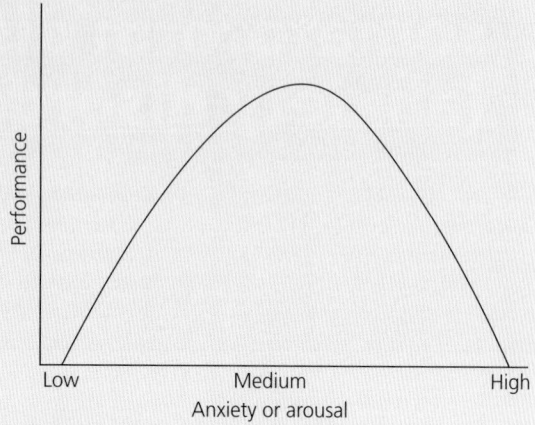

Figure 7.1 The Yerkes–Dodson curve.

ICD-10 classification of neurotic, stress-related, and somatoform disorders (principal diagnostic categories)

F40 Phobic anxiety disorders
   .0　Agoraphobia
      .0　Without panic disorder
      .1　With panic disorder
   .1　Social phobias
   .2　Specific (isolated) phobias
F41 Other anxiety disorders
   .0　Panic disorder
   .1　Generalised anxiety disorder
   .2　Mixed anxiety and depressive disorder
   .3　Other mixed anxiety disorders
F42 Obsessive-compulsive disorder
   .0　Predominantly obsessional thoughts
   .1　Predominantly compulsive acts
   .2　Mixed obsessional thoughts and acts
F43 Reaction to severe stress and adjustment disorders
   .0　Acute stress reaction
   .1　Post-traumatic stress disorder
   .2　Adjustment disorders
F44 Dissociative (conversion) disorders
   .0　Dissociative amnesia
   .1　Dissociative fugue
   .2　Dissociative stupor
   .3　Trance and possession disorders
   .4　Dissociative motor disorders
   .5　Dissociative convulsions
   .6　Dissociative anaesthesia and sensory loss
   .7　Mixed dissociative disorders
   .8　Other dissociative disorders
      .80　Ganser's syndrome
      .81　Multiple personality disorder
      .82　Transient dissociative disorders occurring in childhood and adolescence
F45 Somatoform disorders
   .0　Somatisation disorder

   .1　Undifferentiated somatoform disorder
   .2　Hypochondriacal disorder
   .3　Somatoform autonomic dysfunction
   .4　Persistent somatoform pain disorder
F48 Other neurotic disorders
   .0　Neurasthenia
   .1　Depersonalisation–derealisation syndrome

DSM-IV classification of anxiety disorders
Agoraphobia without a history of panic disorder
Panic disorder with agoraphobia
Panic disorder without agoraphobia
Social phobia
Specific phobia
Generalised anxiety disorder
Anxiety disorder due to a general medical condition
Substance-induced anxiety disorder
Obsessive-compulsive disorder
Acute stress disorder
Adjustment disorders
Post-traumatic stress disorder

DSM-IV classification of dissociative disorders
Dissociative amnesia
Dissociative fugue
Depersonalization disorder
Dissociative identity disorder

DSM-IV classification of somatoform disorders
Somatisation disorder
Conversion disorder
Pain disorder
Hypochondriasis

Symptoms of anxiety

Table 7.1 lists the psychological and physical symptoms of anxiety. In mild anxiety, physical symptoms arise from the body's 'fight-or-flight response', a state of high arousal that results from a surge of adrenaline. These physical symptoms include dry mouth, tremor, sweating, tachycardia, and hyperventilation. In severe anxiety, hyperventilation can lead to a fall in the concentration of carbon dioxide in the blood. This gives rise to an additional set of physical symptoms, including chest tightness, numbness or tingling around the mouth and in the extremities, dizziness, and faintness.

Epidemiology

Anxiety disorders generally have their onset in early adulthood or, less commonly, in middle age. Although very common, their prevalence is difficult to estimate because many cases do not present to medical attention. Those that do may be difficult to diagnose or may be misdiagnosed as a depressive disorder or as a medical disorder. According to the US National Comorbidity Survey (NCS) carried out in the early 1990s, anxiety disorders affect 18.6% of adults in the United States. Females are more affected than males by a ratio of about 2:1, **but in social phobia and obsessive–compulsive disorder this ratio is closer to 1:1.** Depressive symptoms are common in anxiety disorders (and *vice versa*), and if the diagnostic criteria for both depressive disorder and generalised anxiety disorder are fulfilled, a diagnosis of 'mixed anxiety and depressive disorder' (ICD-10) can be made. Other psychiatric disorders are also common in anxiety disorders, including other anxiety disorders, personality disorders, and substance misuse.

Table 7.1 Symptoms of anxiety.

Psychological symptoms	Feelings of fear and impending doom, feelings of dizziness and faintness, restlessness, exaggerated startle response, poor concentration, irritability, insomnia and night terrors, depersonalisation and derealisation
	Globus hystericus or *globus* is the irritating feeling of having a lump in the throat. It leads to forced swallowing and a characteristic gulping sound that is often mimicked in children's cartoons to signal fear
Physical symptoms	Physical symptoms arise from autonomic arousal, hyperventilation, and muscle tension
Cardiovascular	Palpitations, tachycardia, chest discomfort
Gastrointestinal	Dry mouth, feeling of a lump in the throat, nausea, abdominal discomfort, frequent or loose motions
Respiratory	Hyperventilation, difficulty in catching breath, chest tightness
Genitourinary	Urinary frequency, failure of erection, amenorrhoea
Other/general	Hot flushes or cold chills, tremor, sweating, headache and muscle pains, numbness and tingling sensations around the mouth and in the extremities, dizziness, faintness

7

Table 7.2 Prevalence of anxiety disorders (best estimate).

Disorder	Prevalence (%)
Phobic anxiety disorders:	
Agoraphobia	4.9
Social phobias	2.0
Specific (simple) phobias	8.3
Panic disorder	1.6
Generalised anxiety disorder	3.4
Obsessive–compulsive disorder	2.4
PTSD	3.6

PTSD, post-traumatic stress disorder.
Source: *Mental Health: A Report of the Surgeon General* (1999).

ICD-10 and DSM-IV. DSM-IV defines them as 'recurrent, locality-specific patterns of aberrant behaviour and troubling experience that may or may not be linked to a particular DSM-IV category'. Many culture-bound syndromes may be local variations of neurotic, stress-related, and somatoform disorders. Some of the more recognised ones are described in Table 7.3.

> **!** As a general point, it is important to remember that psychiatric symptoms may be modified by cultural factors. For example, in many traditional societies:
> - Acute and catatonic forms of schizophrenia are more highly prevalent
> - 'Depression' is more frequently experienced as somatic symptoms than as depressed mood
> - Some forms of behaviour, such as brief reactive psychosis, trance, and dissociative states may be considered normal.
>
> Culture is also an important determinant of the content of dreams and psychotic experiences.

Culture-bound syndromes

Culture-bound syndromes are mental disorders that only occur in certain cultures or ethnic groups and that are not easily accommodated by psychiatric classifications such as

Table 7.3 Some culture-bound syndromes.

Syndrome	Principal region/ population affected	Description
Amok	Malaysia ♂	Outburst of violent, aggressive, and sometimes homicidal acts after a period of brooding or depression. This is followed by deep sleep, amnesia for the episode and, in some cases, suicide. First described by Captain Cook
Brain Fag	West Africa, New Guinea ♂	Cognitive difficulties, blurred vision, and head and neck pain. Most commonly affects male students who complain of 'too much thinking'
Dhat	India and South Asia ♂	Severe anxiety about loss of semen in the urine, whitish discolouration of the urine, sexual dysfunction, and feelings of weakness and exhaustion. Attributed to excessive masturbation or intercourse
Koro	South-West Asia ♂	Sudden and intense fear of the penis retracting into the body and causing death. Mainly occurs at night and in the context of sexual guilt. Sometimes occurs in local epidemics. Penises may be fastened to prevent their retraction
Latah	Malaysia and Indonesia ⚥	Echolalia, coprolalia, echopraxia, automatic obedience, and dissociative or trance-like behaviour in response to a sudden fright or trauma
Susto	Latin American populations	Loss of the soul from the body after a sudden fright, leaving the body vulnerable to disease. Also called *perdida de la sombra* or 'loss of the shadow'
Anorexia nervosa	Occidental and occidentalised societies ⚥	It has been suggested that anorexia nervosa is a culture-bound syndrome. Can you think of other ICD-listed conditions that may be culture-bound?

Aetiology

Psychiatric and medical conditions

Anxiety may be associated with an anxiety disorder, or with a broad range of psychiatric and medical conditions. Psychiatric conditions associated with anxiety include mood disorders, psychotic disorders, somatoform disorders, and eating disorders. Medical conditions associated with anxiety include endocrine disorders such as hyperthyroidism, Cushing's disease, phaeochromocytoma, and hypoglycaemia, and drug and alcohol intoxication or withdrawal.

Genetic factors

Genetic factors play a predisposing role in the aetiology of anxiety disorders, and may be manifested as 'neurotic' personality traits or neurotic cluster (cluster C) personality disorders (see below and Chapter 8).

Neurochemical abnormalities

Noradrenergic neurons originating in the *locus cœruleus* and serotonergic neurons originating in the raphe nuclei act on the limbic system to increase anxiety, and an imbalance in these neurotransmitters, and in gamma aminobutyric acid (GABA), may contribute to the symptoms of anxiety disorders. This imbalance may result either from biological factors or from psychological factors, or from both.

Environmental factors

Anxiety disorders may be triggered and perpetuated by stressful events, especially those involving a threat. They may also result from stressful or traumatic events in childhood such as parental indifference or physical abuse.

Psychological theories

According to cognitive-behavioural theories, anxiety disorders result from inappropriate thought processes (see Figure 7.2). According to psychoanalytical theory, anxiety disorders have their origins in childhood events such as separation and loss, and in unresolved childhood conflicts of psychosexual development. Phobias in particular may have their origins in the displacement of subconscious fears onto an unrelated object or situation, and are perpetuated through avoidance behaviour that is negatively reinforced through reduction of fear.

Neurosis

'Neurosis' is an old-fashioned but useful term that derives from the Ancient Greek *neuron* (nerve) and loosely means 'disease of the nerves'. The core feature of neurosis is anxiety, but neurosis can manifest as a range of other problems such as irritability, depression, perfectionism, obsessive–compulsive tendencies, and even personality disorders such as anankastic personality disorder. Although neurosis in some form or other is very common, it can prevent us from enjoying the moment, adapting usefully to our environment, and developing a richer, more complex and more fulfilling outlook on life. The psychiatrist Carl Jung (1875–1961) believed that neurotic people fundamentally had issues with the meaning and purpose of their life. In his autobiography of 1961, *Memories, Dreams, Reflections* he noted that 'The majority of my patients consisted not of believers but of those who had lost their faith'. Interestingly, Jung also believed that neurosis could be beneficial to some people despite its debilitating effects. In *Two Essays on Analytical Psychology*, he wrote:

The reader will doubtless ask: What in the world is the value and meaning of a neurosis, this most useless and pestilent curse of humanity? To be neurotic – what good can that do? (…) I myself have known more than one person who owed his whole usefulness and reason for existence to a neurosis, which prevented all the worst follies in his life and forced him to a mode of living that developed his valuable potentialities. These might have been stifled had not the neurosis, with iron grip, held him to the place where he belonged.

Anxiety disorders

Phobic anxiety disorders

A phobia is defined as **a persistent irrational fear that is usually recognised as such and that produces anticipatory anxiety for and avoidance of the feared object, activity, or situation.** Exposure to the feared object, activity, or situation triggers intense anxiety that may take the form of a panic attack (see later). There are three types of phobic anxiety disorders: agoraphobia, social phobia, and specific phobias.

Agoraphobia derives from the Greek *phobia* ('fear') and *agora* ('market or marketplace') and so literally means 'fear of the market place'. Contrary to popular belief agoraphobia does *not* describe a fear of open places, but a fear of places that are difficult or embarrassing to escape from, such as places that are confined, crowded, or far from home. In time, people with agoraphobia may have to rely on trusted companions to accompany them to feared places and, in severe cases, may end up unable to leave their home. A number of studies have uncovered a link between agoraphobia and poor spatial orientation, suggesting that spatial disorientation, particularly in places where visual cues are sparse, may contribute to the development of agoraphobia. Agoraphobia may respond to cognitive-behavioural techniques such as graded exposure and anxiety management (often complemented by cognitive therapy), and to antidepressant drugs. Relapse is common.

Social phobia is fear of being judged by others and of being embarrassed and humiliated, either in most social situations or in specific social situations such as dining or public speaking. Social phobia has many features in common with shyness, and distinguishing between the two can be a cause for debate and controversy. Some critics have gone so far as to suggest that 'social phobia' is nothing more than a convenient label used to pass off a personality trait as a mental illness, and thereby to legitimise its medical 'treatment'. However, it can be argued that social phobia is different from shyness in that it starts at a later age and is more severe and debilitating. Social phobia may respond to cognitive-behavioural techniques such as graded exposure and anxiety management, and to antidepressant drugs. Alcohol and benzodiazepine misuse are more common than in other phobic anxiety disorders.

The third and last type of phobic anxiety disorder, specific phobia, is by far the most common. Specific phobia is, as its name implies, fear of a specific object or situation. Common specific phobias involve enclosed spaces (claustrophobia), heights (acrophobia), darkness (achluophobia), storms (brontophobia), animals (zoophobia), and blood (haematophobia). Unlike other anxiety disorders, specific phobias tend to begin in early childhood, and there seems to be an innate predisposition to developing certain specific phobias such as phobias of spiders (arachnophobia) or snakes (ophidiophobia). Such innate predispositions are intended to protect us from the potential dangers commonly faced by our ancestors, and so to increase our chances of surviving and reproducing. Today man-made dangers such as motor vehicles and electric cables are far more likely to strike us than natural dangers such as spiders and snakes, but most phobias are still for natural dangers. This may be because man-made dangers are comparatively recent arrivals and so have not had sufficient time to imprint themselves onto our genomes. Specific phobias may respond to cognitive-behavioural techniques such as graded exposure and anxiety management, flooding, and modelling.

Panic disorder

Panic attacks are characterised by rapid onset of severe anxiety lasting for about 20–30 minutes. They may occur in panic disorder, phobic anxiety disorders, generalised anxiety disorder, obsessive–compulsive disorder, post-traumatic stress disorder, separation anxiety disorder, depressive disorders, and organic disorders (e.g. substance misuse, hyperthyroidism, hypoglycaemia, phaeochromocytoma). **In panic disorder, panic attacks occur recurrently and unexpectedly.** There is fear of the implications and consequences of a panic attack, e.g. having a heart attack, losing control, 'going crazy', and this fear in itself triggers further panic attacks. A vicious circle takes hold, resulting in panic attacks becoming more frequent and more severe, and even occurring completely out of the blue (Figure 7.2). This can in some cases lead to the development of 'secondary' agoraphobia, in which the person avoids leaving the home so as to minimise the risk and consequences of having a panic attack. Panic disorder may respond to cognitive-behavioural therapy, and to drugs including serotonin-selective reuptake inhibitors (SSRIs), tricyclic antidepressants (TCAs), and benzodiazepines.

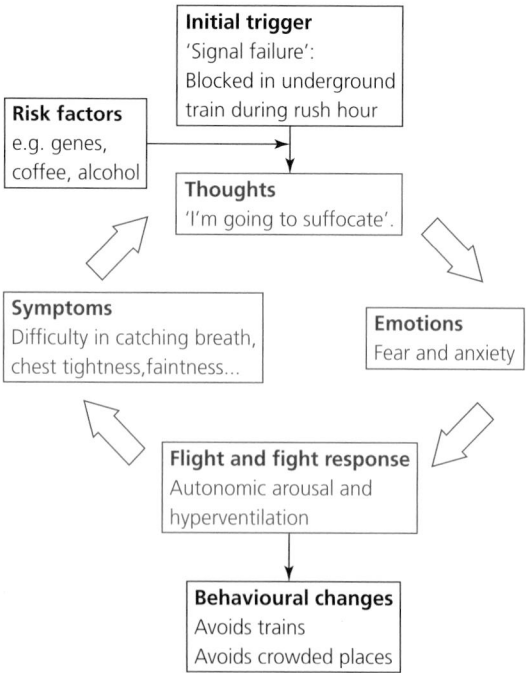

Figure 7.2 Cognitive-behavioural model for panic disorder.

The story of Mrs AB

Mrs AB is a 33-year-old part-time secretary presenting to a community mental health centre after having read a magazine article on hypochondriasis. Ten years ago, while attending a postnatal exercise class following the birth of her only child, Mrs AB noticed a dramatic increase in her heart rate. Terrified that she was going to die from a heart attack, she became aware of a series of other symptoms including difficulty catching breath, chest tightness, and tingling in the hands. She left her baby at the class and ran to the nearby A&E department for help. An ECG was administered but no abnormality was found.

Since then Mrs AB has begun a pattern of experiencing pal-

pitations and seeking medical help. She currently experiences the palpitations about three or four times a month and, as they come on unexpectedly, she feels unable to leave her home alone without her mobile phone or go to places such as cinemas and crowded shopping centres where medical help may be difficult to obtain. As a result, she no longer goes on holiday and her relationship with her husband has come under severe strain.

Diagnosis: Panic disorder with agoraphobia (DSM-IV)
Adapted from Clinical Research Unit for Anxiety and
Depression (www.crufad.com)

Generalised anxiety disorder

Generalised anxiety disorder is characterised by long-standing free-floating anxiety that may fluctuate but that is neither situational (phobic anxiety disorders) nor episodic (panic disorder) (Table 7.4). There is apprehension about a number of events far out of proportion to the actual likelihood or impact of the feared events. Other common symptoms include symptoms of autonomic arousal, irritability, poor concentration, muscle tension, tiredness, and sleep disturbances. Depressive symptoms can also occur, and depression and 'mixed anxiety and depressive disorder' (ICD-10) are important differential diagnoses that may in fact lie on a single spectrum of disorders. Generalised anxiety disorder may respond to counselling, cognitive and behavioural techniques, and drugs including SSRIs, SNRIs, sedative antidepressants such as amitriptyline and trazodone, buspirone (a 5-HT$_{1A}$ partial agonist), and benzodiazepines (see below). Drugs are best prescribed on a short-term basis as an adjunct to psychological treatment. Benzodiazepines in particular should not be prescribed on a long-term basis because of the risk of dependence.

Psychopharmacology: Benzodiazepines

The Austrian scientist Leo Sternbach serendipitously discovered the first benzodiazepine in 1954, and they soon replaced barbiturates as the drug of choice for the treatment of anxiety and insomnia. Benzodiazepines act at the GABA$_A$–BDZ receptor complex to enhance the inhibitory action of GABA, and they have anxiolytic, hypnotic, anticonvulsant, muscle relaxant, and amnesic properties.

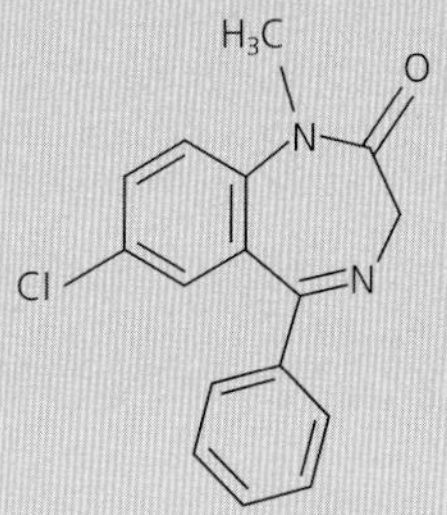

Figure 7.3 Molecular structure of diazepam.

Continued...

Table 7.4 Features distinguishing the three types of anxiety disorder.

	Phobic anxiety	Panic disorder	Generalised anxiety disorder
Occurrence of anxiety	Situational	Episodic	Free-floating
Associated cognitions	Fear of situation	Fear of symptoms	Fear of future
Associated behaviour	Avoidance	Escape	Inhibition

Benzodiazepines have found clinical use in the following indications:

- Disabling anxiety disorders
- Severe acute anxiety
- Agitation
- Insomnia
- Detoxification from alcohol
- Convulsive disorders
- Spastic disorders
- Involuntary movement disorders
- Surgical pre-medication.

The choice of benzodiazepine is principally determined by its indication, as potency and half-life vary considerably from one drug to another.

High potency, short half-life	Alprazolam, lorazepam
High potency, long half-life	Clonazepam
Low potency, short half-life	Oxazepam, temazepam
Low potency, long half-life	Chlordiazepoxide

Commoner adverse effects of benzodiazepines include psychomotor retardation, memory impairment (anterograde amnesia), and paradoxical or disinhibitory reactions. Tolerance (including cross-tolerance to other benzodiazepines and to alcohol) and dependence may develop, so it is generally preferable to prescribe short courses and to avoid repeat prescriptions. Once tolerance has been achieved, abrupt discontinuation may lead to anxiety-like symptoms and to rebound insomnia and, rarely, to depression, psychosis, seizures, and *delirium tremens* (see Chapter 11). Benzodiazepines are relatively safe in overdose but toxic effects are enhanced by a number of drugs, including alcohol. The antidote to benzodiazepines is the benzodiazepine antagonist **flumazenil**.

Reactions to severe stress and adjustment disorders

Acute stress reaction

Acute stress reaction is an acute response to a highly threatening or catastrophic experience (e.g. road accident, criminal assault, natural catastrophe) that subsides in a matter of hours or days. Individual vulnerability plays an important role in the occurrence and severity of an acute stress reaction, as does physical exhaustion and organic factors, for instance, in the elderly. Symptoms are variable but typically include an initial state of shock and symptoms of anxiety and depression. Management is by removal of the stressor, reassurance, and support. A short course of benzodiazepines may also be helpful.

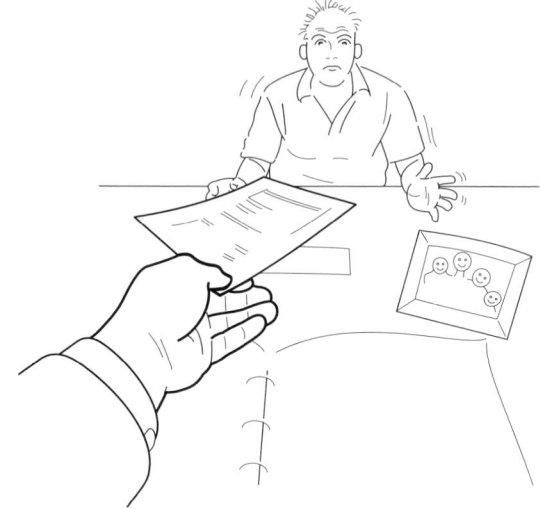

"Here's a prescription for some sedatives. The side effects are anxiety, agitation, and sleeplessness."

Figure 7.4

Post-traumatic stress disorder

Post-traumatic stress disorder (PTSD) is a protracted and sometimes delayed response to a highly threatening or catastrophic experience, most commonly combat exposure in males and sexual assault in females. It is characterised by numbing, detachment, flashbacks, nightmares, partial or complete amnesia for the event, avoidance of (and distress at) reminders of the event, and prominent anxiety symptoms. Associated psychiatric disorders are very common, especially depressive disorders, anxiety disorders, and alcohol and substance misuse. There is no evidence to suggest that PTSD can be prevented through 'debriefing' in the aftermath of the traumatic event. PTSD may respond to supportive psychotherapy, cognitive-behavioural therapy (in the form of cognitive therapy and exposure therapy and relaxation), group therapy, and antidepressants. Benzodiazepines should be avoided because of the high risk of dependence. Prognosis is generally good but in some cases PTSD may persist for years. Historical epithets for PTSD include 'shell shock', 'combat neurosis', and 'survivor syndrome'.

Adjustment disorder

Adjustment disorder is a protracted response to a significant life change or life event such as change of job, migration, divorce, or separation that occurs in persons vulnerable to the disorder. It is characterised by depressive symptoms and/or anxiety symptoms that are not severe enough to meet a diagnosis of depressive disorder or anxiety disorder, but that nevertheless lead to an impairment in social functioning. There is usually a feeling of inability to cope or continue in the present situation that is sometimes accompanied by angry outbursts. Supportive psychotherapy may be helpful, but adjustment disorders have a good prognosis and do not usually last for more than six months.

Abnormal bereavement reaction

Bereavement refers to the grief that occurs after the loss of a loved one, but that can also happen after the loss of a pet or national figure, or the loss of an asset such as health or social status. A bereavement reaction in such cases is normal, and varies greatly in length and severity from one set of circumstances to another, from one individual to another, and from one culture to another. Various stages or phases of grief after bereavement have been suggested, but they are neither consistent nor universal. Sudden and unexpected loss tends to lead to a longer and more severe bereavement reaction, as does the loss of a person who was particularly close, or with whom the patient had a dependent or ambivalent relationship. A bereavement reaction is considered abnormal if it is either unusually intense or unusually prolonged, that is, if it meets the criteria for a depressive disorder or if it lasts for more than six months. It is also considered abnormal if it is delayed, inhibited, or distorted. In such cases, it can be classified as a form of adjustment disorder (ICD-10).

Obsessive–compulsive disorder

According to ICD-10, obsessive–compulsive disorder (OCD) can be classified as predominantly obsessional thoughts, predominantly compulsive acts, or mixed obsessional thoughts and acts.

An obsessional thought is a recurrent idea, image, or impulse that is perceived as being senseless, that is unsuccessfully resisted and that results in marked anxiety and distress. Unlike passivity phenomena (e.g. thought insertion) it is recognised as being a product of one's own mind, even though it may be violent or obscene. Common obsessional thoughts involve doubt, contamination, orderliness and symmetry, safety, physical symptoms, aggression, and sex. According to the 'thought avoidance paradox', the more one tries to stop thinking about something, the more one is likely to do so. For example, try not to think about a pink elephant. Paradoxically, the only way not to think about a pink elephant is actually to think about one!

A compulsive act is a recurrent stereotyped behaviour that is not useful or enjoyable but that reduces anxiety and distress. It is usually perceived as being senseless but is unsuccessfully resisted. A compulsive act may be a response to an obsessive thought or according to rules that must be applied rigidly. Common compulsive acts include washing and cleaning, arranging and ordering, checking, and other ritualistic behaviours; and mental rituals such as counting or repeating a phrase. Compulsive acts are portrayed by Leonardo di Caprio in the film *The Aviator* about the real-life aviator, film director, and rebel billionaire Howard Hughes (di Caprio).

> **Clinical skills: Key features of obsessions and compulsions**
>
> **An obsession**
> - Is a recurrent idea, image, or impulse
> - Is recognised as being a product of one's own mind
> - Is usually perceived as being senseless
> - Is unsuccessfully resisted
> - Results in marked anxiety and distress/impairment of functioning
>
> **A compulsion**
> - Is a recurrent stereotyped behaviour
> - Reduces anxiety but is neither useful nor enjoyable
> - Is usually perceived as being senseless
> - Is unsuccessfully resisted
> - Results in marked distress/impairment of functioning

According to biological models, OCD results from pathology in the caudate nucleus, which fails to suppress signals from the orbitofrontal cortex. As a result, the thalamus becomes overexcited and sends strong signals back to the orbitofrontal cortex, and so on. Such a neuronal loop model of OCD is supported by MRI and PET studies, and by the documented associations between OCD and Tourette's syndrome and Sydenham's chorea (St Vitus' dance), which both involve pathology of the basal ganglia.

The differential diagnosis of OCD includes depressive disorders, anankastic personality disorder, Tourette's syndrome, other anxiety disorders, psychotic disorders, and organic mental disorders. Comorbid mental disorders, especially depressive disorders, are common.

OCD may respond to cognitive-behavioural techniques such as exposure and response prevention (ERP) or to medication in the form of high doses of an SSRI or clomipramine (a TCA that also acts as a serotonin reuptake inhibitor), and adjuncts such as gabapentin, lamotrigine, and olanzapine and risperidone. Evidence suggests that the combination of cognitive-behavioural therapy and an SSRI is more effective than CBT alone. Obsessive–compulsive symptoms are common in depressive disorders and treatment of the underlying depressive disorder may lead to improvement in the obsessive–compulsive symptoms. OCD may run a relapsing and remitting course, but untreated prognosis is poor. In severe and refractory cases, neurosurgery, usually in the form of anterior cingulotomy or capsulotomy, can be considered.

The story of Mr MD

Mr MD is a 30-year-old father of two children presenting with a 9-year history of obsessions and compulsions. He is terrified of being inadvertently responsible for harm befalling his loved ones and so checks 'dangerous' appliances repeatedly to be sure that they are safely turned off. Over the years the doubt that he has turned off all the appliances has gradually strengthened, and simply looking at the stove is no longer reassuring enough. He must stare at each knob on the stove to make sure it is aligned in the off position, and say to himself 'it's off' over and over again. Then he must place his hand on each hotplate and count to 10 to be sure that each hotplate is cold. If this ritual is interrupted, or if he loses his concentration, he has to start all over again, and it can take up to 15 minutes just to check the stove. After checking the stove he also has to check the kettle, toaster, and iron to make sure that they are all turned off and unplugged. He also checks repeatedly to make sure that all doors and windows are locked. Getting out of the house can take up to an hour, and the rituals leave him feeling anxious and exhausted. He is constantly running late and as a result has been asked to resign from his job. Although he recognises that his rituals are senseless, he becomes extremely distressed if he tries to resist them.

Diagnosis: Obsessive–compulsive disorder
Adapted from Clinical Research Unit for Anxiety and Depression (www.crufad.com)

Clinical skills: Cognitive-behavioural techniques for anxiety disorders

Cognitive-behavioural therapy (CBT) is commonly used in the treatment of anxiety disorders. CBT for phobias involves the patient making a list of problems to overcome, and then breaking each problem down into a series of tasks that can be attempted in ascending order of difficulty. For example, a patient with arachnophobia may first think about spiders, then look at pictures of spiders, then look at real spiders from a safe distance, and so on. Relaxation techniques may also be taught to help the patient manage his or her anxiety and cope with each task more comfortably. One common and effective relaxation technique, called 'deep breathing', involves regulating breathing by:

- Breathing in through the nose and holding the air in for several seconds
- Pursing the lips and gradually letting out as much air as possible

- Repeating this cycle *ad lib*.

CBT for panic disorder also involves such graded exposure and relaxation training, but there is an added emphasis on cognitive therapy. For example, the patient may learn to interpret a fast heart rate in terms of the symptoms of anxiety, rather than 'catastrophically' in terms of having a heart attack. The patient may also be taught how to control his or her breathing so as to prevent hyperventilation, and thus to prevent the potentially alarming symptoms that hyperventilation can give rise to. CBT for OCD typically involves exposure and response prevention: the patient is taught to delay responding to his or her compulsive urges, and to distract himself or herself for increasingly long periods from the tension and anxiety that this gives rise to. Other psychological treatments for anxiety disorders include supportive therapy, counselling, psychodynamic therapy, and family therapy.

Dissociative (conversion) disorders

In a dissociative disorder a traumatic event results in a disruption of the usually integrated functions of consciousness, memory, identity, or perception of the environment. Dissociative disorders are sometimes called conversion disorders, reflecting the theory that they result from the conversion of anxiety into more tolerable symptoms (primary gain) that attract the benefits of the sick role (secondary gain). Note, however, that in DSM-IV, 'conversion disorder' refers to a more limited group of disorders (motor loss, sensory loss, and convulsions) that are classified under 'somatoform disorders' (Table 7.5). Another name for dissociative disorders is hysteria but this term has largely been abandoned, notably because of its sexist and pejorative connotations. According to ICD-10, dissociative disorders may involve amnesia, fugue, stupor, trance and possession, motor loss, sensory loss, convulsions, Ganser's syndrome, and multiple personalities (Table 7.5). The patient may deny the impact of the traumatic event and/or have a lack of concern for his or her disability. Such an unnatural lack of concern is sometimes referred to as *la belle indifférence*. The differential diagnosis of dissociative disorders is from physical causes for these disorders, other psychiatric disorders including somatoform disorder and substance misuse, factitious disorder, and malingering. It is important to exclude physical disorders but this may be difficult and may involve extensive investigations. Management involves acceptance and support, physical rehabilitation if indicated, and treatment of comorbid psychiatric disorders. Prognosis is good.

Table 7.5 Dissociative disorders listed in ICD-10.

Dissociative amnesia		Loss of memory, most commonly for a traumatic or stressful event
Dissociative fugue		Sudden, unexpected journey that may last several months. There is memory loss and confusion about personal identity or assumption of another identity. Once the fugue ends, the memory of it is lost
Dissociative stupor		Although conscious, the patient is motionless and mute and does not respond to stimulation. Important differential diagnoses include affective disorders, schizophrenia, and organic brain diseases
Trance and possession disorders		Temporary replacement of a patient's identity by a spirit, ghost, deity, other person, animal, or inanimate object that is *not* accepted by the patient's culture as a normal part of a collective cultural or religious experience
DSM-IV: Classified under somatoform disorders as 'conversion disorder'	**Dissociative motor disorders**	Dissociative motor disorders may include the full range of organic motor disorders and more, but most commonly involve paralysis of muscle groups, e.g. paralysis of a limb or hemiparesis. *Atasia abasia* is a type of dissociative motor disorder involving an inability to stand or walk
	Dissociative anaesthesia/ sensory loss	Dissociative sensory loss may accompany dissociative motor disorders and is most commonly of the 'glove and stocking' distribution. Less common are hemi-anaesthesia and loss of the special senses
	Dissociative convulsions	Pseudoseizures that have no organic basis. A serum prolactin taken 10–20 minutes after the event is not raised, as might be expected after a generalised tonic-clonic seizure or complex partial seizure
Ganser's syndrome		A very rare syndrome characterised by *vorbeireden* or 'approximate answers' (e.g. 2 + 2 = 5), absurd statements, confusion, hallucinations, and psychogenic physical symptoms. First described in three prisoners by Sigbert Ganser in 1898, it has been suggested that Ganser's syndrome might be best understood in terms of a factitious disorder
Multiple personality disorder		Two or more distinct identities that recurrently take control of a shared body, and memory loss of each identity for the other. The rare disorder is thought to result from childhood trauma at a time before the personality is fixed

7

Personality disorders

8

Key learning objectives

- Definition of personality disorder
- Clusters of personality disorders in DSM-IV
- Description of each of the personality disorders
- Differential diagnosis of personality disorders

- Assessment of personality
- Management of personality disorders
- Recognition of ego defence mechanisms

Watson here will tell you that I can never resist a touch of the dramatic.

Sherlock Holmes

A brief history of personality disorders

The study of human personality or 'character' dates back at least to antiquity. In his 'Characters', Tyrtamus (371–287 BC) – nicknamed 'Theophrastus' or 'divinely speaking' by his contemporary Aristotle – divided the people of the Athens of the fourth century BC into 30 different personality types (Table 8.1). The 'Characters' exerted a strong influence on subsequent studies of human personality such as those of Thomas Overbury (1581–1613) in England and Jean de la Bruyère (1645–1696) in France.

The concept of **personality disorder** itself is much more recent and tentatively dates back to the French psychiatrist Philippe Pinel's 1801 description of *manie sans délire*, a condition which he characterised as outbursts of rage and violence ('manie') in an absence of any signs of psychotic illness such as delusions and hallucinations ('délires'). In the UK, the English physician J. C. Pritchard (1786–1848) coined the term 'moral insanity' in 1835 to refer to a larger group of people characterised by 'morbid perversion of the natural feelings, affections, inclinations, temper, habits, moral dispositions and natural impulses', but the term – probably considered too broad and non-specific – soon fell into disuse.

About 60 years later, in 1896, the German psychiatrist Emil Kraepelin (1856–1926) described seven forms of antisocial behaviour under the umbrella of 'psychopathic personality'. This term was later broadened by Kraepelin's younger colleague Kurt Schneider (1887–1967) to include those who 'suffer from their abnormality'. Schneider's seminal volume, *Psychopathic Personalities* (1923), still forms the basis of current classifications of personality disorders.

Psychiatry, 2e. By Neel Burton. Published 2010 by Blackwell Publishing.

Flattery	Unseasonableness	Grossness	Meanness	
Complaisance	Officiousness	Garrulity	Avarice	
Surliness	Unpleasantness	Loquacity	Cowardice	
Arrogance	Offensiveness	Newsmaking	Superstition	
Irony	Stupidity	Evil-speaking	Patronage of rascals	
Boastfulness	Boorishness	Grumbling	The aristocratic temper	
Petty ambition	Shamelessness	Distrustfulness		
Late-learning	Recklessness	Penuriousness		

Table 8.1 Theophrastus' 30 character types.

Introduction

Personality is the supreme realisation of the innate idiosyncrasy of a living being. It is an act of high courage flung in the face of life, the absolute affirmation of all that constitutes the individual, the most successful adaption to the universal conditions of existence coupled with the greatest possible freedom for self-determination.

C. G. Jung

Being an individual man is a thing that has been abolished, and every speculative philosopher confuses himself with humanity at large; whereby he becomes something infinitely great, and at the same time nothing at all ... To be a particular individual is world-historically absolutely nothing, infinitely nothing – and yet, this is the only true and highest significance of a human being, so much higher as to make every other significance illusory.

Søren Kierkegaard (1813–1853)

The majority of people with a personality disorder never come into contact with psychiatric services, and those who do usually do so in the context of another psychiatric disorder or at a time of personal crisis, e.g. after harming themselves or committing a criminal offence. Nevertheless, personality disorders are important to psychiatrists and doctors in general because they predispose to other psychiatric disorders, and affect both their presentation and their treatment. They also (by definition) result in considerable distress and impairment, and may therefore need to be addressed 'in their own right'. Whether this should be the remit of the medical profession is a subject of debate and controversy, especially given that some personality disorders predispose to criminal activity.

DSM-IV defines personality disorder as an enduring pattern of inner experience and behaviour that deviates markedly from cultural expectations, is inflexible and pervasive, has an onset in adolescence or early adulthood, is stable over time, and leads to distress or impairment.

ICD-10 similarly defines personality disorder as 'a severe disturbance in the personality and behavioural tendencies of the individual; not directly resulting from disease, damage, or other insult to the brain, or from another psychiatric disorder; usually involving several areas of the personality; nearly always associated with considerable personal distress and social disruption; and usually manifest since childhood or adolescence and continuing throughout adulthood'.

These definitions are of necessity rather imprecise and arbitrary, as are the descriptions of the specific personality disorders themselves, which are more the product of historical observation than of scientific study. For this reason, personality disorders rarely present in their 'textbook' form, and have a marked tendency to blur into one another. Their division into three clusters (A, B, and C) in DSM-IV is intended to reflect this tendency, with a given personality disorder most likely to blur with other personality disorders within its own cluster.

Characterising the 10 recognised personality disorders is difficult enough, but diagnosing them reliably is even more so. For example, how far from cultural expectations must personality traits deviate before they can be counted as a personality disorder? To what extent must they lead to distress or impairment? And what should count as 'distress or impairment'? Whatever the answers to these questions, they are bound to include a large part of subjectivity, and so a psychiatrist may be more likely to diagnose a person with a personality disorder if he or she has a dislike for or a prejudice against him or her. For this reason chiefly, it has been argued that a diagnosis of 'personality disorder' is little more than a convenient psychiatric label for undesirables and social deviants.

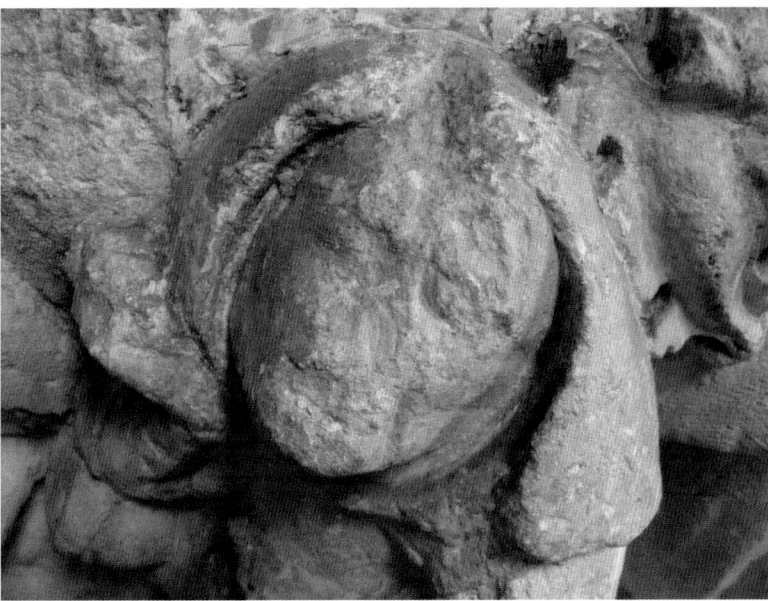

Figure 8.1 The term 'personality' derives from the Ancient Greek *persona*, meaning 'mask'. Photo by Neel Burton.

Classification

ICD-10 of personality disorders

F60 Specific personality disorders
 F60.0 Paranoid personality disorder
 F60.1 Schizoid personality disorder
 F60.2 Dissocial personality disorder
 F60.3 Emotionally unstable personality disorder (not
      included in DSM-IV)
 F60.4 Histrionic personality disorder
 F60.5 Anankastic personality disorder
 F60.6 Anxious (avoidant) personality disorder
 F60.7 Dependent personality disorder
 F60.8 Other specific personality disorders including
      narcissistic personality disorder
F61 Mixed and other personality disorders
F62 Enduring personality changes, not attributable to brain
    damage and disease

Table 8.2 DSM-IV classification of personality disorders.

Cluster	Description	Personality disorders in the cluster
A	Odd, bizarre, eccentric	Paranoid Schizoid Schizotypal*
B	Dramatic, erratic	Antisocial Borderline Histrionic Narcissistic
C	Anxious, fearful	Avoidant Dependent Obsessive–compulsive

* In ICD-10, schizotypal personality disorder is no longer included under personality disorders but alongside schizophrenia as 'schizotypal disorder'. Multiple personality disorder is classified under dissociative disorders in both ICD-10 and DSM-IV.

DSM-IV classification of personality disorders

In DSM-IV personality disorders are classified on a different 'axis' (Axis II) from mental illnesses and are grouped into three 'clusters' (see Table 8.2).

Epidemiology

It is estimated that personality disorders affect about 10% of the population, and up to 50% of psychiatric in- and out-patients, although these figures ultimately depend on where psychiatrists draw the line between a 'normal personality' and an abnormal one. The high prevalence of personality disorders amongst psychiatric patients underscores the importance of assessing personality as part of the psychiatric history (see Chapter 1). Almost all epidemiological studies reveal an excess of personality disorder in males, younger adults, and urban communities.

Aetiology

The aetiology of personality disorders is unclear, but they are generally thought to arise from an interplay of genetic factors and early life experiences, such as parental loss or emotional, physical, or sexual abuse. There is mounting evidence for an association between certain behaviours and neurochemical imbalances: the most robust evidence so far is for impulsive behaviour and reduced CSF serotonin. Although personality is usually acquired or 'fixed' in childhood and adolescence, profound and enduring personality change can sometimes occur in adulthood after exposure to a highly threatening or catastrophic experience, or after recovery from a mental illness. Another cause is brain disease and head injury, but this is classified under organic mental disorders.

Clinical features

Paranoid personality disorder

Paranoid personality disorder is characterised by a pervasive distrust of others, including friends and partner. As a result the person is guarded and suspicious and constantly on the lookout for clues or suggestions to confirm his fears. He has a strong sense of self-importance and personal rights, is overly sensitive to setbacks and rebuffs, easily feels shame and humiliation, and persistently bears grudges. As a result he finds it difficult to engage in close relationships and may have a tendency to withdraw from others. The principal ego defence mechanism used is projection (see later). The disorder is more common in males. Prevalence is 0.6%.

Schizoid personality disorder

Coined by Bleuler in 1908, the term 'schizoid' describes a natural tendency to direct attention toward one's inner life and away from the external world. In schizoid personality disorder, the person is detached and aloof and prone to introspection and fantasy. He has no desire for social or sexual relationships, is indifferent to others and to social norms and conventions, and lacks emotional response. In extreme cases, he may appear cold and callous. Treatment is often not provided because people with schizoid personality disorder are generally able to function well despite their reluctance to form close relationships, and are not concerned by the fact that they may be seen to have a mental disorder. It has been suggested that people with schizoid personality disorder not only have a rich inner life but are quite sensitive and experience a deep longing for intimacy. However, they find initiating and maintaining interpersonal relationships too difficult or too distressing and so retreat into their inner worlds. Prevalence is 0.4%.

Schizotypal personality disorder

Schizotypal personality disorder is characterised by oddities of appearance, behaviour, and speech, and anomalies of thinking similar to those seen in schizophrenia. Anomalies of thinking may include odd beliefs, magical thinking (e.g. thinking that stepping on a crack in the pavement leads to a misfortune), suspiciousness, obsessive ruminations, and unusual perceptual experiences. People with schizotypal personality disorder often fear social interaction and see other people as harmful. This may lead to the development of ideas (but *not* delusions) of reference, in which they believe that events are somehow related to them or relevant to them, even though they know that this is irrational. Thus, whereas both people with schizotypal personality disorder and people with schizoid personality disorder avoid social interaction, in the former it is because they fear other people, whereas in the latter it is because they have no desire to interact with other people or find interacting with other people too difficult. Compared to the average person, people who suffer from schizotypal personality disorder have a relatively high probability of 'converting' to schizophrenia at some time in the future. For this reason, ICD-10 classifies schizotypal personality disorder alongside schizophrenia as 'schizotypal disorder'. Prevalence is 0.6%.

At Vanderbilt University, Folley and Park conducted two experiments to compare the creative thinking processes of schizophrenia sufferers, 'schizotypes' (people with schizotypal traits), and normal control subjects. In the first experiment, subjects were asked to make up new functions for household objects. Whilst the schizophrenia sufferers and the normal control subjects performed similarly to one another, the schizotypes performed better than either. In the second experiment, subjects were once again asked to make up new functions for household objects as well as to perform a basic control task while the activity in the prefrontal lobes was monitored by a brain scanning technique called near-infrared optical spectroscopy. Whilst all three groups used both brain hemispheres for creative tasks, the right hemispheres of the schizotypes showed hugely increased activation compared to the schizophrenia sufferers and the normal controls. For Folley and Park, these results support the idea that increased use of the right hemisphere and thus increased communication between the brain hemispheres may be related to enhanced creativity in psychosis-prone populations.

B. S. Folley and S. Park (2005) Verbal creativity and schizotypal personality in relation to prefrontal hemispheric laterality: a behavioural and near-infrared optical imaging study. *Schizophrenia Research* 80(2–3):271–282

Dissocial/antisocial personality disorder

Until Schneider broadened the concept of personality disorder to include those who 'suffer from their abnormality', personality disorder was more or less synonymous with antisocial personality disorder. Antisocial personality disorder is far more common in men than in women, and is characterised by a callous unconcern for the feelings of others. The person disregards social rules and obligations, is irritable and aggressive, acts impulsively, lacks guilt, and fails to learn from experience. In many cases he has no difficulty finding relationships, and can even appear superficially charming (the so-called 'charming psychopath'), but his relationships are usually fiery, turbulent, and short-lived. As antisocial personality disorder is the mental disorder that is the most highly correlated with crime, he is likely to have a criminal record or to have a history of being in and out of prison. Although a personality disorder cannot be diagnosed before adulthood, the presence of three types of behaviour in children – sometimes referred to as MacDonald's triad – is thought to predict the later development of antisocial personality

Table 8.3 Possible findings in the history of a person with antisocial personality disorder.

- History of cruelty to animals, fire-setting (pyromania), and bedwetting (enuresis)
- History of truanting, bullying others, being expelled or suspended from school, or leaving school early
- Poor employment history with several changes of job and long periods of unemployment
- Convictions of assault and damage to property
- Brief relationships, often with violence to partners
- Substance misuse (especially sedatives such as alcohol and benzodiazepines)

disorder: bedwetting, cruelty to animals, and pyromania (impulsive fire setting for the purposes of gratification or relief). Other possible findings in the history of a person with antisocial personality disorder are listed in Table 8.3. Prevalence is 1.9%.

> ! Note that 'antisocial personality disorder' is not synonymous with 'psychopathy' or 'psychopathic disorder', which is a considerably narrower concept that is not recognised in either ICD-10 or DSM-IV. Only about 20% of people with antisocial personality disorder also meet the criteria for psychopathy, as defined by Hare's Psychopathy Checklist-Revised (PCL–R). PCL-R is a clinical rating scale of 20 items, each scored on a three-point scale. In addition to lifestyle and criminal behaviour, it assesses aspects such as grandiosity, callousness, impulsivity, lack of remorse, pathological lying, and glib and superficial charm.

Emotionally unstable/borderline personality disorder

In borderline personality disorder, the person essentially lacks a sense of self and as a result experiences feelings of emptiness and fears of abandonment. There is a pattern of intense but unstable relationships, emotional instability, outbursts of anger and violence (especially in response to criticism), and impulsive behaviour. Suicidal threats and acts of self-harm are common, for which reason people with borderline personality disorder are often seen by GPs, A&E doctors, and psychiatrists. Borderline personality disorder was so-called because it was thought to lie on

8

the 'borderline' between neurotic (anxiety) disorders and psychotic disorders such as schizophrenia and bipolar affective disorder. It has been suggested that borderline personality disorder often results from childhood sexual abuse, and that the reason why it is about three times more common in women than in men is because women are more likely to be victims of childhood sexual abuse. However, feminists have argued that borderline personality disorder is so common in women because women presenting with angry and promiscuous behaviour tend to be diagnosed with borderline personality disorder, whereas men presenting with identical behaviour tend to be diagnosed with antisocial personality disorder. The principal ego defence mechanisms used are splitting, projection, and projective identification (see later). Prevalence is 1.6%.

> **Typical case of borderline personality disorder as seen through the eyes of an A&E doctor**
>
> Twenty-eight-year-old Miss GL was brought into A&E after taking an impulsive overdose after an argument with her boyfriend, during which he threatened to leave her. Miss GL's boyfriend tells the A&E doctor that she took an overdose of 16 paracetamol just as he had his foot in the front door, screaming out, 'I hate you! Look at me, I'm going to die and it's all your fault!' Old medical records reveal that she last took an overdose only three months ago, after having had a similar argument. They also reveal that she has used all kinds of drugs, and that she had a road traffic accident only nine months ago. She has dropped out of three university courses and has never held down a job for more than six months. By the time she leaves A&E she is no longer angry but excited at the prospect of being taken out for a meal by her boyfriend.

Histrionic personality disorder

People with histrionic personality disorder lack a sense of self-worth, for which they depend on the attention and approval of others. They often seem to be dramatising or 'playing a part' ('histrionic' derives from the Latin *histrionicus*, 'pertaining to the actor') in a bid to attract and manipulate attention. They may take great care of their physical appearance and behave in a manner that is overly charming or inappropriately seductive. As they crave excitement and act on impulse or suggestion, they may put themselves at risk of having an accident or being exploited. Their dealings with other people often seem insincere or superficial, which can impact on their social and romantic relationships. This is especially distressing for them, because they are very sensitive to criticism and rejection and react badly to loss or failure. A vicious circle may form in which the more rejected they feel the more histrionic they become, and the more histrionic they become the more rejected they feel. Interestingly, it can be argued that a vicious circle of such a kind exists for every personality disorder and, indeed, for every mental disorder. Prevalence is 2.0%.

Narcissistic personality disorder

In narcissistic personality disorder the person has a grandiose sense of self-importance, a sense of entitlement, and a need to be admired. He is envious of others and expects them to be the same of him. He lacks empathy and readily exploits others to achieve his goals. To others he may seem self-absorbed, controlling, intolerant, selfish, and insensitive. If he feels slighted or ridiculed, he may be provoked into a fit of destructive anger and revenge-seeking. Such a reaction is sometimes referred to as 'narcissistic rage', and can result in disastrous consequences for those to whom it is directed. The principal ego defence mechanisms used are denial, distortion, and projection (see later). Narcissistic personality disorder is not specifically described in ICD-10. Prevalence is less than 1.0%.

Anankastic personality disorder

Anankastic personality disorder is characterised by excessive preoccupation with details, rules, lists, order, organisation, or schedules; perfectionism so extreme that it prevents a task from being completed; and devotion to work and productivity at the expense of leisure and relationships. A person with anankastic personality disorder is typically doubting and cautious, rigid and controlling, humourless, and miserly. His underlying high level of anxiety arises from a perceived lack of control over a universe that evades his understanding, and the more he tries to exert control the more out of control he feels. As a natural consequence, he has little tolerance for grey areas and tends to simplify the universe by seeing actions and beliefs as either absolutely right or absolutely wrong. His relationships with friends, colleagues, and family tend to be strained by the unreasonable demands that he makes on them. People with anankastic personality disorder tend to view their obsessions as rational and consistent with their self-image ('egosyntonic'), whereas people with OCD tend to view their obsessions as irrational and inconsistent with their self-image ('egodystonic'). Prevalence is 1.7%.

Anxious–avoidant personality disorder

In avoidant personality disorder, the person is persistently tense because he believes that he is socially inept, unappealing, or inferior, and as a result fears being embarrassed, criticised, or rejected. He avoids meeting people unless he is certain of being liked, is restrained even in his intimate relationships and avoids taking risks. Avoidant personality disorder may be associated with actual or perceived rejection by parents or peers during childhood, but is also strongly associated with anxiety disorders. Research suggests that people with avoidant personality disorder excessively monitor their internal reactions and the internal reactions of other people. This prevents them from engaging naturally and fluently in a social situation. A vicious circle may form in which the more they monitor internal reactions, the more inept they feel, and the more inept they feel the more they monitor internal reactions. Prevalence is 0.7%.

Dependent personality disorder

Dependent personality disorder is characterised by a lack of self-confidence and an excessive need to be taken care of. The person needs a lot of help to make everyday decisions and needs important life decisions to be taken for him. He greatly fears abandonment and may go through considerable lengths to secure and maintain relationships. A person with dependent personality disorder sees himself as inadequate and helpless, and so abdicates self-responsibility and turns his fate to one or more protective others. He imagines that he is at one with his protective others whom he idealises as being competent and powerful, and towards whom he behaves in a manner that is ingratiating and self-effacing. People with dependent personality disorder are particularly suited to people with a cluster B personality disorder, who feed on the unconditional high-regard in which they are held. Overall, people with dependent personality disorder maintain a naïve and child-like attitude, and have limited insight into either themselves or others. This not only reinforces their lack of self-confidence and excessive need to be taken care of, but also leaves them particularly vulnerable to being abused or exploited. Prevalence is 0.7%.

8

Successful psychopaths

Whilst personality disorders can lead to 'distress and impairment', they can also enable a person to achieve very highly within certain fields. In 2005, B. J. Board and K. F. Fritzon at the University of Surrey (Disordered personalities at work. *Psychology, Crime and Law* (2005), 11, 17–32.) found that high-level British executives were more likely to have one of three personality disorders compared to criminal psychiatric patients at the high security Broadmoor Hospital. These were histrionic personality disorder, narcissistic personality disorder, and anankastic personality disorder. It is certainly possible to envisage that people could benefit from certain strongly ingrained and potentially maladaptive personality traits. For example, people with histrionic personality disorder may be adept at charming and manipulating others, and therefore at building and exercising business relationships. People with narcissistic personality disorder may be highly ambitious, confident, and self-focused, and able to exploit people and situations to their best advantage. People with anankastic personality disorder may get quite far up the corporate and professional ladders simply by being so devoted to work and productivity. Even people with borderline personality disorder can at times be bright, witty, and the very life of the party, suggesting that a personality disorder might simply be seen as 'too much of a good thing' or 'a good thing out of control'. In their study Board and Fritzon described the executives with a personality disorder as 'successful psychopaths' and the criminals as 'unsuccessful psychopaths', and it may be that creative visionaries and disturbed psychopaths have more in common than first meets the eye. As the American psychologist and philosopher William James (1842–1910) put it, 'When a superior intellect and a psychopathic temperament coalesce … in the same individual, we have the best possible condition for the kind of effective genius that gets into the biographical dictionaries'.

Ego defence mechanisms

In Freudian psychoanalytic theory, ego defence mechanisms are unconscious processes that we use to defuse the anxiety that arises when who we really are (our unconscious 'id') comes into conflict with who we would like to be or think we should be (our conscious 'superego'). For example, at an unconscious level a man may find himself attracted to another man, but at a conscious level he may find this attraction completely unacceptable. To defuse the anxiety that arises from this conflict, he may use one or several of a number of defence mechanisms. For example,

he may refuse to admit to himself that he is attracted to this man; or he may superficially adopt ideas and behaviours that are diametrically opposed to the fact that he is attracted to this man, e.g. go out for several pints with the lads, speak in a gruff voice, and bang his fists on the counter; or he may project his attraction onto somebody else and then berate *him* for being 'gay'. In each scenario he has used one of three common ego defence mechanisms which are, respectively, denial, reaction formation, and projection. A broad range of such ego defence mechanisms are recognised, and the combination in which they are used reflects on our personality. Whilst we cannot escape using ego defence mechanisms, we can gain some understanding of how they are used and of how we use them. Such self-knowledge gives us much better insight not only into what is happening to us and to other people, but also into objective reality. Note that the list of ego defence mechanisms provided in Table 8.4 is not exhaustive.

Differential diagnosis

The principal differential diagnosis of personality disorder is from affective disorders, substance misuse, psychotic disorders, anxiety disorders (especially phobia and panic disorder), obsessive–compulsive disorder, learning disability, dementia, and autism.

Management, course, and prognosis

Personality disorders are lifelong disorders but in many cases naturally tend to mitigate in middle and old age, as people grow and gain wisdom. For example, at 15-year follow-up, most patients with borderline personality disorder no longer meet the criteria for the condition. Important complications of personality disorder include depressive disorder, substance misuse, accidents, and deliberate self-harm and suicide, not to omit social complications such as unemployment, homelessness, and crime.

In terms of management, a long-term management plan that states realistic and mutually agreed goals should be communicated to all staff potentially involved in the patient's care. This plan may, for example, involve emotional and practical support, psychological therapies, monitoring, and crisis intervention. Psychological therapies may be delivered in the form of individual therapy, group therapy, or 'milieu therapy'. Milieu therapy places

Table 8.4 Ego defence mechanisms.

Denial	The refusal to admit to certain unacceptable aspects of external reality
Repression	The 'forgetting' of unacceptable ideas, affects, emotions, memories, and drives
Distortion	The reshaping of external reality to suit inner needs
Isolation	The separation of an idea from its associated affects and behaviours
Splitting	The division of ideas, objects, and persons into good and bad by selectively focussing on positive or negative attributes
Idealisation	The overestimation of positive attributes and underestimation of negative attributes of an idea, object, or person
Displacement	The redirection of feelings for a person or thing to another, less important person or thing, e.g. a man who is angry at his boss vents his anger by kicking his dog
Conversion	The transformation of unacceptable ideas into more acceptable somatic symptoms
Compensation	The overemphasis of one sphere of activity to compensate for a lack of success in another, e.g. a schoolboy who is bad at sports makes himself popular by playing the buffoon
Dissociation	The splitting off of a group of ideas or behaviours from the mainstream of consciousness, e.g. a politician who is committed to fighting against poverty and social injustice evades income tax on a sizeable proportion of his income
Undoing	The thinking of a thought or carrying out of an act that negates a previous, unacceptable thought or act, e.g. a woman throws a plate at her husband then 'makes up for it' by smothering him in kisses
Reaction formation	The adoption of ideas and behaviours that are diametrically opposed to one's own, e.g. a man who finds himself attracted to another man treats him with contempt
Projection	The attribution of one's unacceptable ideas or behaviours to others, e.g. the man in the above example believes that the man he is attracted to is in fact attracted to him
Projective identification	A primitive, non-verbal mode of relating to others that involves the projection of parts of the self onto others such that they feel pressured to think, feel, and act in accordance with the projection
Rationalisation	The use of feeble but seemingly plausible arguments either to justify one's shortcomings (sour grapes) or make them seem 'not so bad after all' (sweet lemons), e.g. an SHO in surgery says he failed his exams because of a biased examiner (sour grapes), but that failing his exams has given him more time in training or more time to think about his career options (sweet lemons)
Intellectualisation	The use of abstract terms that are devoid of feeling to think about one's instinctual drives, e.g. thinking of love in terms of idealisation!
Sublimation	The channelling of instinctual drives into constructive activities such as study, sport, or art. Like altruism, humour, ascetism, and anticipation, sublimation is considered to be one of the more mature defence mechanisms
Altruism	Controversially thought of as a form of sublimation in which a person diffuses his or her anxiety by stepping outside him- or her-self and helping others. Many people in careers such as nursing or teaching are able to put their needs into the background by focussing on the needs of others. Similarly, many people who care for a disabled or elderly person value their carer role, and can experience profound anxiety and distress when this role is removed from them
Humour	By seeing the absurd or ridiculous aspect of an emotion, event, or situation, a person is able to put it into a less threatening context and thereby to diffuse the anxiety that it provokes in him or her. The things that people laugh about most are their errors and inadequacies; the difficult challenges that they face such as personal identity, social and sexual relationships, and death; and meaninglessness or absurdity. Freud famously noted that 'there is no such thing as a joke'
Ascetism	The denial of the importance of what we normally fear and strive for, and so the denial of the very grounds for anxiety
Anticipation	Arguably the most mature defence mechanism of all. It involves finding self-knowledge and using this self-knowledge to predict or 'anticipate' our feelings and reactions

8

emphasis on the patient's treatment environment and everyday events and interactions, and is epitomised by the therapeutic communities pioneered at the Cassel and Henderson Hospitals (see later). Dialectical behavioural therapy (DBT) in particular is an effective psychological therapy for the treatment of borderline personality disorder and recurrent self-harm that is based on Buddhist teachings, cognitive and behavioural theory, and dialectics. Psychotropic drugs and inpatient admissions should play only a very limited role in the management of personality disorders, although both may be helpful in the management of comorbid psychiatric symptoms and disorders. In many cases it is helpful to agree to some boundaries around their use.

Complex Needs Service

The Complex Needs Service (CNS) is for people with long-standing and hard to resolve emotional problems or interpersonal difficulties; these are often, although not invariably, people who have been diagnosed with a personality disorder.

A person may be referred to the CNS by his or her psychiatrist, but in many cases he or she may be encouraged to self-refer by calling, writing to, or emailing the CNS. The person then meets with a member of the CNS staff to discuss the CNS and his or her problems and needs. After this initial meeting, the person may decide to join a weekly 'options' group which aims to prepare him or her for joining a therapeutic community (TC). He or she may attend the options group for up to one year, during which time he or she can decide whether or not to join a TC.

Joining a TC involves a commitment to attend a daily programme every weekday for a period of 18 months. This is a very significant commitment, and demands a very high level of self-motivation. The idea behind a TC is that a person is best able to change by interacting positively with other people, that is, by forming relationships with other people in an atmosphere of trust and security, and by feeling mutually accepted, valued, and supported.

A TC is governed by a set of values and beliefs about the way people should treat each other; these are based on self-awareness, interdependence, deep mutual respect, and the assumption of personal responsibility. There is a busy daily programme that involves formal and informal therapeutic activities, including group therapy, individual therapy, creative therapies, social or cultural events, and educational or work placements. Members also participate in the running of the TC, and may even become involved in daily activities such as cooking, cleaning, gardening, and administration. Members and staff meet together regularly to receive feedback from one another, discuss the running of the community, and make decisions about it.

People who have spent time in a TC tend to use less medication and healthcare services than they used to, and also tend to require fewer hospital admissions.

Forensic psychiatry

The prevalence of personality disorders in the prison population has been estimated at up to 75%, with antisocial personality disorder being by far the most common one. Often described as the interface between mental health and the law, forensic psychiatry is the sub-specialism of psychiatry concerned with the assessment, treatment, and rehabilitation of mentally disordered people who have come into contact with the criminal justice system or, in some cases, who are likely to come into contact with the criminal justice system. These are amongst the most interesting, but also the most disturbed and difficult to manage patients. Forensic psychiatrists care for their inpatients in locked wards, including the national high security hospitals: Ashworth, Broadmoor, and Rampton in England, and Carstairs in Scotland. They may also be involved in outpatient care in prisons and communities, and may advise local general adult psychiatrists on such matters as risk and the management of antisocial behaviours. An important aspect of their job is to give evidence in court and prepare legal reports on medicolegal issues such as fitness to plead, diminished responsibility, and management of mentally disordered offenders.

Recommended reading

Games People Play (1973) Eric Berne. Penguin Books.
Solitude (1997) Anthony Storr. HarperCollins.
Jung: A Very Short Introduction (2001) Anthony Stevens. Oxford Paperbacks.
Lost in the Mirror: An Inside Look at Borderline Personality Disorder (2001) Richard A. Moskovitz. Taylor Trade Publishing.
The Siren's Dance: My Marriage to a Borderline: A Case Study (2003) Anthony Walker. Rodale Press.

Summary

Definition
- DSM-IV defines personality disorder as an enduring pattern of inner experience and behaviour that deviates markedly from cultural expectations, is inflexible and pervasive, has an onset in adolescence or early adulthood, is stable over time, and leads to distress or impairment.

Classification
- In DSM-IV personality disorders are classified on a different 'axis' (Axis II) from mental disorders and are grouped into three 'clusters':
  - Odd, bizarre, eccentric (cluster A) – paranoid, schizoid, and schizotypal personality disorders
  - Dramatic, erratic (cluster B) – antisocial, borderline, histrionic, and narcissistic personality disorders
  - Anxious, fearful (cluster C) – avoidant, dependent, anankastic personality disorders.

Prevalence
- The overall prevalence of personality disorders is about 10–15%, but the prevalence in outpatient and inpatient psychiatric patients is up to 50%.

Differential diagnosis
- The principal differential diagnosis of personality disorder is from affective disorders, substance misuse, psychotic disorders, anxiety disorders (especially phobia and panic disorder), obsessive–compulsive disorder, learning disability, dementia, and autism.

Prognosis and management
- Personality disorders are lifelong disorders but many tend to improve in middle and old age.
- Important complications include depressive disorder, substance misuse, and deliberate self-harm and suicide.
- The mainstay of management is psychotherapy but evidence as to its effectiveness is lacking.

Self-assessment

Answer with true or false. Answers on p. 218.

1. In DSM-IV personality disorders are classified on Axis II.
2. In DSM-IV cluster B is described as odd, bizarre, eccentric.
3. Anankastic personality disorder is a cluster C personality disorder.
4. Personality disorders are clear-cut, discrete disorders that do not blur.
5. The prevalence of personality disorders in outpatient and inpatient psychiatric patients is about 10–15%.
6. Personality disorders usually have their onset in childhood or adolescence.
7. Personality disorders are lifelong disorders but tend to improve in middle and old age.
8. Drugs play an important role in the treatment of certain personality disorders.
9. Important complications of personality disorders include depressive disorder, substance misuse, and deliberate self-harm.
10. Schizoid personality disorder is characterised by eccentric behaviour and anomalies of thinking and affect similar to those seen in schizophrenia.
11. Dissocial personality disorder is significantly more common in males.
12. In dissocial personality disorder, the person has difficulty in finding relationships.
13. Borderline personality disorder is more common in females.
14. In paranoid personality disorder, the person is suggestible, especially to those in a position of authority.
15. Anankastic personality disorder is related to obsessive–compulsive disorder.
16. Anxious-avoidant personality disorder is characterised by a lack of self-confidence and an excessive need to be taken care of.
17. The main ego defence mechanism in paranoid personality disorder is splitting.
18. The main ego defence mechanisms in borderline personality disorder are splitting, projection, and projective identification.

8

Organic psychiatric disorders (delirium and dementias)

9

Key learning objectives

- Definition of delirium and clinical features
- Prevalence of delirium amongst hospital inpatients over the age of 65
- Principal causes of delirium
- Differential diagnosis of delirium
- Key investigations in delirium
- Prevention and management of delirium
- Complications of delirium

- Definition of dementia and principal clinical features
- Common types of dementia and their differentiating factors
- Differential diagnosis of dementia, including 'mild cognitive impairment'
- Key investigations in dementia
- Management of dementia, including management of functional and social problems

Pray, do not mock me:
I am a very foolish fond old man,
Four score and upward, not an hour more nor less;
And, to deal plainly,
I fear I am not in my perfect mind.
Methinks I should know you, and know this man;
Yet I am doubtful: for I am mainly ignorant
What place this is; and all the skill I have
Remembers not these garments; nor I know not
Where I did lodge last night. Do not laugh at me;
For, as I am a man, I think this lady
To be my child Cordelia.
Shakespeare, *King Lear*, Act IV, Scene 7, 60–70

Psychiatry, 2e. By Neel Burton. Published 2010 by Blackwell Publishing.

Introduction

Organic psychiatric disorders are so-called because they result from biological causes such as pathological lesions, medical disorders, and drugs (although substance misuse is by convention classified separately). Organic psychiatric disorders are contrasted to so-called 'functional' psychiatric disorders such as schizophrenia and bipolar affective disorder that have historically been thought of as resulting from altered 'functioning' of the brain. This organic/functional dichotomy has played an important historical role in delineating neurology and psychiatry, although mounting evidence for a biological basis of 'functional' disorders suggests that neurology and psychiatry may be the same specialty after all. It is interesting to note that the brain is the only organ for which there are two medical specialties. It seems that the disorders that fall under the remit of neurology tend to principally affect motor and sensory function, whereas those that fall under the remit of psychiatry tend to principally affect the higher functions such as emotion, belief, and volition. There are, however, a number of exceptions and grey areas.

Organic disorders can sometimes present as a 'functional' psychiatric disorder, e.g. hypothyroidism can present as a depressive disorder or a brain tumour can present as a psychotic disorder. These 'functional' presentations of organic disorders are not classified under mood disorders or psychotic disorders, but under organic psychiatric disorders as 'organic mood disorder due to hypothyroidism' or 'organic delusional disorder due to a brain tumour'. Although 'functional' presentations of organic disorders are relatively uncommon, they are very important to exclude. They are covered in the chapters on 'functional' psychiatric disorders.

Delirium

> ! Delirium is a condition that sits on the border of general medicine, geriatrics, psychiatry, and neurology, as a result of which no one takes full responsibility for teaching about it. However, delirium is both very common and very deadly, and all medical students and junior doctors need to have a thorough understanding of it.

Definition

Delirium (Latin, 'off the track'), or acute confusional state, is common in hospitalised patients, and particularly in young children and in the elderly. **Delirium occurs in up to 40% of over-65s during hospitalisation**. It is defined by ICD-10 as 'an aetiologically non-specific syndrome characterised by concurrent disturbances of consciousness and attention, perception, thinking, memory, psychomotor behaviour, emotion, and the sleep–wake cycle [that is] transient and of fluctuating intensity …'

Classification

ICD-10 classification of delirium

F05   Delirium, not induced by alcohol and other
      psychoactive substances
      F05.0   Delirium, not superimposed on dementia
      F05.1   Delirium, superimposed on dementia
      F05.8   Other delirium

DSM-IV classification of delirium

Delirium due to a general medical condition
Substance intoxication delirium
Substance withdrawal delirium
Delirium due to multiple aetiologies

Aetiology

Table 9.1 lists the commoner causes of delirium. Almost anything can cause delirium, which ultimately results from excessive neurotransmitter release (especially acetylcholine and dopamine) and abnormal signal conduction.

Table 9.1 Causes of delirium (NB: This list is non-exhaustive).

Drugs (commonest cause)	Alcohol, opiates, sedatives, anticholinergics, diuretics, steroids, digoxin, anticonvulsants, lithium, TCAs, MAOIs, L-dopa, 'polypharmacy'
Metabolic	Renal failure, hepatic failure, respiratory failure, cardiac failure, disorders of electrolyte balance (especially hyponatraemia and hypercalcaemia), dehydration, porphyria
Infective	Urinary tract infection (remove urinary catheters that are no longer necessary), pneumonia, septicaemia, endocarditis, encephalitis, meningitis, cerebral abscess, HIV, malaria
Endocrine	Hypoglycaemia, diabetic ketoacidosis, hypothyroidism, hyperthyroidism, Cushing's syndrome
Neurological	Stroke, subarachnoid haemorrhage, head injury, space-occupying lesions, epilepsy
Other	Other hypoperfusion states (e.g. anaemia, cardiac arrhythmias), postoperative states, stress and sleep deprivation, change in environment, faecal impaction, urinary retention, vitamin deficiencies (B_1 thiamine, B_3 niacin, B_{12} cyanocobalamin)

TCA, tricyclic antidepressant; MAOI, monoamine oxidase inhibitor.

Clinical features

Delirium usually has a rapid onset (hours to days). Duration is typically days to weeks, but can last months, especially in certain conditions such as chronic liver disease, carcinoma, or subacute bacterial endocarditis. In many cases the course is diurnally fluctuating, with the patient relatively settled during the daytime and most agitated in the evening ('sundowning'). In some cases the patient may not be agitated at all (so-called 'hypoactive delirium'), in which case the diagnosis may be difficult to make.

Delirium is characterised by:

- Impaired consciousness and difficulty focusing, maintaining, and shifting attention
- Impairment of abstract thinking and comprehension and, in some cases, transient delusions
- Impairment of immediate recall and recent memory, with remote memory being relatively spared
- Disorientation in time and, in severe cases, also in place and person
- Perceptual abnormalities (distortions, illusions, and hallucinations – often in the visual modality)
- Hyperactivity or hypoactivity, and unpredictable shifts from one to the other
- Disturbance and, in severe cases, reversal of the sleep–wake cycle
- Emotional disturbances.

Table 9.2 Differentiating delirium from dementia.

Feature	Delirium	Dementia
Onset	Rapid	Insidious
Course	Fluctuating	Progressive
Duration	Days to weeks (reversible)	Months to years (irreversible)
Consciousness	Altered	Clear
Attention	Impaired	Usually normal
Memory	Immediate recall impaired	Immediate recall usually normal
Pyschomotor changes	Hyperactivity or hypoactivity	Usually none
Sleep–wake cycle	Disturbed	Usually normal

Differential diagnosis

- Delirium superimposed on dementia (dementia is an important risk factor for delirium)
- Dementia (Table 9.2)
- Substance misuse
- Affective disorder
- Psychotic disorder

Investigations

It is important to maintain a high degree of suspicion for delirium in susceptible patients, and to carry out daily assessments of their cognitive and mental status. If delirium is suspected, a psychiatric history, mental state

9

The story of Mrs DV

Mrs DV, a 73-year-old lady, is admitted in an acute confusional state after taking an overdose of eight tablets of temazepam 10 mg. She has no significant medical or psychiatric history, but her son says that her dog died three months ago and that she has been severely affected by its death. Urine dipstick reveals a urinary tract infection and so she is started on antibiotics.

The medical team ask for a psychiatric opinion as to Mrs DV's suicidal risk. The psychiatrist arrives as 6 pm to find her very agitated. She says she is seeing spiders on the curtains and implores the psychiatrist to 'call the firemen before the petrol station shuts'. The psychiatrist is clearly unable to make an accurate assessment of her suicidal risk, so he asks the medical team to call him back once she is more of her normal self. Unfortunately, she dies from septicaemic shock three days later.

Diagnosis: delirium (probably) due to multiple aetiologies – old age, bereavement, temazepam overdose, change in environment, urinary tract infection

Table 9.3 Investigations in delirium (mandatory, first-line investigations are in bold).

Blood tests	**FBC, U&Es**, LFTs, TFTs, glucose, thiamine level, blood drug screen
Infection screens	**Urinary dipstick, MSU**, sputum samples, blood cultures, lumbar puncture
Imaging	**CXR**, AXR, CT head, MRI head
Other	**ECG**, EEG*, urinary drug screen

* Characteristic changes in delirium include slowing of the posterior dominant rhythm and generalised slow-wave activity.

examination, full physical examination (including vital signs), and delirium screen (Table 9.3) need to be carried out. This should help to confirm the diagnosis and to identify one or more physical causes, although in a minority of cases no causes can be found.

Management and prognosis

Delirium should be actively prevented in susceptible patients. Prevention can be achieved by simple measures that are unfortunately often overlooked. These include:

- Routine cognitive assessment
- Rationalising the drug chart
- Ensuring that sensory aids such as spectacles and hearing aids are in place
- Encouraging fluids and nutrition, and correcting any electrolyte imbalances and nutritional deficiencies
- Encouraging mobilisation
- Encouraging family members to spend time at the bedside.

If delirium supervenes despite these preventive measures, the cause of the delirium must be found and treated.

The patient should be nursed in a consistent, comfortable, and familiar environment on a medical (rather than a psychiatric) ward. The family should be educated about their relative's condition and encouraged to remain at the bedside to reorient and reassure him or her. Clocks, calendars, and familiar objects from home can be brought in to act as memory cues.

Tranquillisers should be avoided but can find a role in management if the patient is agitated or psychotic. Haloperidol is the drug of choice (except if delirium is caused by alcohol or benzodiazepines, in which case it is a benzodiazepine) because of its minimal anticholinergic side-effects. Doses should be kept to a minimum (e.g. haloperidol 0.5 mg QDS, but *not* 'as required' to avoid

precipitating alternating episodes of agitation and sedation), and stopped as soon as it is felt that it is no longer indicated.

Complications of delirium can sometimes be prevented, but if they cannot they should be actively sought out and addressed. They include:

- Prolonged hospital stay and increased risk of nosocomial infections
- Accelerated cognitive decline
- Aspiration pneumonia
- Fluid and electrolyte imbalance
- Malnutrition
- Falls
- Injuries
- Decreased mobility
- Pressure sores.

Mortality is high, both in hospital and after discharge – one-year mortality has been estimated to be as high as 50%.

Dementia

Definition

*Dementia is a syndrome due to disease of the brain, usually of a chronic or progressive nature, in which there is disturbance of multiple higher cortical functions, including memory, thinking, orientation, comprehension, calculation, learning capacity, language, and judgement. **Consciousness is not clouded** … Dementia produces an appreciable decline in intellectual functioning, and usually some interference with personal activities of daily living, such as washing, dressing, eating, personal hygiene, excretory, and toilet activities.*

ICD-10

Diagnosis

*The primary requirement for diagnosis is **evidence of a decline in both memory and thinking sufficient to impair personal activities of daily living**, as described above. The impairment of memory typically affects the registration, storage, and retrieval of new information, but previously learned and familiar material may also be lost, particularly in later stages. Dementia is more than dysmnesia: there is also impairment of thinking and reasoning capacity, and a reduction in the flow of ideas.*

ICD-10

The diagnosis of the type of dementia (e.g. Alzheimer's disease versus vascular dementia or mixed dementia) is made on clinical grounds and can only be verified by brain biopsy or at postmortem.

Clinical features

The principal clinical features of dementia are described in Table 9.4. They vary not only according to the severity of the dementia, but also according to the type of dementia, as different types of dementia tend to affect different parts of the brain (Figure 9.1 and Table 9.5).

Table 9.4 Principal clinical features of dementia (ranked according to approximate order of progression in Alzheimer's disease, from 1 to 7).

1. Memory loss	Short-term memory is more affected than long-term memory, leading to impaired learning and disorientation (first in time and then in place and person)
2. Impaired thinking	Poor judgement, decreased fluency, dyscalculia, concrete thinking and impaired abstraction, lack of ability to plan or sequence behaviour, delusions
3. Language impairments	Expressive and receptive dysphasia/aphasia
4. Deterioration in personal functioning	Deterioration in occupational functioning, social functioning, and self-care (activities of daily living). Severe senile self-neglect is referred to as Diogenes syndrome after the ancient ascetic Greek philosopher. Diogenes syndrome may be accompanied by syllogomania, a tendency to hoard rubbish
5. Disturbed personality and behaviour	Euphoria and emotional lability or apathy and irritability, disinhibition leading to aggressive and socially inappropriate behaviour, inattention and distractibility, obsessive and stereotyped behaviours
6. Perceptual abnormalities	Visual and auditory agnosia, visuospatial difficulties, body hemineglect, inability to recognise faces (prosopagnosia), illusions, hallucinations (often visual), cortical blindness
7. Motor impairments	Apraxia, spastic paresis, urinary incontinence

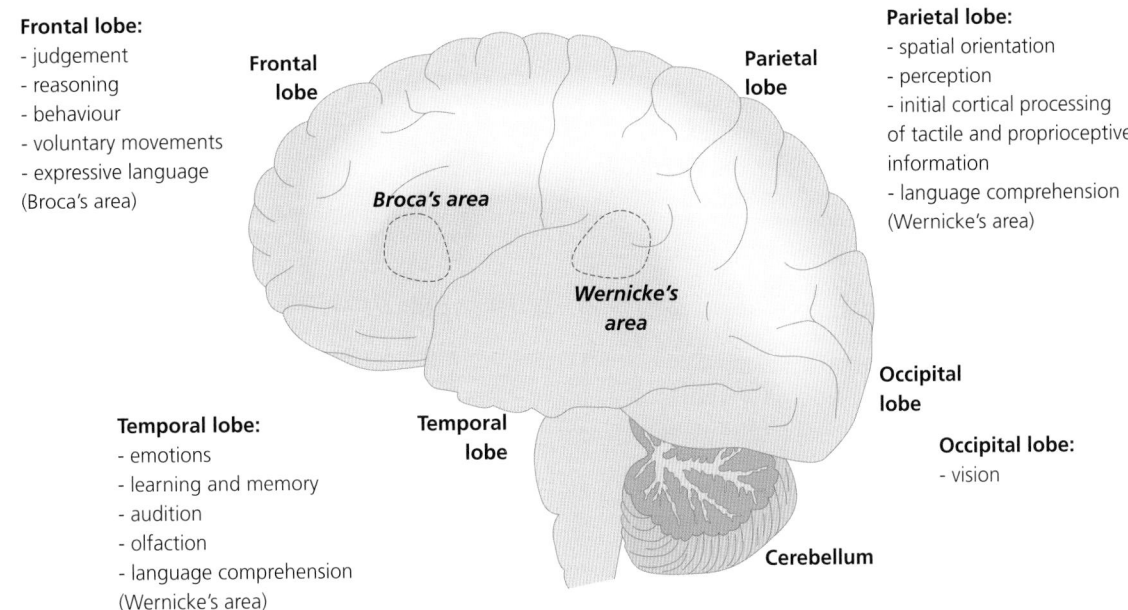

Frontal lobe:
- judgement
- reasoning
- behaviour
- voluntary movements
- expressive language
(Broca's area)

Parietal lobe:
- spatial orientation
- perception
- initial cortical processing of tactile and proprioceptive information
- language comprehension
(Wernicke's area)

Temporal lobe:
- emotions
- learning and memory
- audition
- olfaction
- language comprehension
(Wernicke's area)

Occipital lobe:
- vision

Figure 9.1 Localisation of cerebral function.

Table 9.5 Focal lobe deficits.

Frontal lobe	**Orbitofrontal syndrome**: disinhibition, aggressive and socially inappropriate behaviour, obsessive or repetitive stereotyped behaviours, euphoria, emotional lability, poor insight
	Dorsolateral prefrontal syndrome: apathy, irritability, lack of ability to plan or sequence behaviour, decreased fluency, impaired abstraction
Temporal lobe	**Dominant (left) temporal lobe**: verbal agnosia, visual agnosia, receptive aphasia, hallucinations
	Non-dominant (right) temporal lobe: visuospatial difficulties, inability to recognise faces (prosopagnosia), hallucinations
	Bilateral disease: apathy, Korsakov's syndrome, Klüver–Buçy syndrome – a rare syndrome consisting of hyperorality, hypersexuality, and blunted emotional reactivity
Parietal lobe	**Dominant (left) parietal lobe**: receptive aphasia, agnosia, apraxia, Gerstmann's syndrome – finger agnosia, dyscalculia, dysgraphia, left–right disorientation
	Non-dominant (right) parietal lobe: body hemineglect, visuospatial difficulties, anosognosia or denial of deficits, constructional apraxia
	Bilateral disease: visuospatial imperception, spatial disorientation, Balint's syndrome – a rare disorder of visuospatial processing
Occipital lobe	Visual perception defects such as visual agnosia, alexia, and prosopagnosia, progressing to cortical blindness, illusions, and visual hallucinations, and to Anton's syndrome – a form of anosognosia involving the denial of cortical blindness

Frontal lobe syndrome and the story of Phineas Gage

Phineas Gage (1823–1860) was working on the construction of the Rutland and Burlington Railroad when he accidentally ignited gunpowder with a large tamping iron. The tamping iron was blown through his head with such force that it landed several yards behind him. Although Gage survived (he was even talking and walking immediately after the accident), his friends described him as 'no longer Gage'. The local doctor, JM Harlow, reported that:

Gage was fitful, irreverent, indulging at times in the grossest profanity (which was not previously his custom), manifesting but little deference for his fellows, impatient of restraint or advice when it conflicts with his desires, at times pertinaciously obstinate, yet capricious and vacillating, devising many plans of future operations, which are no sooner arranged than they are abandoned in turn for others appearing more feasible. A child in his intellectual capacity and manifestations, he has the animal passions of a strong man. Previous to his injury, although untrained in the schools, he possessed a well-balanced mind, and was looked upon by those who knew him as a shrewd, smart businessman, very energetic and persistent in executing all his plans of operation. In this regard his mind was radically changed, so decidedly that his friends and acquaintances said he was 'no longer Gage'.

J. M. Harlow, 'Passage of an iron rod through the head',
Boston Medical and Surgical Journal (1848), 39, 389–393

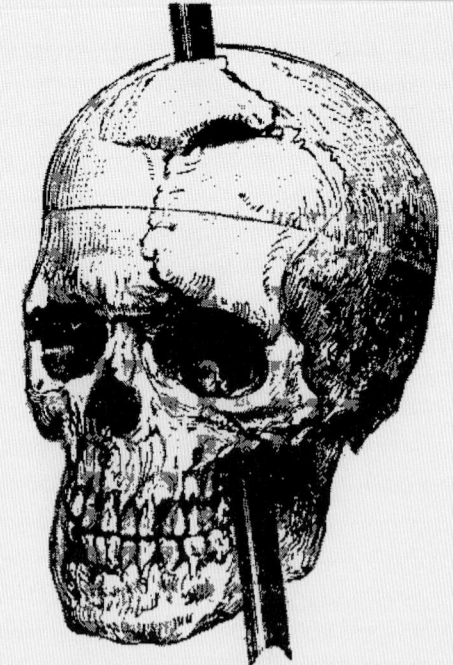

Figure 9.2 The iron bar passed through the ventromedial areas of the prefrontal cortex. (From J. M. Harlow, Recovery from the passage of an iron bar through the head. *Publications of the Massachusetts Medical Society* (1868), 2, 327–347.)

Types

Dementias can be classified as either primary (or degenerative) or secondary. Note that this primary/secondary dichotomy is as confusing and problematic as the organic/functional dichotomy discussed earlier in this chapter, and for similar reasons.

The principal primary (degenerative) dementias are:
- Alzheimer's disease
- Dementia with Lewy bodies and Parkinson's disease
- Pick's disease and other frontotemporal dementias
- Huntington's disease.

Secondary dementias are listed in Table 9.6.

The commonest dementias are Alzheimer's disease, dementia with Lewy bodies, vascular dementia, and frontotemporal dementias.

Table 9.6 Secondary dementias.

Vascular (common)	Vascular dementia
Infective	AIDS, Lyme disease, neurosyphilis, prion diseases, encephalitis
Inflammatory	Systemic lupus erythematosus, cranial arteritis, encephalopathy, multiple sclerosis
Neoplastic	Primary or secondary tumour, paraneoplastic syndrome
Metabolic	Cardiac, hepatic, and renal failure, anaemia, chronic hypoglycaemia, vitamin B_{12} deficiency, thiamine deficiency (Wernicke–Korsakov syndrome), Wilson's disease
Endocrine	Hyper- and hypo-thyroidism, hyper- and hypo-parathyroidism, Addison's disease, Cushing's syndrome
Toxic	Alcohol, heavy metals, organic solvents, organophosphates
Traumatic	Severe single head injury, repeated head injury (punch-drunk syndrome, *dementia pugilistica*), subdural haematoma
Other	Normal pressure hydrocephalus, radiation, anoxia

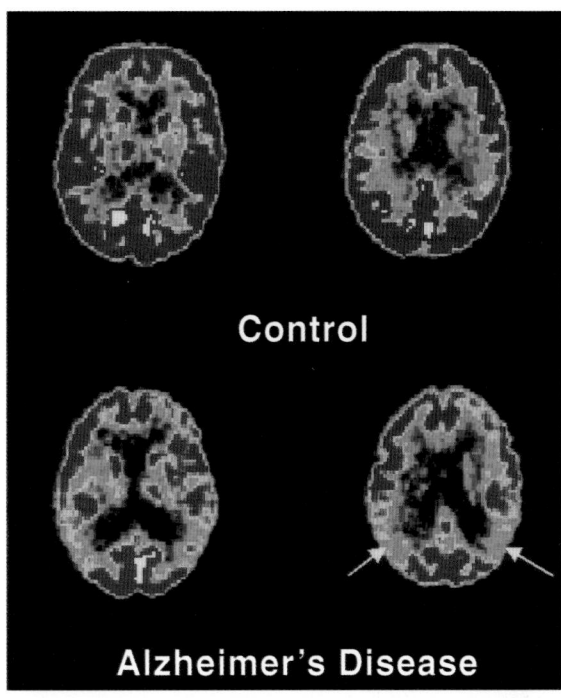

Figure 9.3 PET scans taken with the glucose metabolic tracer 18F-fluorodeoxyglucose (FDG). The two upper parts of the image show the normal distribution of glucose metabolism in a control subject at two different homographic levels. The lower parts of the image show hypometabolism in the parietal lobes (arrows) and temporoparietal cortex in a patient with Alzheimer's disease. (Reproduced with permission from N. Qizilbash, H. Broadaty, H. Chui and J. Kaye (eds) *Evidence based Dementia Practice* (2002), Blackwell Science.)

Alzheimer's disease

Epidemiology

Alzheimer's disease (AD) is the commonest cause of dementia, accounting for more than 50% of all cases of dementia and affecting about 500,000 people in the UK. Its prevalence rate approximately doubles for every five years of age from the age of 65 (prevalence 1%) to the age of 90 (prevalence 30–40%). It is more common in females, even after taking into account their longer life expectancy.

Neuropathology

Selective neuronal and synaptic loss leads to neurochemical abnormalities (notably a cholinergic deficit) and

9

symmetrical cortical atrophy that is initially more pronounced in the temporal and parietal lobes (Figure 9.3). Extracellular senile plaques and intracellular neurofibrillary tangles are seen in normal ageing, but they are more numerous in AD and they are closely related to the degree of cognitive impairment.

- Senile plaques consist of a core of beta-amyloid surrounded by filamentous material.
- Neurofibrillary tangles consist of coiled filaments of abnormally phosphorylated microtubule-associated protein tau (note that tau is also found in Pick bodies, see later).

Other histopathological findings include glial proliferation, granulovascular degeneration, and Hirano inclusion bodies.

Aetiology

Risk factors for AD include:

- Age (up to about age 90)
- Female sex (the female-to-male ratio is 2 : 1)
- Family history (overall relative risk of 4)
- Down's syndrome
- Head injury
- Dialysis (due to aluminium-containing dialysis fluids). In terms of genetics:
- **Inheritance of the ε4 allele of apolipoprotein E on chromosome 19** is a risk factor for the common sporadic, late-onset form of the disease. The ε2 allele on the other hand is protective
- **Mutations in the *beta-amyloid precursor protein (APP)* gene on chromosome 21, in the *presenilin-1* gene on chromosome 14, and in the *presenilin-2* gene on chromosome 1** are involved in rare, early-onset or 'pre-senile' familial forms of the disease. The inheritance pattern is autosomal dominant.

Factors that may protect against late-onset AD include a healthy and engaged lifestyle, high educational attainment (although this may simply delay detection), non-steroidal anti-inflammatory drugs (NSAIDs), hormone replacement therapy (HRT), and vitamins C and E.

Clinical features

AD is characterised by insidious onset and progression of memory loss and personality changes. Other spheres of cognitive and non-cognitive impairment are added over the course of several years (see Table 9.4). Life expectancy

from the time of diagnosis is about eight years. The experience of Alzheimer's disease is faithfully depicted by Dame Judi Dench in the film *Iris*, about the life of the writer and philosopher Iris Murdoch.

Dementia with Lewy bodies

Epidemiology

Dementia with Lewy bodies (DLB) is an entity that has only relatively recently been recognised and that overlaps with Alzheimer's disease and parkinsonian dementia. It is the second commonest cause of dementia, and accounts for about 20% of all cases.

Neuropathology

Both subcortical and cortical structures are involved:

- **Lewy bodies are intracellular eosinophilic inclusions consisting of abnormally phosphorylated neurofilament proteins aggregated with ubiquitin and alpha-synuclein;**
- There is associated neuronal loss leading to cholinergic deficit and other chemical abnormalities. There is, however, only minimal cortical atrophy;
- Compared to Alzheimer's disease, senile plaques may be present but neurofibrillary tangles are not a marked feature.

Aetiology

Aetiology is unclear. DLB may form part of a spectrum of Lewy-body disorders that includes Parkinson's disease. In DLB, Lewy bodies are more numerous in cortical areas (especially in cortical layers V and VI of the temporal lobe, the cingulate gyrus, and the insular cortex), whereas in Parkinson's disease they are more numerous in the basal ganglia.

Clinical features

DLB is especially characterised by:

- Marked fluctuations in cognitive impairment and alertness
- Vivid visual hallucinations and other psychotic symptoms
- Early parkinsonism and neuroleptic sensitivity
- Frequent faints and falls

Note that memory loss may not be a marked feature in the early stages of DLB. Life expectancy from the time of diagnosis is about six years.

9

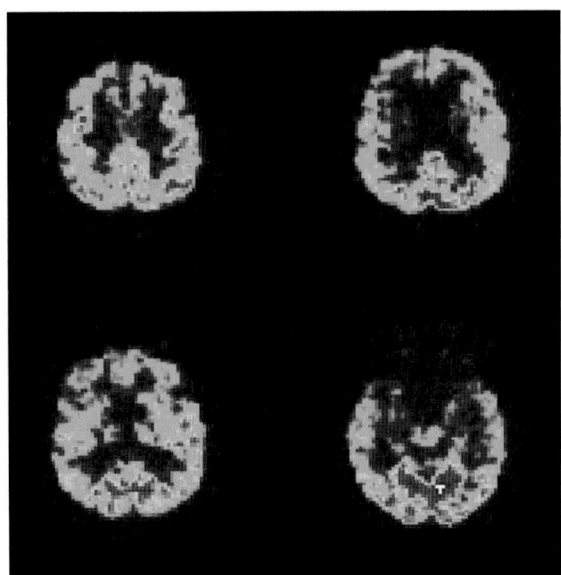

Figure 9.4 PET 18F-fluorodeoxyglucose (FDG) image from a patient with frontotemporal dementia. Glucose metabolism is reduced in the frontal and anterior temporal brain regions. See Figure 9.3 for control images. (Reproduced with permission from N. Qizilbash, H. Broadaty, H. Chui, and J. Kaye (eds) *Evidence based Dementia Practice* (2002), Blackwell Science.)

Frontotemporal dementias (using Pick's disease as the archetypal form)

Epidemiology

Pick's disease is a type of frontotemporal dementia accounting for about 5% of all cases of dementia. It is more common in females than in males, and the peak age of onset is 45–60 years, that is, in middle age.

Neuropathology

There is selective, often asymmetrical, 'knife-blade' atrophy, neuronal loss, and gliosis affecting the frontal and temporal lobes (Figure 9.4). **There are characteristic 'ballooned' neurons called Pick cells and tau-positive neuronal inclusions called Pick bodies.** There are, however, no senile plaques or neurofibrillary tangles as in Alzheimer's disease.

Aetiology

Aetiology is unclear. Familial forms exist and are more common in people of Scandinavian descent.

Clinical features

The clinical features involve insidious and progressive dementia characterised by early and prominent personality changes and behavioural disturbances, eating disturbances, mood changes, cognitive impairment, language abnormalities, and motor signs.

Huntington's disease

Epidemiology

The prevalence of Huntington's disease, or Huntington's chorea, in Caucasians is 5–10 per 100,000. Onset is usually in the fourth or fifth decade, but in some cases it can be in childhood or old age.

Neuropathology

Abnormal huntingtin protein leads to the degeneration of neurons, notably in the caudate nucleus and putamen and in the cerebral cortex. Degeneration in the caudate nucleus and putamen leads to movement disorders; degeneration in the cerebral cortex leads to dementia.

Aetiology

Huntington's disease is an **autosomal dominant neurodegenerative disorder resulting from 36 or more CAG trinucleotide repeats that encode glutamine in the huntingtin gene on chromosome 4.** The age of onset decreases as the number of CAG trinucleotide repeats increases. This happens from one generation to the next in the paternal line, a phenomenon referred to as 'anticipation'.

Clinical features

Huntington's disease is characterised by choreiform (dance-like) movements, progressive dementia, and other psychiatric disturbances, notably early depression and behavioural disturbances. The later stages in particular are marked by increasing dementia with cognitive impairment, behavioural changes, and depressive symptoms. Insight is often retained until late, as a result of which the suicide rate is very high, in the order of about 10%.

9

Vascular dementia

Epidemiology

Vascular dementia is the third commonest cause of dementia after Alzheimer's disease and dementia with Lewy bodies, accounting for about 20% of all dementias. In Japan it is the commonest cause of dementia, accounting for about 50% of all dementias. In so-called 'mixed dementia' there is evidence of both Alzheimer's disease and vascular dementia. Vascular dementia is more common in males.

Neuropathology

Focal disease may result from single or, more commonly, from multiple thrombotic or embolic infarcts. Small vessel disease leads to diffuse disease (Binswanger's disease and lacunar state). Note that focal and diffuse disease often coexist.

Aetiology

Risk factors include:
- Older age
- Male sex
- Cardiovascular disease
- Cerebrovascular disease
- Valvular disease
- Hypercoagulation disorders
- Hypertension
- Hypercholesterolaemia
- Diabetes
- Smoking
- Alcohol.

Clinical features

Vascular dementia classically has an abrupt onset and step-wise progression (Figure 9.5). Clinical features are variable and depend on the location of the infarcts, but mood and behavioural changes are common. Insight is usually retained until late. Significant comorbidity leads to a shorter mean life expectancy than in Alzheimer's disease.

Other dementias and amnestic syndrome

Normal pressure hydrocephalus

Normal pressure hydrocephalus is a potentially, partially reversible form of dementia that accounts for about 5% of

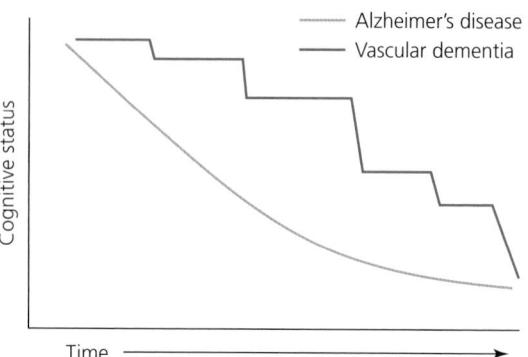

Figure 9.5 Compared to Alzheimer's disease, vascular dementia classically has an abrupt onset and step-wise progression.

all cases of dementia. It is thought to be a form of communicating hydrocephalus with impaired CSF reabsorption at the arachnoid villi. Formation of CSF eventually equilibrates with reabsorption, and so intracranial pressure is only slightly raised. For this reason, the classic signs of raised intracranial pressure such as headache, vomiting, and altered consciousness are absent. Instead, the classic triad in normal pressure hydrocephalus consists of gait disturbance and ataxia, dementia, and urinary incontinence (in that order of progression). Lumbar puncture and lumbar tapping and head imaging are useful in reaching the diagnosis. A ventriculoperitoneal shunt can be surgically implanted to drain excess CSF to the abdomen where it is absorbed.

HIV-related dementia

HIV-related dementia or AIDS dementia complex is usually observed in the late stages of AIDS in one-quarter to one-third of AIDS patients. It is in fact a metabolic encephalopathy that results from a direct effect of the HIV virus. The HIV enters the CNS by infecting macrophages and monocytes that cross the blood–brain barrier. These cells then provoke an inflammatory response that ultimately results in neuronal loss. This is in addition to other brain-related complications of HIV infection such as opportunistic infections, cerebral lymphoma and metastasis of AIDS-related cancers, toxic effects of drug treatments, and malnutrition. Clinical features include cognitive impairment progressing to dementia, behavioural changes, and motor involvement.

Creutzfeld–Jakob disease and other prion-related diseases

Prions are protein particles that do not contain RNA or DNA, but that can nevertheless be infectious. Prion diseases are a group of related neurodegenerative diseases that affect both humans and animals and that result from the deposition of the prion protein (PrP) in the form of amyloid sheets. In humans they include Creutzfeld–Jakob disease (CJD), Gerstmann–Sträussler syndrome (GSS), and kuru. Prion diseases can occur sporadically, as in most cases of CJD which result from spontaneous PrP^{C} to PrP^{Sc} conversion or somatic mutation; or they can be inherited, as in the case of GSS which results from the autosomal dominant inheritance of a mutation in the PrP gene on chromosome 20; or they can be contracted by infection, as in the case of new variant CJD (nvCJD) which results from the ingestion of bovine spongiform encephalopathy (BSE)-infected beef products, or in the case of kuru which results from the cannibalism of neural tissue, described in the Fore people of New Guinea. All these human prion diseases are very rare: the most common by far is CJD, which has an incidence of one in a million. Prion diseases tend to affect grey matter, producing neuronal loss, gliosis, and characteristic spongiform change. In CJD there is rapidly progressive dementia associated with myoclonic jerks and a variable constellation of pyramidal, extrapyramidal, and cerebellar signs. The mean age of onset is 62 years and death occurs in about eight months. In contrast, the mean age of onset for vCJD is just 28 years. The first cases of nvCJD were reported in 1995, and so far most cases have been circumscribed to the UK. In contrast to sporadic CJD, psychiatric symptoms are common at the time of first presentation, and there are no characteristic EEG changes. Death occurs in about 12 months.

Amnestic syndrome

Amnestic syndrome is rare and results from damage to the mamillary bodies, hippocampus, or thalamus. The most common cause is thiamine deficiency secondary to chronic alcoholism (see Wernicke–Korsakov syndrome, Chapter 11), and other causes include thiamine deficiency due to other causes, head injury, hypoxia, carbon monoxide poisoning, herpes simplex encephalitis, and brain tumours. There is selective loss of recent memory with disorientation and confabulation, and relative sparing of immediate and long-term memory and other intellectual faculties. Amnestic syndrome is usually irreversible.

Differential diagnosis

Dementia is a clinical diagnosis, and its differential diagnosis includes:

- Amnestic syndrome (see above)
- Mild cognitive impairment (see below)
- Delirium
- Delirium superimposed upon dementia
- Depressive disorder ('pseudodementia'). Note however that depressive disorders and anxiety disorders affect about 50% of patients with dementia
- Late-onset schizophrenia (paraphrenia)
- Learning difficulties (mental retardation)
- Substance misuse
- Iatrogenic causes, particularly drugs
- Dissociative disorder
- Factitious disorder
- Malingering.

Mild cognitive impairment refers to subtle but measurable memory difficulties that are more severe than those seen in normal ageing but less severe than those seen in Alzheimer's disease. There is no deterioration in overall thinking and judgement or in level of functioning. **However, the risk of conversion to Alzheimer's disease is about 15% per year.**

Investigations

A physical examination should be carried out to identify any underlying causes of dementia (see Table 9.6) and any complications of dementia such as malnutrition, burns, or falls.

Physical investigations in dementia should include FBC, U&Es, calcium, serum cholesterol, LFTs, TFTs, serum B_{12} and folate, serum glucose, and CXR. Neuroimaging such as CT and MRI can be helpful, particularly to exclude potentially treatable causes such as tumour, subdural haematoma, and hydrocephalus. Further investigations should be ordered on a case-by-case basis and may include HIV testing, syphilis serology, vasculitic, autoimmune, neoplastic, and toxicological screens,

9

copper studies, CSF examination, and genetic testing. Brain biopsy itself is rarely indicated.

Detailed neurocognitive testing by a clinical psychologist can be helpful in identifying cognitive impairments and in confirming a diagnosis. The Mini Mental State Examination (MMSE) is often used as a screening and monitoring tool.

Management

In secondary dementias, the dementia may be partially reversed if the underlying cause is treated. If the dementia cannot be reversed, the aim of management is to improve or maintain the quality of life of the patient and carer(s). This involves treating the symptoms and complications of dementia, addressing functional problems, addressing social problems, and providing education and support for carers. There may be a limited role for drug treatment, principally in the form of a cholinesterase inhibitor (see later).

Symptoms and complications

In Alzheimer's disease and dementia with Lewy bodies, a cholinesterase inhibitor should usually be tried first. Other drugs should be used as infrequently and sparingly as possible:
- A benzodiazepine such as diazepam or lorazepam for anxiety and agitation
- A serotonin-selective reuptake inhibitor (SSRIs) such as citalopram for depressive symptoms
- An antipsychotics such as quetiapine for psychosis. Special care should be taken in DLB and in some fronto-temporal dementias so as to avoid severe extrapyramidal side-effects. Antipsychotics should *not* be used to manage behavioural problems as they may hasten cognitive decline and increase the risk of stroke.

Medical complications such as chest infection and urinary tract infection should be sought out and treated.

Cholinesterase inhibitors

Cholinesterase inhibitors include donepezil, rivastigmine, galantamine, and tacrine, although the latter is not licensed in the UK. They act by increasing cholinergic neurotransmission and can modestly and temporarily ameliorate cognitive performance and behavioural problems in a minority of patients with mild to moderate Alzheimer's disease and dementia with Lewy bodies. Dose-related gastrointestinal side-effects are common; other side-effects are relatively rare. The National Institute for Health and Clinical Excellence (NICE) recommends that an anticholinesterase inhibitor should initially be prescribed after thorough assessment in a specialist clinic if the MMSE is 10 or greater. The prescription should be reassessed after 2–4 months and continued only if there is demonstrable improvement or lack of decline. Thereafter the prescription should be reassessed at six-month intervals.

Other drugs that are sometimes used to offset cognitive decline include NSAIDs and antioxidants such as selegiline and vitamin E. Memantine is a recently approved N-methyl-d-aspartate (NMDA) receptor antagonist that protects neurones from glutamate-mediated neurotoxicity and that has been demonstrated to be effective in moderate to severe Alzheimer's disease.

Functional problems

The first step is careful assessment of the patient's functional abilities and exposure to risk. Care should be taken to ensure personal hygiene and adequate nutrition. Functional abilities can be maintained and even improved by a regular daily routine, environmental modifications, and graded assistance. The patient should be reoriented and reassured, and encouraged to partake in physical and mental activity. Memory aids such as clocks, calendars, notebooks, and photographs, and reality orientation and reminiscence therapies may also be helpful, particularly in the early stages of the disease.

Social problems

Areas to consider include accommodation, social isolation, and financial and legal matters such as power of attorney, curatorship, and wills.

Carer education and support

Carers should be educated about the condition and given advice about its management, including about financial and legal affairs. Caring for a person with dementia is very physically and emotionally demanding and carers should be encouraged to seek psychological support from a carer support group. Day care, respite care, or long-term care in a residential or nursing home may in time be necessary.

What do they think has happened, the old fools,
To make them like this? Do they somehow suppose
It's more grown-up when your mouth hangs open and
*　　drools,*
And you keep on pissing yourself, and can't remember
Who called this morning? Or that, if they only chose,
They could alter things back to when they danced all night,
Or went to their wedding, or sloped arms some September?
Or do they fancy there's really been no change,
And they've always behaved as if they were crippled or tight,
Or sat through days of thin continuous dreaming
Watching the light move? If they don't (and they can't),
*　　it's strange;*
Why aren't they screaming?
　　　　　　　　　From *The Old Fools* by Philip Larkin

Recommended reading

Dancing with Dementia: My Story of Living Positively with Dementia (2005) Christine Bryden. Jessica Kingsley Publishers.
Who Will I Be When I Die (2004) Christine Astley Boden. HarperCollins. (A first hand account of what it's like to be an Alzheimer sufferer.)

Summary

Delirium
Aetiology
- Occurs in 20–30% of over-65s during hospitalisation.
- The commonest cause is drugs. Other causes are listed in Table 9.1.

Clinical features
- Onset is usually rapid, course diurnally fluctuating, and duration days to weeks.
- Clinical features include impaired consciousness, impairment of abstract thinking and comprehension, impairment of immediate recall and recent memory, perceptual abnormalities, hyperactivity or hypoactivity, disturbance of the sleep–wake cycle, and emotional disturbances.

Differential diagnosis
- Differential diagnosis includes delirium superimposed on dementia, dementia, affective disorders, and psychotic disorders.
- Mandatory first-line investigations to search for a cause include FBC, U&Es, urinary dipstick, MSU, CXR, and ECG.

Prognosis
- Complications include prolonged hospital stay and increased risk of nosocomial infections, accelerated cognitive decline, aspiration pneumonia, fluid and electrolyte imbalance, malnutrition, falls, injuries, decreased mobility, and pressure sores.
- One-year mortality has been estimated at 50%.

Dementia
Clinical features
- Clinical features vary not only according to the severity of the dementia, but also according to the type of dementia, as different types of dementia affect different parts of the brain. They include (in approximate order of progression for Alzheimer's disease) memory loss, impaired thinking, language impairments, deterioration in personal functioning, disturbed personality and behaviour, perceptual abnormalities, and motor impairments.

Types
- The commonest dementias are Alzheimer's disease, dementia with Lewy bodies, vascular dementia, and frontotemporal dementias. Each has distinct aetiopathological and clinical features.
- Alzheimer's disease, the commonest type of dementia, is characterised by insidiously progressive memory loss and personality changes. Other spheres of cognitive and non-cognitive impairment are added over the course of several years.
- Dementia with Lewy bodies is a recently recognised entity that overlaps with Alzheimer's disease and parkinsonian dementias. It is the second commonest cause of dementia, and is characterised by marked fluctuations in cognitive impairment and alertness, vivid visual hallucinations, early parkinsonism, and frequent falls.

Continued...

9

- Vascular dementia classically has an abrupt onset and step-wise progression. Clinical features are variable and depend on the location of infarcts, but mood and behavioural changes are common. Significant comorbidity leads to a shorter survival than in Alzheimer's disease.
- Pick's disease is a frontotemporal dementia characterised by early and prominent personality changes and behavioural disturbances, eating disturbances, mood changes, cognitive impairment, language abnormalities, and motor signs. Onset is in middle age and loss of memory may not be a prominent feature.

Differential diagnosis
- The differential diagnosis of dementia is principally from mild cognitive impairment, delirium, delirium superimposed upon dementia, depressive disorder, and late-onset schizophrenia.

Management
- If the dementia cannot be reversed, the aim of management is to improve the quality of life of the patient and carer(s). This involves treating symptoms and complications of dementia, addressing functional problems, and providing education and support for carers.
- Anticholinesterase inhibitors include donepezil, rivastigmine, galantamine, and tacrine. They act by increasing cholinergic neurotransmission and can modestly and temporarily ameliorate cognitive performance and behavioural problems in some patient's with Alzheimer's disease and dementia with Lewy bodies.

Self-assessment

Simply answer with true or false. Answers on p. 219.

1. The commonest cause of delirium is infective.
2. Urinary retention and faecal impaction can cause delirium.
3. In delirium, consciousness is not clouded.
4. In delirium, recent memory is relatively spared.
5. In delirium, the patient is typically most agitated during the daytime and improves at night.
6. Simple measures that can prevent delirium, such as rationalisation of the drug chart and correction of electrolyte disturbances, are all too often overlooked.
7. In delirium, haloperidol is the drug of choice if tranquillisers cannot be avoided. Doses should be kept to a minimum and the drug should be stopped as soon as it is felt that it is no longer required.
8. Delirium superimposed upon dementia can accelerate cognitive decline.
9. In delirium, prognosis after discharge from hospital is good.
10. To make a diagnosis of dementia there should be evidence of a decline in either memory or thinking sufficient to impair activities of daily living.
11. In dementia, lesions in the non-dominant temporal lobe can lead to verbal agnosia, visual agnosia, receptive aphasia, and hallucinations.
12. In dementia, lesions in the non-dominant parietal lobe can lead to body hemineglect and visuospatial disorders.
13. Risk factors for Alzheimer's disease include age, male sex, family history, and head injury.
14. Inheritance of the ε2 allele of apolipoprotein E on chromosome 19 is a risk factor for the common sporadic, late-onset form of Alzheimer's disease.
15. Neurofibrillary tangles seen in Alzheimer's disease consist of a core of beta-amyloid surrounded by filamentous material.
16. In mild cognitive impairment, the risk of conversion to Alzheimer's disease is about 15% a year.
17. Dementia with Lewy bodies is a recently recognised entity that overlaps with Alzheimer's disease and parkinsonian dementias, and that may form part of a spectrum of Lewy-body disorders that includes Parkinson's disease.
18. Dementia with Lewy bodies classically has an abrupt onset and step-wise progression.
19. A person has mental capacity so long as he or she has the ability to understand and retain relevant information for long enough to reach a reasoned decision, regardless of the actual decision reached.
20. If capacity is lacking, the next-of-kin has the responsibility to act in the best interests of the patient, although it is good practice for him or her to involve the doctor in charge and other carers and relatives in the decision-making.

Mental retardation (learning disabilities) 10

Key learning objectives

- Definition of mild, moderate, severe, and profound mental retardation and level of care and support needed for each
- Genetic, prenatal, perinatal, and postnatal causes of mental retardation

- Clinical features of mental retardation, especially definitions of impairment, handicap, and disability

Definition and classification

'Mental retardation' (MR, the term used by ICD-10 for the preferred term 'learning disabilities') is not a mental disorder *per se*, but a label for identifying groups of people in need of care and support, and at special risk of developing behavioural disturbances and psychiatric disorders.

Idiocy is not a disease, but a condition in which the intellectual faculties are never manifested; or have never been developed sufficiently to enable the idiot to acquire such an amount of knowledge as persons of his own age and placed in similar circumstances with himself are capable of receiving.

Esquirol 1845, quoted in Gelder *et al*,
Shorter Oxford Textbook of Psychiatry (2001)

In DSM-IV MR is classified alongside personality disorders on Axis II, and is defined as:

- IQ of 70 or less
- Significant limitations in adaptive functioning in at least two areas
- Onset before the age of 18.

Psychiatry, 2e. By Neel Burton. Published 2010 by Blackwell Publishing.

DSM-IV and ICD-10 divide MR into mild, moderate, severe, and profound subtypes (Table 10.1).

! It is important to bear in mind that people from deprived socioeconomic backgrounds or from different cultural or linguistic backgrounds, as well as people with sensory, motor, or communication handicaps, may obtain spuriously depressed IQ scores. Therefore, a diagnosis of MR should be withheld in people who are not otherwise functionally impaired.

Epidemiology

The prevalence rate of MR is about 2–3%. Decreases in incidence have been matched by increases in life expectancy, leading to large changes in the age structure of the patient population, but only to small changes in the overall prevalence rate. Of all cases of MR, mild MR accounts for about 85% of cases, moderate MR for about 10% of cases, and severe and profound MR for about 5% of cases. The male-to-female ratio for severe MR is 6:5, but is higher for mild MR mostly because males have a larger variance in IQ than females.

ICD-10 code	IQ	Mental age	Level of care and support
F70 Mild	50–69	9 to under 12	Limited, can become self-sufficient and live independently
F71 Moderate	35–49	6 to under 9	Variable, can live in a supervised environment such as a group home
F72 Severe	20–34	3 to under 6	Continuous, can master basic self-care and communication skills
F73 Profound	<20	Under 3	Continuous, not capable of self-care

Table 10.1 Subtypes of mental retardation.

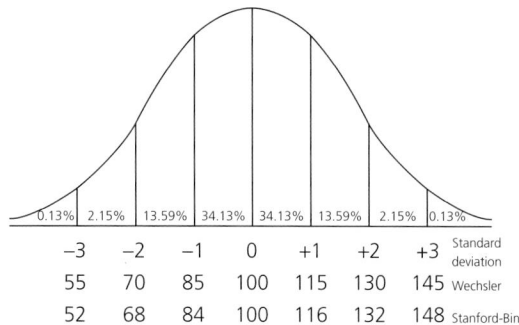

Figure 10.1 IQ distribution, standard deviations, and corresponding scores.

Table 10.2 Specific causes of mental retardation (this list is not fully exhaustive).

Genetic	See Table 10.3
Prenatal	Pre-eclampsia
	Placental insufficiency
	Foetal alcohol syndrome (see Chapter 11)
	Congenital hypothyroidism
	Infections such as rubella, toxoplasmosis, cytomegalovirus, syphilis, and HIV
	Myelomeningocoele
	Hydrocephalus
Perinatal	Brain trauma and hypoxia
	Intraventricular haemorrhage
	Hyperbilirubinaemia
	Infections
Postnatal	Head injury
	Brain infections
	Brain tumours
	Hypoxia
	Chronic lead poisoning
	Poverty
	Neglect and abuse

Aetiology

Most cases of mild mental retardation represent the tail end of the normal distribution curve (Figure 10.1) and result from an interaction of genetic factors and environmental factors such as psychosocial deprivation and nutritional deficiency. A specific cause is more commonly found in severe MR. Specific causes can be classified as genetic, prenatal, perinatal, and postnatal (Tables 10.2 and 10.3).

10

Clinical skills: Definitions of impairment, disability, and handicap

Impairment	Any loss or abnormality of psychological, physiological, or anatomical structure or function
Disability	Any restriction or lack (resulting from an impairment) of ability to perform an activity in the manner or within the range considered normal for a human being
Handicap	A disadvantage for a given individual, resulting from an impairment or disability, that limits or prevents the fulfilment of a role that is normal, depending on age, sex, social and cultural factors, for that individual

Source: World Health Organization, Geneva

Table 10.3 Genetic causes of mental retardation (MR).

Cause	Notes
Chromosomal abnormalities	
Trisomy 21 (Down's syndrome)	Down's syndrome is the commonest cause of MR. Incidence is about 1 in 700 births overall, but increases to about 1 in 30 births in mothers aged 45. 95% of cases result from non-disjunction of chromosome 21, and the remaining 5% from Robertsonian translocations (4%) or mosaicism (1%). MR is accompanied by characteristic physical abnormalities including oblique or almond-shaped palpebral fissures, Brushfield spots on the irises, flat nasal bridge, protruding tongue, short neck, shortened limbs, and single transverse palmar creases ('simian creases'). There is increased risk of deafness, cataracts, respiratory infections, cardiovascular malformations, gastrointestinal abnormalities, haematological abormalities, hypothyroidism, epilepsy, and early-onset Alzheimer's disease
Fragile X syndrome (Martin–Bell syndrome)	Martin–Bell syndrome is the second commonest cause of MR. Incidence is about 1 in 1500 births. Results from CGG trinucleotide repeats in the *FMR* gene on the long arm of chromosome X, and is therefore commoner in males. MR is accompanied by characteristic physical abnormalities including elongated face, large and/or protruding ears, prognathism, macro-orchidism, and hypotonia. As in all trinucleotide repeat disorders, e.g. Huntington's disease and Lesch Nyhan syndrome, disease severity increases in successive generations. This phenomenon is referred to as 'anticipation'
Other chromosomal abnormalities	Other chromosomal abnormalities include other trisomies and deletions such as *cri du chat* syndrome (deletion of the short arm of chromosome 5). Note that numerical sex chromosome abnormalities such as Klinefelter's syndrome, triple X syndrome, and Turner's syndrome do not typically produce MR
Single gene disorders	
Phenylketonuria	Phenylketonuria is the commonest metabolic disorder, with an incidence of about 1 in 10,000 births. It results from the autosomal recessive inheritance of a defect in the phenylalanine hydroxylase enzyme, which results in a high serum phenylalanine. MR is accompanied by short stature, hyperactivity and irritability, epilepsy, lack of pigment, and eczema. Treatment is by diet control
Other metabolic disorders	Other metabolic disorders include other disorders of amino acid metabolism such as homocysteinuria, disorders of carbohydrate metabolism such as galactosaemia, disorders of lipid metabolism such as Tay Sachs disease, and mucopolysaccharidoses such as Hunter's syndrome and Hurler's syndrome
Neurofibromatosis	The incidence of neurofibromatosis is about 1 in 3000 births. A mutation in the *NF1* gene on chromosome 17 (type I neurofibromatosis or Von Recklinghausen's syndrome) leads to mild MR accompanied by *café au lait* spots, multiple neurofibromas, and other abnormalities of the skin, soft tissues, nervous system, and bone. Joseph Merrick, the 'Elephant Man', probably suffered from type I neurofibromatosis and Proteus syndrome, not elephantiasis (as depicted in the excellent film directed by David Lynch and starring Anthony Hopkins)
Tuberous sclerosis	The incidence of tuberous sclerosis is about 1 in 6000 births. It results from the autosomal dominant inheritance of, or a mutation in, the *TSC1* gene on chromosomes 9 or the *TSC2* gene on chromosome 16. Both these genes are tumour suppressor genes. Penetrance is variable: there may be MR accompanied by autism, epilepsy, characteristic skin changes, and tumours of the brain and other organs

10

Clinical features

In MR there are uniformly impaired cognitive, language, motor, and social skills, and failure to meet expected developmental milestones (although in some cases the condition does not present until preschool years). Alternatively behavioural disturbances such as hyperactivity, aggression, inattention, and abnormal movements, including repeated self-harming behaviours, may dominate the clinical picture. Physical disorders including sensory and motor disabilities, epilepsy, and incontinence are common, but the full range of physical disorders

Table 10.4 Possible presentations of mental illness in a person with mental retardation.

Schizophrenia	Deterioration from previous level of functioning
	Behaviour that seems out of character
	Evidence of hallucinations and delusions, even though these may be poorly formed
Hypomania	Overactivity
	Giggling
	Disinhibition
Depression	Loss of appetite
	Sleep disturbance
	Speech and motor retardation
	Anhedonia

depends on the underlying cause of MR. **Mental disorders such as schizophrenia, affective disorders, anxiety disorders, adjustment disorders, dissociative disorders, delirium, dementia, and autism are all more common than in the normal population,** but are more difficult to diagnose because symptoms may be modified or may not be articulated by the patient. For example, in psychosis hallucinations and delusions may be less elaborate, and may have to be diagnosed on the basis of behavioural changes such as fearfulness and head- or ear-banging (Table 10.4). The patient with MR may be both highly impulsive and highly suggestible, for which reasons criminal behaviours such as arson and exhibitionism are more likely to be engaged in.

Assessment

The aim of assessment is not only to diagnose mental MR, but also to determine its aetiology (assistance from a paediatric neurologist may be required), associated physical conditions, associated psychiatric disorders, and functional skills. If a diagnosis of MR has already been made, the patient may have been referred to a psychiatrist to investigate suspected mental illness or a decline in functioning, or to carry out a forensic or risk assessment related to criminal behaviour. Assessment of MR requires patience and tolerance of uncertainty. **The approach to the patient should be flexible and modified according to his or her cognitive abilities and communication skills, and greater emphasis should be placed on direct observation and informant histories (particularly from parents)** than in non-mentally retarded patients. In the history, particular attention should be paid to obstetric complications, neurodevelopmental delays, and behavioural disturbances. Other important areas of the history include the past medical history, family history, and social history. The mental state examination, if not already covered, is carried out at the end of the medical history. Physical examination should encompass sensory assessment, developmental assessment, and functional behavioural assessment. Selected investigations may include standardised assessment instruments, metabolic studies, cytogenetic studies, and neuroimaging.

Management

The management of moderate to severe MR usually involves an individualised and multidisciplinary habilitation plan coordinated by a community learning disability team. The modalities of this habilitation plan depend upon the patient's medical problems, developmental and educational status, emotional and behavioural problems, and family resources. Healthcare professionals that may be co-opted into the patient's care include psychiatrists and other medical professionals, educational psychologists, specialist teachers, speech and language therapists, occupational therapists, behavioural therapists, and family therapists. Social services may also be involved, particularly if the family's resources are limited. Medical management is seldom useful, except in certain cases such as phenylketonuria. Psychotropic drugs are used in the management of psychiatric disorders and behavioural problems, as in other patient groups. Although care in the community is to be encouraged, day care may be required to provide respite to the family, and a small minority of patients may need to be taken into residential care.

Prevention of MR involves improved obstetric and perinatal care, earlier detection of genetic disorders through amniocentesis and chorionic villus sampling, and, if appropriate, genetic counselling.

Self-assessment

Simply answer with true or false. Answers on p. 219.

1. Mental retardation has historically been regarded as a form of mental illness.
2. In DSM-IV mental retardation is classified on Axis II.
3. Onset before the age of 18 is necessary for a diagnosis of mental retardation to be made (DSM-IV).
4. With reference to IQ, about 85% of people lie within two standard deviations of the mean.
5. Moderate mental retardation describes an IQ in the range of 35–49.
6. Mild mental retardation accounts for 85% of all cases of mental retardation.
7. The prevalence rate of mental retardation is about 1%.
8. The male-to-female ratio in severe mental retardation is about 2 : 1.
9. Decreases in the incidence of mental retardation have lead to large changes in the overall prevalence rate.
10. Specific causes of mental retardation can be divided into genetic, prenatal, perinatal, and postnatal causes.
11. Martin–Bell or Fragile X syndrome is the commonest cause of mental retardation and results from trinucleotide repeats in the *FMR* gene on the long arm of chromosome X.
12. 5% of cases of Down's syndrome result from non-disjunction of chromosome 21.
13. Brushfield spots describe small white or greyish/brown spots on the periphery of the iris, and are seen in Down's syndrome.
14. *Cri du chat* syndrome results from a disorder of amino acid metabolism.
15. Turner's syndrome is a common cause of mild mental retardation in females.
16. Phenylketonuria can be treated by diet control.
17. Acoustic neuromas are typical of type I neurofibromatosis or Von Recklinghausen's syndrome.
18. 'Handicap' refers to any restriction or lack (resulting from an impairment) of ability to perform an activity in the manner or within the range considered normal for a human being.
19. In mental retardation, different areas of cognitive functioning are uniformly impaired.
20. In some cases of mental retardation, behavioural disturbances such as hyperactivity, aggression, inattention, and abnormal movements (including repeated self-injurious behaviours) may dominate the clinical picture.

10

Substance misuse

11

Key learning objectives

- The recommended limits for alcohol consumption
- Features of alcohol dependence
- Symptoms of alcohol withdrawal
- Key features of *delirium tremens* and Wernicke–Korsakov syndrome
- Other complications of alcohol misuse and dependence
- Alcohol risk assessment

- Role and limitations of blood tests in alcohol misuse
- Management of alcohol dependence, including detoxification and maintenance treatment
- Routes of administration, mechanism of action, sought-after effects, and undesired effects of commonly used illicit drugs

Classification and diagnosis

In both ICD-10 and DSM-IV the first step in diagnosis is to specify the substance or class of substance involved. In drug users taking more than one substance or class of substance, this is the most important substance used. If the most important substance used is unclear or if substance use is indiscriminate, a diagnosis of **disorder due to multiple drug use** (ICD-10) or **polysubstance-related disorder** can be made.

Step 1: Specify the substance or class of substance involved

ICD-10		DSM-IV
F10	Alcohol	Alcohol
F11	Opioids	Opioids
F12	Cannabinoids	Cannabis
F13	Sedatives or hypnotics	Sedatives, hypnotics, or anxiolytics
F14	Cocaine	Cocaine
F15	Other stimulants, including caffeine	Amphetamines
F16	Hallucinogens	Caffeine
F17	Tobacco	Hallucinogens
F18	Volatile solvents	Phencyclidine
F19	Multiple drug use and other	Nicotine
		Inhalants
		Polysubstance
		Other

Psychiatry, 2e. By Neel Burton. Published 2010 by
Blackwell Publishing.

Step 2: Specify the type of disorder involved

ICD-10		**DSM-IV**
.0	Acute intoxication	Intoxication
.1	Harmful use	Abuse
.2	Dependence syndrome	Dependence
.3	Withdrawal state	Withdrawal
.4	Withdrawal state with delirium	Withdrawal delirium
.5	Psychotic disorder	Psychotic disorders
.6	Amnesic syndrome	Amnestic disorder
.7	Residual and late-onset psychotic disorder	Dementia
.8	Other mental and behavioural disorders	Mood disorders
		Anxiety disorders
		Sexual dysfunctions
		Sleep disorders

The second step in diagnosis is to **specify the type of disorder** involved.

For example, for heroin dependence the ICD-10 coding is F11.2 (opioids, dependence syndrome), for Othello syndrome it is F10.5 (alcohol, psychotic disorder), and for Korsakov syndrome it is F10.6 (alcohol, amnestic syndrome).

Alcohol

Edgar Allen Poe

And the raven, never flitting, still is sitting, still is sitting
On the pallid bust of Pallas just above my chamber door;
And his eyes have all the seeming of a demon's that is
  dreaming,
And the lamp-light o'er him streaming throws his shadow
  on the floor;
And my soul from out that shadow that lies floating on the
  floor
Shall be lifted – nevermore!
    Edgar Allen Poe (1809-1849), final stanza of *The Raven*

On 3 October 1849, Poe was found on the streets of Baltimore, delirious and 'in great distress, and … in need of immediate assistance', according to the man who found him. Poe died in hospital 4 days later, at the age of only 40. The cause of his death remains a mystery but, every year, on the morning of his birthday, his grave is visited by an unknown man who, draped in black and holding a silver-tipped cane, kneels down for a toast of Martel cognac.

Epidemiology

The recommended daily limits for alcohol consumption are **3–4 units a day in males (up to 21 units a week) and 2–3 units a day in females (up to 14 units a week)**. Beyond this there is a significant risk of alcohol-related health and social problems. A unit is about 8 g of alcohol, equivalent to half a pint of ordinary beer, one glass of table wine, one conventional glass of sherry or port, or one single bar measure of spirits. As a rough guide, one bottle of wine is equivalent to about 12 units, and one bottle of spirits to about 40 units.

In the USA a study found the lifetime prevalence of alcohol dependence to be 14%, and the one-year prevalence to be 7%. **In the UK the prevalence of alcohol dependence is about 7% in males and 2% in females,** but these figures mask higher rates of harmful drinking and hazardous drinking (Figure 11.3). Perhaps more tellingly, about 25% of emergency hospital admissions and about 10% of psychiatric admissions are alcohol related, and the number of alcohol-related deaths recorded has more than doubled since 1979 – and still continues to increase. In 1999, alcohol-related deaths – the majority from liver disease – accounted for 1 in 40 deaths. Although alcohol misuse is most prevalent amongst young males, in recent years there has been a disproportionate increase in the numbers of females and adolescents misusing alcohol. Compared to males, females have a stronger genetic predisposition to alcohol dependence, and are also more likely to suffer from the physical complications of alcohol misuse. The prevalence of alcohol misuse is particularly high among the divorced/separated, the unemployed, and

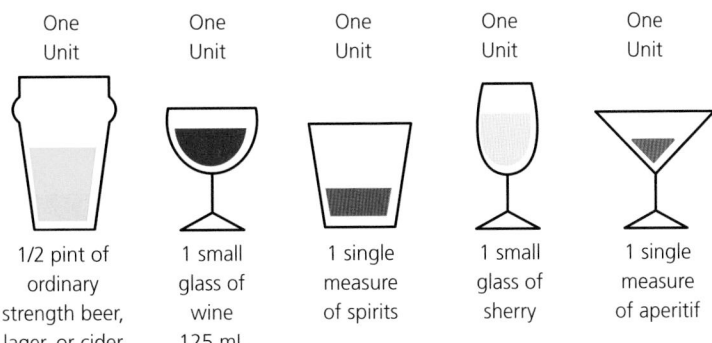

One Unit	One Unit	One Unit	One Unit	One Unit
1/2 pint of ordinary strength beer, lager, or cider	1 small glass of wine 125 mL	1 single measure of spirits	1 small glass of sherry	1 single measure of aperitif

Figure 11.1 Equivalences for one unit of alcohol.

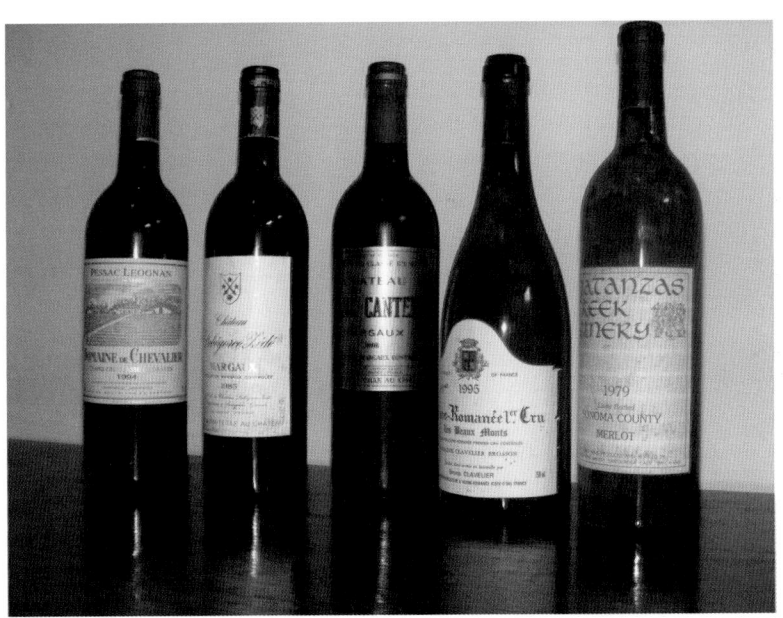

Figure 11.2 A bottle of claret or burgundy typically contains about 12 units of alcohol, but a bottle of red wine from the New World (right) is likely to contain more. Photo by Neel Burton.

11

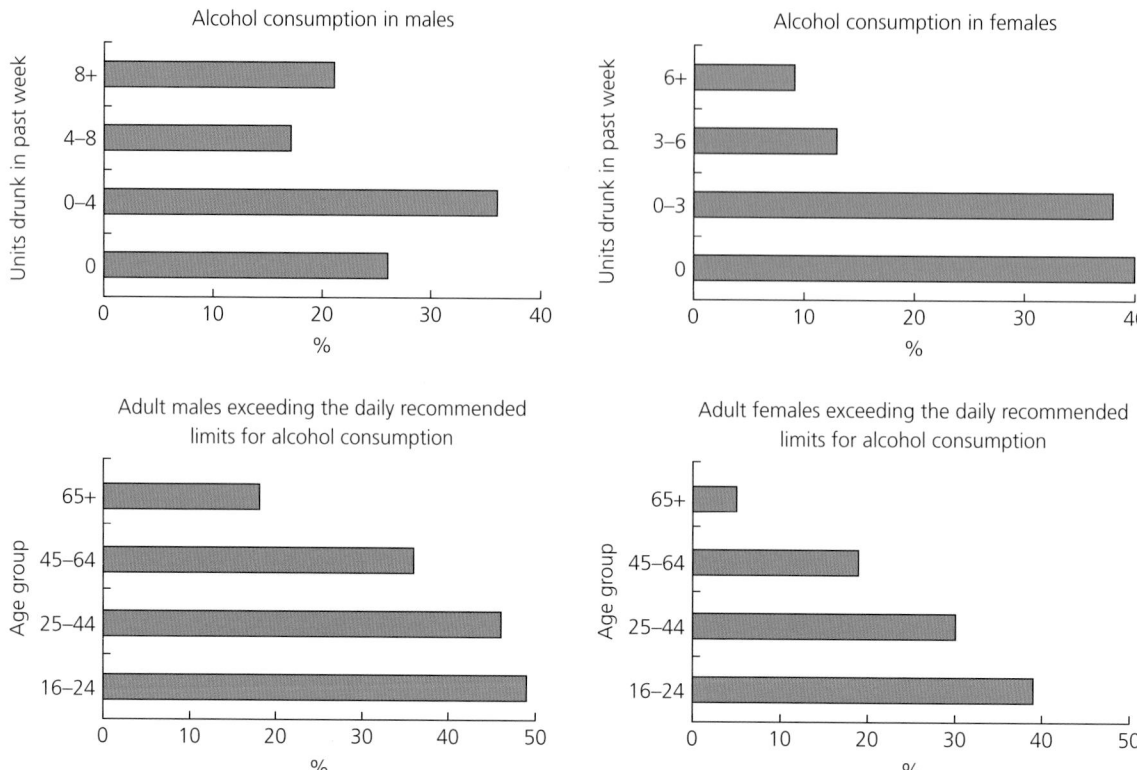

Figure 11.3 Alcohol consumption among people aged 16 and over in England by sex; and adults exceeding daily recommended limits for alcohol consumption in Great Britain on their heaviest drinking day in the last week by age and sex. In studying these charts it should be remembered that alcohol consumption is typically under-reported. (Source: *General Household Survey 2001–02*, ONS).

the homeless. There are important international variations in the prevalence of alcohol misuse and dependence. Generally speaking, as compared to the UK, alcohol misuse is more prevalent in Russia, Latin America, and the Caribbean, and less so in Africa and South-East Asia.

Aetiology

The user's perspective

I have absolutely no pleasure in the stimulants in which I sometimes so madly indulge. It has not been in the pursuit of pleasure that I have periled life and reputation and reason. It has been in the desperate attempt to escape from torturing memories, from a sense of insupportable loneliness, and a dread of some strange impending doom.
Edgar Allan Poe on alcohol, quoted in Meyers (1989)

Genetics

The concordance rate for alcohol dependence in monozygotic twins is 70% in males and 43% in females, versus 43% in males and 32% in females in dizygotic twins. First-degree relatives of alcohol-dependent persons have an approximately seven-fold increased risk of developing alcohol dependence, and adoption studies of sons of alcohol-dependent parents suggest that this increased risk is to a large extent maintained after adoption by non-alcohol dependent parents. The genetic influence in alcohol dependence may exert itself through heritable personality factors or through single genes that modulate the body's response to alcohol. East-Asian populations, for example, are much less likely to develop alcohol dependence because they have an isoenzyme of aldehyde dehydrogenase that, upon drinking alcohol, leads to an accumulation of acetaldehyde and unpleasant symptoms such as

11

flushing, nausea, palpitations, and headache (this is the so-called 'flushing reaction').

Neurochemical abnormalities

Alcohol has a variety of effects on a number of neurotransmitters, including GABA, dopamine, serotonin, and glutamate. The euphoriant and reinforcing effects of alcohol are mediated by GABA, dopamine, and serotonin. In alcohol dependence there is a compensatory upregulation of glutamate to compensate for the (GABA-ergic) CNS depressant effects of alcohol. Suddenly withdrawing alcohol therefore leads to symptoms of CNS hyperexcitability.

Psychological theories

There is no such thing as an 'alcoholic personality', although anxiety disorders, borderline personality disorder, antisocial personality disorder, and a history of childhood conduct disorder are particularly associated with alcohol misuse. According to cognitive-behavioural theories, alcohol dependence may result from positive reinforcement (seeking out the pleasant effects of alcohol) and negative reinforcement (avoiding the negative effects of alcohol withdrawal), from a conditioned response to one or more circumstances (e.g. a pub or nightclub), or from modelling the drinking behaviour of relatives, peers, and 'celebrities'. According to psychodynamic theories, alcohol dependence may result from maternal deprivation, childhood sexual abuse, or unconscious gains resulting from intoxication and personal damage caused.

Social factors/other

- **Life events:** life events such as separation, bereavement, or loss of employment may lead to alcohol misuse and dependence.
- **Occupation:** certain occupational groups are at a higher risk of alcohol dependence, e.g. publicans and bar staff, salesmen, entertainers, journalists, and doctors. Generally speaking, alcohol dependence is more prevalent in the unskilled manual social class and in the unemployed.
- **Population levels of alcohol consumption:** the average level of alcohol consumption in a given population is closely related to the level of alcohol-related disorders, e.g. to the number of deaths from cirrhosis. The average level of alcohol consumption in a population

can be controlled through three factors: price, availability, and social attitudes to alcohol.

Comorbidity

Other psychiatric disorders – especially depressive disorders, anxiety disorders, and stress-related disorders – and medical disorders (e.g. chronic pain and terminal illness) commonly lead to alcohol misuse and dependence. Equally, alcohol misuse commonly leads to other psychiatric disorders and medical disorders (see Table 11.1). The term *dual diagnosis* refers to the co-occurrence of both a psychiatric disorder and substance misuse (alcohol or illicit drugs), although it does not strictly speaking encompass psychiatric states that result directly from, or are fully contingent upon, substance misuse (e.g. paranoid ideation or hallucinations that occur after taking cocaine). The failure to recognise comorbid substance misuse in a patient can lead to an incorrect diagnosis and to an inappropriate management plan.

Clinical features and complications

Key features of alcohol dependence

The following are seven key features of alcohol dependence:
1. Compulsion to drink
2. Primacy of drinking over other activities
3. Stereotyped pattern of drinking
4. Increased tolerance to alcohol
5. Repeated withdrawal symptoms
6. Relief drinking to avoid withdrawal symptoms
7. Reinstatement after abstinence.

   For a diagnosis of alcohol dependence to be made, DSM-IV requires at least three from a similar list of seven features occurring at any time during a 12-month period.

Withdrawal symptoms

Withdrawal symptoms usually occur after several years of heavy drinking and range from mild anxiety and sleep disturbance to life-threatening *delirium tremens*. They are most likely to occur first thing in the morning, which is why some people with alcohol dependence sleep with a straw in their mouth. Common symptoms include agitation, tremor (the 'shakes'), sweating, nausea, and retching. If these symptoms are not relieved by alcohol or

11

Table 11.1 Other complications of alcohol misuse and dependence.

Psychiatric	● Mood and anxiety disorders – may be either complications or, less commonly, aetiological factors
	● Suicide and deliberate self-harm
	● Alcoholic hallucinosis – auditory hallucinations, first of fragmentary sounds then of derogatory voices, usually in the third person. These auditory hallucinations can persist even after several months of abstinence, in some cases leading to secondary delusions. They are notoriously unresponsive to antipsychotic medication
	● Othello syndrome (pathological jealousy, delusions of infidelity) – often compounded by sexual problems and the spouse's lack of interest in a drunken partner. If treatment is failing it may be necessary for the couple to separate so as to protect the spouse
	● Cognitive impairment – may be partially reversible if drinking is stopped
	● Pathological intoxication (*manie à potu*) – an uncommon idiosyncratic reaction to alcohol marked by maladaptive changes in behaviour
Neurological	● Episodic anterograde amnesia
	● Seizures
	● Perhipheral neuropathy
	● Cerebellar degeneration
	● Optic atrophy (rare)
	● Central pontine myelinosis (rare)
	● Marchiafava–Bignami disease – demyelination of corpus callosum, optic tracts, and cerebral peduncles manifesting as dysarthria, ataxia, seizures, and impaired consciousness, and eventually dementia and limb paralysis (rare)
Gastrointestinal	● Oesophagitis
	● Oesophageal varices
	● Gastritis
	● Peptic ulceration
	● Acute and chronic pancreatitis
	● Alcoholic hepatitis
	● Cirrhosis: 10–20% of alcohol-dependent people develop cirrhosis
	● Cancer of the oesophagus, stomach, and liver
Cardiovascular	● Hypertension – increased risk of stroke and ischaemic heart disease
	● Cardiac arrhythmias
	● Cardiomyopathy
Other medical	● Episodic hypoglycaemia
	● Vitamin deficiencies and anaemia
	● Accidents, especially head injury
	● Hypothermia
	● Respiratory depression
	● Aspiration pneumonia
	● Increased susceptibility to infections
	● Sexual problems: decreased libido, impotence
Social	● Family and marital difficulties
	● Employment difficulties
	● Accidents
	● Financial problems
	● Vagrancy and homelessness
	● Crime and its repercussions

11

medical treatment (see later), they may last for several days and progress to include transient perceptual distortions and hallucinations, seizures, and *delirium tremens*.

After acute alcohol intoxication, 'hangover' effects peak several hours after drinking and subside within 8–24 hours. Hangover effects are thought to result from dehydration, the toxic effects of the alcohol metabolites acetaldehyde and acetate and of congeners (impurities produced during alcohol fermentation), irritation of the gastric lining, hypoglycaemia, and vitamin B_{12} deficiency. They include thirst, headache, lethargy and sleep disturbance, dizziness and vertigo, increased sensitivity to light and sound, irritability, anxiety, dysphoria, sympathetic hyperactivity, red eyes, muscle ache, and hypothermia. There is no compelling evidence for any of the interventions currently used for preventing or treating hangovers, and the best approach is probably one involving fluids, food, and sleep. NSAIDs and paracetamol should be avoided because their effects on the stomach lining and liver (respectively) are compounded by alcohol. Caffeine may increase the effect of analgesics used, but it is also a diuretic and promotes dehydration. Note that the medical term for 'hangover' is veisalgia.

Delirium tremens (the 'DTs')

Delirium tremens is a medical emergency that occurs in about 5% of alcohol-dependent people at 1–3 days after stopping alcohol. It is therefore relatively common, and especially so in hospital inpatients. It is a delirious disorder characterised by:

- Clouding of consciousness
- Disorientation in time and place
- Impairment of recent memory
- Fear, agitation, and restlessness
- Vivid hallucinations (most commonly visual) and delusions (most commonly paranoid)
- Insomnia
- Autonomic disturbances (tachycardia, hypertension, hyperthermia, sweating, dilated pupils)
- Coarse tremor
- Nausea and vomiting
- Dehydration and electrolyte imbalances
- Seizures.

Important differentials include hypoglycaemia, drug overdose, and other causes of delirium, e.g. urinary tract infection. *Delirium tremens* should also be differentiated from alcohol hallucinosis and Wernicke's encephalopathy (see below). Prevention and treatment involve benzodiaz-

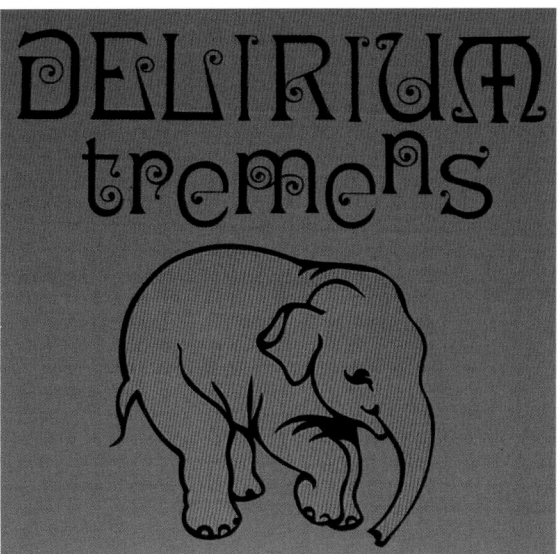

Figure 11.4 Delirium tremens is also the name of a brand of Belgian beer that contains 9% alcohol. Brewery Huyghe NV, Melle, Belgium. Reproduced with permission.

epines, correction of fluid and electrolyte imbalances, treatment of concurrent infections, and parenteral multivitamin injections. *Delirium tremens* often complicates other medical emergencies such as infection and injury, and fever and signs of shock are poor prognostic signs. **Its untreated mortality rate is in the order of 10%.**

Wernicke–Korsakov syndrome (Wernicke's encephalopathy and Korsakov's syndrome)

Wernicke's encephalopathy is a medical emergency. It is a disorder of acute onset characterised by impaired consciousness and confusion, episodic memory impairment, ataxia, nystagmus, abducens and conjugate gaze palsies, pupillary abnormalities, and peripheral neuropathy (the 'classical triad' that students are often asked about consists of confusion, ataxia, and ocular palsy). **It results from thiamine (vitamin B_1) deficiency, most commonly secondary to alcohol dependence, and can therefore be prevented by thiamine supplementation.** Other causes include starvation, malabsorption, hyperemesis, and carbon monoxide poisoning. The differential diagnosis is principally from hypoglycaemia, hepatic encephalopathy, and subdural haemorrhage. Treatment involves parenteral thiamine, but only 20% of sufferers recover, and 10% die from haemorrhages in the brainstem and hypo-

11

thalamus. The remainder go on to develop Korsakov's syndrome (amnestic syndrome), an irreversible syndrome of prominent impairment of recent memory and, to a lesser extent, remote memory resulting from neuronal loss, gliosis, and haemorrhage in the mamillary bodies and damage to the dorsomedial nucleus of the thalamus. Confabulation – the falsification of memory in clear consciousness – may be a marked feature, but immediate recall, perception and other cognitive functions are usually intact. 'The Lost Mariner' is a case study of Korsakov's syndrome recounted by Oliver Sacks in *The Man Who Mistook His Wife for a Hat*.

Alcohol in pregnancy

The amount of alcohol that can be safely drunk in pregnancy is uncertain, so it is probably best to avoid it altogether. Drinking alcohol in pregnancy increases the rate of stillbirths and other obstetric complications. It can also lead to foetal alcohol syndrome (FAS). FAS affects 1–2 live births per 1000 and is characterised by growth retardation, dysmorphology (particularly midfacial anomalies), and CNS involvement (cognitive impairment, learning disabilities, and impulsiveness). Milder forms of FAS, sometimes referred to as foetal alcohol effects (FAE), are thought to be more common and principally circumscribed to CNS involvement.

Management and prognosis

Alcohol misuse is common and clinicians in all specialties should maintain a high index of suspicion for it and routinely ask about alcohol intake. Rapid screening questionnaires such as the CAGE questionnaire may be useful in this context, although they are not as sensitive as a comprehensive alcohol risk assessment. If drinking habits are difficult to assess, take an informant history or ask the patient to keep an alcohol diary.

Clinical skills/OSCE: Alcohol risk assessment

Before starting
- Introduce yourself to the patient and establish a rapport.
- Explain to him that you are going to ask him some questions about his drinking habits and ask for his consent to do this. Remember to be sensitive in your questioning.

Alcohol history
- Ask about alcohol intake e.g. in a typical day:
  - Type (enquire separately into beer, wine, and spirits)
  - Amount
  - Place
  - Time.
- Ask about features of alcohol dependence:
  - Compulsion to drink
  - Primacy of drinking over other activities
  - Stereotyped pattern of drinking, e.g. narrowing of drinking repertoire
  - Increased tolerance to alcohol
  - Withdrawal symptoms, e.g. anxiety, sweating, tremor, nausea, fits, *delirium tremens*
  - Relief drinking to avoid withdrawal symptoms
  - Reinstatement after abstinence.

Psychiatric/medical history
Ask about depression and the common medical complications of alcohol abuse, e.g. peptic ulceration, pancreatitis, liver disease, ischaemic heart disease, peripheral neuropathy.

Drug history
Note that:
- Substance abuse is common in alcoholics
- Alcohol potentiates the effects of certain drugs such as phenytoin.

Social history
Cover employment, housing, marital problems, financial problems, and legal (forensic) problems.

Informant history
An informant history can often give a clearer and more accurate account of the patient's drinking habits.

After finishing
- Give the patient feedback on his or her drinking habits (e.g. number of units drunk versus recommended number of units) and, if appropriate, suggest ways for him or her to cut down his or her alcohol intake.

11

Clinical skills: CAGE questionnaire

C Have you ever felt you should **C**ut down on your drinking?

A Have people **A**nnoyed you by criticising your drinking?

G Have you ever felt bad or **G**uilty about drinking?

E Have you ever taken a drink first thing in the morning (**E**ye opener)?

Two or more positive replies are said to identify alcohol misuse.

! Antidepressant and antipsychotic drugs may be used to treat associated psychiatric disorders, but it is also important to remember that symptoms of anxiety and depression often resolve with the cessation of drinking.

Blood tests may be helpful in augmenting the findings of screening questionnaires such as the CAGE questionnaire, and in monitoring progress. Gamma-glutamyl-transferase (GGT) is raised in about 80% of heavy drinkers, alkaline phosphatase (ALP) in about 60%, and mean corpuscular volume (MCV) in about 50%. Of the three tests, MCV has the highest specificity for alcohol misuse but, due to the long half-life of red blood cells (120 days), may remain elevated for a long time after the patient has stopped drinking. Carbohydrate-deficient transferrin (CDT) has an even higher specificity than MCV, but is not commonly available in the UK. The sensitivity and specificity of GGT, ALP, and MCV can be improved by ordering them in combination.

Early treatment of alcohol misuse is often delivered in primary care and involves simple advice and support, and appraisal of current medical, psychological, and social problems. It may also be useful to devise a goal-oriented management plan that is tailored to the patient's needs and that can be mutually agreed upon.

If alcohol misuse has already reached the stage of dependence, **detoxification** is required. This involves a reducing course of a benzodiazepine *in lieu* of alcohol, e.g. chlordiazepoxide 20 mg QDS reducing daily over 5–7 days and supplemented by thiamine 200 mg OD (often in the form of a multivitamin preparation). Detoxification can usually be carried out in the community either by the GP practice or the local substance misuse service, but hospital admission should be considered if the patient has a comorbid medical or psychiatric disorder (including drug misuse), a history of convulsions or *delirium tremens*, or a lack of social support. Note that a similar drug regimen to the one outlined above can also be used for the early stages of alcohol withdrawal.

After detoxification the patient should be advised to abstain from alcohol as abstention has a better prognosis than controlled drinking, especially if the patient has suffered physical damage from alcohol or is aged 40 or over. Abstention can be encouraged by maintenance treatments such as the opiate antagonist naltrexone (not currently licensed in the UK), acamprosate (Campral), and disulfiram (Antabuse). Acamprosate is an 'anticraving' drug that enhances GABA neurotransmission and therefore mimics the CNS depressant effects of alcohol. Disulfiram on the other hand is an alcohol-sensitising deterrent drug that blocks the oxidation of alcohol by irreversibly inhibiting the enzyme aldehyde dehydrogenase, leading to an accumulation of acetaldehyde and associated symptoms of flushing, palpitations, headache, nausea, and a choking sensation (it can be thought of as a chemical form of aversion therapy). For this reason, it should not be started until the breath alcohol has returned to zero. It is contra-indicated in hypertension, coronary artery disease, and cardiac failure as it can cause cardiac arrhythmias; other side-effects include sedation, constipation, and halitosis (bad breath).

Maintenance treatments require close supervision, often by a nominated 'supervisor' such as the patient's spouse, and are not a substitute to psychosocial interventions. These latter include attendance at groups run by local community alcohol services or Alcoholics Anonymous, supportive psychotherapy (including supportive psychotherapy for carers), cognitive-behavioural therapy, and marital and family therapy. Social skills training is an effective component of substance misuse treatment programmes that aims to impart the skills needed to function more effectively in social situations, and involves a variety of interventions such as role playing in groups (e.g. declining the offer of an alcoholic drink, or going to a bar and ordering a non-alcoholic drink), assertiveness training, and problem solving skills.

Alcohol dependence is a chronic relapsing condition and **only 20–50% of patients remain abstinent one year after detoxification.** Predictors of relapse include poor motivation, lack of employment and social support, and comorbid mental illness.

11

Alcoholics Anonymous

Founded in 1935 in Ohio, Alcoholics Anonymous is a spiritually oriented community of alcoholics whose aim is to stay sober and, through shared experience and understanding, to help other alcoholics to do the same, 'one day at a time', by avoiding that first drink. The essence of the programme involves a 'spiritual awakening' that is achieved by 'working the steps', usually with the guidance of a more experienced member or 'sponsor'. Members attend initially daily meetings in which they share their experiences of alcoholism and recovery, and engage in prayer or meditation. A prayer that is usually recited at every meeting is the Serenity Prayer, the short version of which goes:

God grant me the serenity to accept the things I cannot change,
Courage to change the things I can,
And the wisdom to know the difference.

Illicit drugs

I don't do drugs, I am drugs.

Salvador Dali

A brief history of illicit drugs

Opiates

The Sumerians cultivated the **opium poppy** as early as 3400 BC and referred to it as *Hul Gil* or 'joy plant'. In the 18th century, the British East India Company gained a monopoly on the increasingly important opium trade and in 1839 China's efforts to suppress it triggered a series of belligerent attacks from the British that led to a Chinese defeat. The British thus maintained their opium trade and gained a piece of China called Hong Kong. The first synthetic opiate, diamorphine, appeared at the end of that century. In 1896 Bayer Pharmaceuticals started marketing it under the name of **heroin**, 'the hero of medicines'.

Clinical skills: Motivational interviewing

Scenario A

Doctor: *According to your blood tests, you're drinking too much alcohol.*

Patient: *I suppose I do enjoy the odd drink.*

Doctor: *You're probably having far more than just the odd drink. Alcohol is very bad for you, you need to stop drinking.*

Patient: *You sound like my wife.*

Doctor: *Well, she's right you know. Alcohol can cause liver and heart problems and many other things besides. So you really need to stop drinking, OK?*

Patient: *Yes, doctor, thank you.*

(Patient never returns.)

Scenario B (using motivational interviewing)

Doctor: *We all enjoy a drink now and then, but sometimes alcohol can do us a lot of harm. What do you know about the harmful effects of alcohol?*

Patient: *Quite a bit, I'm afraid. My best friend, well, he used to drink a lot. Last year he spent three months in hospital. I visited him often, but most of the time he wasn't with it. Then he died from internal bleeding.*

Doctor: *I'm sorry to hear that, alcohol can really do us a lot of damage.*

Patient: *It does a lot of damage to the liver, doesn't it?*

Doctor: *That's right, but it doesn't just damage our body, it also damages our lives: our work, our finances, our relationships.*

Patient: *Funny you should say that. My wife's been at my neck …*

(…)

Doctor: *So, you've told me that you're currently drinking about 16 units of alcohol a day. This has placed severe strain on your marriage and on your relationship with your daughter Emma, not to mention that you haven't been to work since last Tuesday and have started to fear for your job. But what you fear most is ending up lying on a hospital bed like your friend Tom. Is that a fair summary of things as they stand?*

Patient: *Things are completely out of hand, aren't they? If I don't stop drinking now, I might lose everything I've built over the past 20 years: my job, my marriage, even my daughter.*

Doctor: *I'm afraid you might be right.*

Patient: *I really need to quit drinking.*

Doctor: *You sound very motivated to stop drinking. Why don't we make another appointment to talk about the ways in which we might support you?*

11

Stimulants

In 1859 Mantegazzo first isolated **cocaine** from the coca leaf, which was chewed upon by native South Americans to relieve fatigue. The drug became so popular as to be included in an American drink called Coca-Cola, or Coke, which only became a 'soft' drink in 1914, after a number of deaths by overdose. In 1887 Edeleano first synthesised 'phenylisopropylamine' or **amphetamine**. By the 1930s amphetamine had found use as an over-the-counter nasal decongestant and in the treatment of narcolepsy and attention-deficit hyperactivity disorder (ADHD, see Chapter 13). It became popular as a drug of abuse in the 1940s, after being given to soldiers to improve their performance. First synthesised in 1912, the psychedelic amphetamine MDMA or **ecstasy** only became available in the 1960s, but soon replaced cocaine as the drug of choice in bars and clubs.

Hallucinogens (psychedelics)

In 1938 Albert Hofman discovered **lysergic acid diethylamide (LSD)**, a derivative of ergot. In 1943 he took it by accident and described the experience as 'an uninterrupted stream of fantastic pictures, extraordinary shapes with intense kaleidoscopelike play of colours [sic]'. The drug quickly established itself as a street drug, but Hofman strongly disapproved of its use in this context. He commented, 'In old times psychedelic substances were considered sacred and they were used with the right attitude and in a ritual and spiritual context. And what a difference if we compare it with the careless and irresponsible use of LSD in the streets and in the discotheques of New York City and everywhere in the West. It is a tragic misunderstanding of the nature and the meaning of these kinds of substances'.

Epidemiology

As illicit drugs are by definition illicit, their epidemiology is more difficult to establish than that of alcohol. According to the 2003–04 British Crime Survey, over 11 million people aged 16–59 in England and Wales have at some point used illicit drugs, and over 4 million have used class A drugs (Figure 11.5). From 1998 to 2003–04 the overall

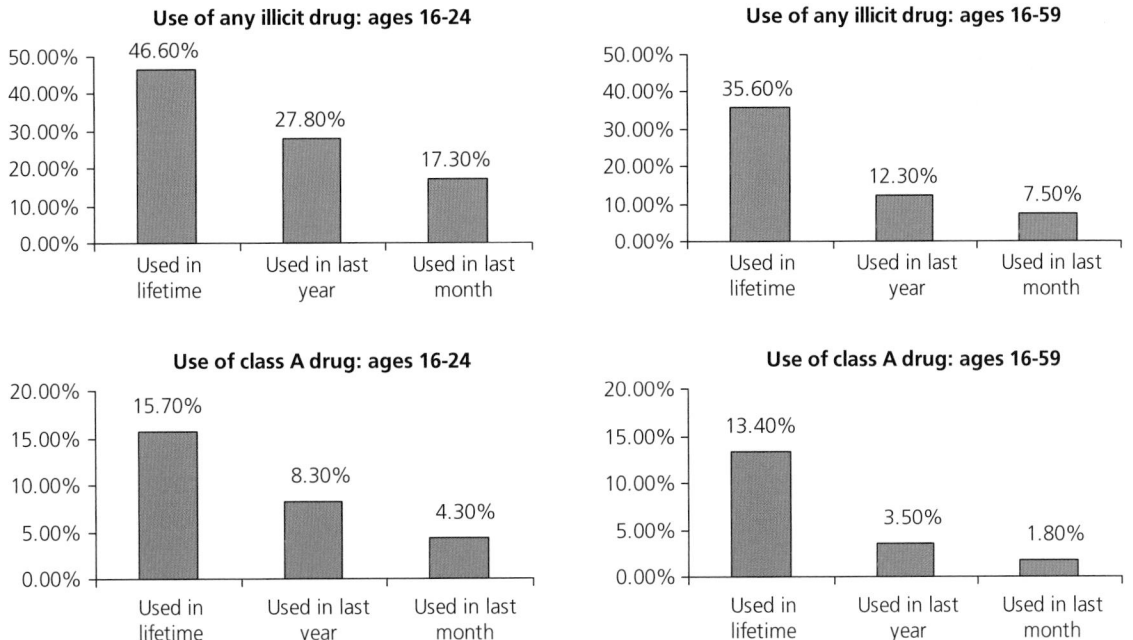

Figure 11.5 Use of any illicit drug and of a class A drug, young people (ages 16–24) and population as a whole (ages 16–59). Source: *British Crime Survey 2003–04.*

Table 11.2 Controlled substances under the Misuse of Drugs Act 1971 (UK).

Class A	Ecstasy, LSD, phencyclidine, psilocybin, magic mushrooms, heroin, morphine, pethidine, opium, methadone, cocaine, crack cocaine, amphetamines (if prepared for injection)
Class B	Amphetamines, methylphenidate (Ritalin), barbiturates, cannabis
Class C	Benzodiazepines, gamma hydroxybutyrate (GHB, 'liquid ecstasy'), ketamine, anabolic steroids

Table 11.3 Some of the street names for commonly used illicit substances.

Heroin	Smack, Hammer, 'H', gear, scag, brown
Cocaine	Charlie, coke, snow, white lady, freebase, crack, rock, 'C'
Amphetamines	Speed, whizz, ice, uppers, go, zip, goey, dexies
Ecstasy	'E', bickies, disco biscuits, love drug, vitamins, XTC, Rolexes, dolphins
LSD	Acid, trips, micro dots, blotters, tabs
Cannabis	Marijuana, pot, dope, grass, weed, leaf, green, smoke, gunga

Table 11.4 Some risk factors for illicit drug use.

- Being young
- Being male
- Being single or divorced, or cohabiting
- Visiting pubs or wine bars three times a week or more
- Going to nightclubs
- Renting accommodation
- Living in a terrace or flat/maisonette
- Living in a council or inner city area
- Living in London
- Having a limiting disability or illness
- Being unemployed
- Earning more than £30,000 a year

Source: *British Crime Survey 2003/04.*

number of people having used 'any drug' in the past year did not change, but the number using cocaine and ecstasy significantly increased and the number using LSD significantly decreased. Amongst young people (16–24 years),

24.6% had used cannabis in the past year, 5.3% had used ecstasy, 4.9% cocaine, 4.4% amyl nitrate (poppers), and 4% amphetamines. Poppers are alkyl nitrite inhalants that produce a euphoric head rush and relax smooth muscle; as a recreational drug they are principally used to enhance the sexual experience.

Aetiology

The user's perspective

Choose a job. Choose a career. Choose a family. Choose a f***ing big television. Choose washing machines, cars, compact disc players and electrical tin openers. Choose good health, low cholesterol, and dental insurance. Choose fixed interest mortgage repayments. Choose a starter home. Choose your friends. Choose leisurewear and matching luggage. Choose a three-piece suit on hire purchase in a range of f***ing fabrics. Choose DIY and wondering who the f*** you are on a Sunday morning. Choose sitting on that couch watching mind-numbing, spirit-crushing game shows, stuffing f***ing junk food into your mouth. Choose rotting away at the end of it all, p***ing your last in a miserable home, nothing more than an embarrassment to the selfish, f***ed up brats you spawned to replace yourselves. Choose your future. Choose life…But why would I want to do a thing like that? I chose not to choose life. I chose something else. And the reasons? There are no reasons. Who needs reasons when you've got heroin?

Renton, quoted in the film *Trainspotting*
(1996), Irvine Welsh

The aetiology of drug misuse is similar to that of alcohol misuse and as such is multifactorial. Social factors such as the availability of the drug and attitudes to drug taking in the peer group are important in determining the likelihood of experimentation. About 10% of experimenters go on to develop problems, usually at a young age. They are more likely to come from a dysfunctional family and to have a history of delinquency or truancy. They are also more likely to have a mental disorder such as depression, anxiety or personality disorder, or certain personality traits such as sensation-seeking and impulsivity.

Drug misuse is reinforced by sought-after effects such as euphoria. These effects are mediated by the midbrain dopamine system that projects from the ventral tegmental area to the forebrain, including to the ***nucleus accumbens*** (the so-called 'craving centre'). Studies have suggested that an allele of the dopamine D_2 receptor may be a risk factor for substance misuse, and other such neurotransmitter system abnormalities are also likely to be involved. Once a pattern of drug misuse is established, neuroadaptive changes in the brain lead to the phenomena of tolerance and withdrawal. As a result, increased amounts of the drug are required to achieve sought-after effects and to avoid withdrawal symptoms.

Clinical features and management

This section describes the sought after and adverse effects of commonly misused drugs, including opioids such as heroin and morphine, cocaine, amphetamines, ecstasy, LSD, cannabis, benzodiazepines, and volatile substances.

In addition to drug-specific adverse effects, drug misuse in general can lead to a number of medical, psychiatric, and social complications. Intravenous drug use carries a risk of local complications such as infection of the injection site and venous thrombosis, and systemic complications such as septicaemia, bacterial endocarditis, hepatitis B and C, and HIV. Drug misuse in early pregnancy can lead to foetal abnormalities, in late pregnancy to dependence in the foetus, and after delivery to withdrawal symptoms in the newborn. Associated psychiatric disorders are common, especially depressive disorders, anxiety disorders, and personality disorders, and are often precipitated and/or perpetuated by drug misuse. An inability to fulfil social obligations results in unemployment, marital problems, and neglect of children. Other social consequences include motoring offences, accidents, and criminal activity.

> **!** The Mental Health Act cannot be invoked for substance misuse and dependence, but associated or secondary mental disorder may constitute grounds for compulsory admission and treatment of that disorder under the Act.

Opioids

- An opioid is any agent that binds to opioid receptors, including endogenous opioid peptides, opium alkaloids such as morphine and codeine, semi-synthetic opioids such as heroin and oxycodone, and fully synthetic opioids such as pethidine and methadone. The term 'opiate' is often used as a synonym of 'opioid', but is more properly restricted to the natural opium alkaloids and the semi-synthetic opioids derived from them.

- Routes of administration: oral, intramuscular, intravenous, subcutaneous ('skin popping'), sniffed ('snorted'). Heroin can also be inhaled ('chasing the dragon').

- Mechanism of action: act at specific opioid receptors. Morphine and heroin are relatively selective for the µ-opioid receptor subtype. As heroin is only detectable in the urine for 1–2 days, taking heroin rather than cannabis gives patients and prisoners a better chance of evading random urine drug screens.

- Effects: euphoria, analgesia, respiratory depression, constipation, anorexia, loss of libido, pruritus, pinpoint pupils (miosis). **Tolerance develops rapidly but diminishes as soon as the drug is stopped, leading to a potentially fatal accidental overdose if the drug is restarted at the previous dose, e.g. after the patient is discharged from hospital.**

- Overdose: respiratory depression and death.

- Withdrawal syndrome: intense craving, restlessness, insomnia, muscle pains, tachycardia, dilated pupils, running nose and eyes, sweating, piloerection (hence the expression 'going cold turkey'), abdominal cramps, vomiting, diarrhoea. **These symptoms begin about 8–12 hours after the last dose, peak at 36–72 hours, and subside over 7–10 days.**

- Management:
  - Detoxification: stop the drug and prescribe reducing doses of a substitute drug such as methadone or buprenorphine (first ensure that the person really is using opioids and not just angling for a substitute drug to misuse or sell off). Provide psychological support, e.g. abstinence/rehabilitation programme and, if need be, social support. Clonidine and lofexidine are centrally acting α2 agonists that can also be used in detoxification. Naltrexone, a long-acting opioid antagonist, can be used to help prevent relapses. However, it induces withdrawal if the patient is still dependent
  - Harm reduction and maintenance therapy: if abstinence is unrealistic, consider substitute prescribing of oral methadone or buprenorphine with the aim of reducing injecting, stabilising drug use and lifestyle, and reducing crime. Needle exchanges and drug education programmes are also good practice, and may lead the addict to consider detoxification
  - Overdose: cardiorespiratory support, IV naloxone. Upon regaining consciousness the addict may not be

11

pleased that you have ruined his or her hit, but the half-life of naloxone is shorter than that of heroin and, unless you bear this in mind and use a continuous infusion, he or she may soon collapse again.

Confessions of an English Opium-Eater

It will occur to you often to ask, Why did I not release myself from the horrors of opium, by leaving it off, or diminishing it! To this I must answer briefly; it might be supposed that I yielded to the fascinations of opium too easily; it cannot be supposed that any man can be charmed by its terrors. The reader may be sure, therefore, that I made attempts innumerable to reduce the quantity. I add, that those who witnessed the agonies of those attempts, and not myself, were the first to beg me to desist.

Thomas de Quincey (1785–1859) in
Confessions of an English Opium-Eater,
which first appeared in *London Magazine* in 1821

Cocaine

- Related compounds: crack or freebase cocaine, speedball (a mixture of cocaine and heroin). Crack cocaine, so named for the sound it makes upon burning, produces a short-lived high that especially encourages dependence.
- Routes of administration: inhaled ('snorted'), injected, smoked (crack cocaine). Inhalation can cause perforation of the nasal septum.
- Mechanism of action: blocks reuptake of serotonin and catecholamines, especially dopamine.
- Effects: euphoria, increased confidence and energy, decreased inhibition, decreased need for food or sleep, dilated pupils, tachycardia, hypertension, hyperthermia. In higher doses, visual and auditory hallucinations, paranoid ideation, aggression – increased dopamine mimics schizophrenia. Formication ('cocaine bugs') describes the feeling of having insects crawling under the skin. Violence is common.
- Overdose: tremor, confusion, seizures, stroke, cardiac arrhythmias, myocardial infarction, myocarditis, cardiomyopathy, respiratory arrest.
- Withdrawal symptoms: generalised malaise, intense craving, dysphoria, anxiety, irritability, agitation, fatigue, hypersomnolence, vivid and unpleasant dreams, suicidal ideation.

- Management: cognitive behavioural therapy and treatment of comorbid psychiatric illness. In acute intoxication consider benzodiazepines and antipsychotics to treat symptoms, and treat complications.

Amphetamines

- Related compounds: methamphetamine, dexamphetamine ('speed'), methylphenidate (Ritalin), ecstasy.
- Routes of administration: oral, injected, inhaled ('snorted'). The pure form of methamphetamine called 'ice' can be smoked or injected.
- Mechanism of action: blocks reuptake of noradrenaline and dopamine. Note that amphetamines are used in the treatment of narcolepsy (see Chapter 12) and hyperactivity disorders (see Chapter 13).
- Effects: over-activity, talkativeness, insomnia, anorexia, dry lips, mouth, and nose (frequent lip licking), pupil dilatation (mydriasis), tachycardia, hypertension, hyperthermia. Adverse effects include dysphoria, anxiety, irritability, insomnia, and confusion. Prolonged use in high doses may lead to stereotyped repetitive behaviour and paranoid psychosis that is almost impossible to differentiate from schizophrenia.
- Overdose: cardiac arrhythmias, severe hypertension, stroke, circulatory collapse, seizures, coma.
- Withdrawal syndrome: dysphoria and decreased energy, and sometimes depression, anxiety, fatigue, and nightmares. There may be intense craving and suicidal ideation.
- Management: cognitive-behavioural therapy, treat comorbid psychiatric illness. In acute intoxication consider benzodiazepines and antipsychotics to treat symptoms. Treat complications.

Ecstasy (3,4 methylenedioxy-methamphetamine or MDMA)

- Related compounds: amphetamines.
- Routes of administration: oral.
- Mechanism of action: increases serotonergic, dopaminergic, and noradrenergic neurotransmission. High lasts 4–6 hours.
- Effects: euphoria, sociability, intimacy, heightened perceptions, loss of appetite, nausea, tachycardia, hypertension, hyperthermia, sweating, dehydration, teeth grinding (bruxism).
- Overdose: still unclear, but similar to amphetamines.

- Withdrawal syndrome: dysphoria and fatigue ('coming down'), which limits abuse potential.
- Management: education to avoid hyperthermia by replacing fluids and taking breaks from dancing (ecstasy is typically used in nightclubs or at rave parties).

Lysergic acid diethylamide (LSD)

- Related compounds: other synthetic hallucinogens include dimethyltryptamine and ecstasy. Naturally occurring hallucinogens include psilocybin (magic or psychedelic mushrooms) and mescaline (peyote cactus). In the UK the Drugs Bill 2005 made psychedelic mushrooms a class A drug.
- Route of administration: oral.
- Mechanism of action: partial agonism at serotonin $5-HT_{2A}$ receptors.
- Effects: pupil dilatation, tachycardia, hypertension, mood changes (euphoria, distress, or anxiety), distortion or intensification of sensory experience, synaesthesia (cross-referencing of the senses, e.g. seeing sounds, hearing colours), and in some cases distortion of body image. Psychological effects last from 8 to 14 hours. 'Bad trips' occur if the user is not relaxed, e.g. if he or she has had a recent argument or is feeling resentful, or if the setting is overly stimulating.
- Overdose: overdose is rare but may result in nausea and vomiting, autonomic overactivity, hyperthermia, coma, and respiratory arrest.
- Withdrawal syndrome: a withdrawal syndrome has not been described, although a minority of users experience disturbing flashbacks. Tolerance can occur but dependence is rare.
- Management: consider benzodiazepines for acute intoxication and for distressing flashbacks.

Cannabis

- Related compounds: cannabis derives from the hemp plant *Cannabis sativa* and refers to marijuana ('grass'), sinsemilla, hashish, or hash oil. The main active chemical in cannabis is Δ9-tetrahydrocannabinol.
- Route of administration: usually smoked but can also be eaten or drunk as an infusion.
- Mechanism of action: acts on a specific cannabinoid receptor in the CNS. The endogenous ligand for this receptor is anandamide.
- Effects: variable according to dose and circumstances; the pre-existing mood tends to be exaggerated. The effects include heightened aesthetic experiences, altered perception of time and space, impaired short-term memory, attention, and motor skills, reddening of the eyes, irritation of the respiratory tract, dry mouth, and tachycardia. Adverse effects include anxiety, paranoid ideation, gynaecomastia, reduced spermatogenesis, and carcinoma of the bronchus. **Cannabis use has been linked with an increased risk of psychotic disorders, conferring an approximate two-fold increase in an individual's relative risk of subsequently developing schizophrenia.** No direct mechanism for this link has been identified.
- Overdose: higher doses may lead to confusion and psychosis.
- Withdrawal syndrome: mild and short-lived symptoms of restlessness, irritability, nausea, anorexia, and insomnia. Tolerance and dependence can occur but are both uncommon.
- Management is aimed at reducing use and promoting abstinence. Advise users not to drive or to operate machinery.

Benzodiazepines

- Related compounds: other sedatives/hypnotics that are often misused include chlormethiazole, chloral, and barbiturates.
- Routes of administration: oral, injected.
- Mechanism of action: benzodiazepines act at the $GABA_A$–BDZ receptor complex to enhance the inhibitory action of GABA.
- Effects: benzodiazepines have anxiolytic, hypnotic, anticonvulsant, muscle relaxant, and amnesic properties. Tolerance develops rapidly. Dependence is common: about one-third of patients taking benzodiazepines for more than six months develop dependence.
- Overdose: oversedation, coma, death. Additive effects with other drugs, including opiates and alcohol.
- Withdrawal syndrome: anxiety, irritability, tremor, disturbed sleep, altered perception and, rarely, depression, psychosis, seizures, and *delirium tremens*. In some cases the withdrawal syndrome may be prolonged for several months.
- Management:
  - Overdose: flumazenil
  - Detoxification: switch from benzodiazepines with a short half-life to benzodiazepines with a long half-life (e.g. diazepam) and taper off over a period of several weeks or months

11

– Prevention: iatrogenic dependence is the commonest form of benzodiazepine dependence, so restrict the use of these drugs and prescribe them for short-term use only
– Advise users not to drive or to operate machinery.

Volatile substances

- Related compounds: household products such as spray paint, permanent markers, correction fluid, glue, lighter fluid, hairspray, and petrol-containing volatile substances such as toluene, ethyl acetate, butane, and propane, amongst others.
- Routes of administration: inhalation ('huffing').
- Mechanism of action: increases GABA-ergic neurotransmission.
- Effects: similar to those of alcohol, but more rapid onset. Euphoria, disorientation, nausea, vomiting, blurring of vision, slurring of speech, incoordination, staggering gait, hallucinations. Adverse effects include cardiac arrhythmias and respiratory depression leading to sudden death. There is a high risk of trauma, asphyxia, and aspiration pneumonia. Chronic misuse may lead to organ damage, peripheral neuropathy, and CNS neurotoxicity.

- Overdose: as above, including coma and death.
- Withdrawal syndrome: although dependence can develop, withdrawal symptoms are unusual.
- Management aims at early detection and the promotion of abstinence.

Recommended reading

A Million Little Pieces (2004) James Frey. John Murray.
Street Drugs (1995) Andrew Tyler. Coronet Books.
Forbidden Drugs: Understanding Drugs and Why People Take Them (1999) Philip Robson. Oxford University Press.
Working with Substance Misusers: A Guide to Theory and Practice (2002) Trudi Peterson and Andrew McBride (eds). Routledge (imprint of Taylor & Francis).

Summary

Alcohol misuse

- The recommended daily limits for alcohol consumption are 3–4 units a day in males and 2–3 units a day in females – a unit is about 8 g of alcohol, equivalent to half a pint of ordinary beer.
- In the UK the prevalence of alcohol dependence is about 7% in males and 2% in females, but these figures mask higher rates of harmful drinking and hazardous drinking.
- The seven key features of alcohol dependence are:
  1. Compulsion to drink
  2. Primacy of drinking over other activities
  3. Stereotyped pattern of drinking
  4. Increased tolerance to alcohol
  5. Repeated withdrawal symptoms
  6. Relief drinking to avoid withdrawal symptoms
  7. Reinstatement after abstinence
- Withdrawal symptoms usually occur after several years of heavy drinking and range from mild anxiety and sleep disturbance to life-threatening *delirium tremens*.
- *Delirium tremens* is a delirious disorder characterised by fear, agitation, and restlessness, coarse tremor, nausea and vomiting, seizures, vivid hallucinations and delusions, insomnia, autonomic disturbances, and dehydration and electrolyte imbalances. The untreated mortality rate is about 5%.

- Wernicke's encephalopathy is a disorder of acute onset characterised by impaired consciousness and confusion, episodic memory impairment, ataxia, nystagmus, abducens and conjugate gaze palsies, pupillary abnormalities, and peripheral neuropathy. Wernicke's encephalopathy often progresses to Korsakov's psychosis, a long-term syndrome characterised by severe memory impairment and confabulation.
- Early treatment of alcohol misuse is often delivered in primary care and involves simple advice and support, and appraisal of current medical, psychological, and social problems.
- Psychological interventions include attendance at groups run by local community alcohol services or Alcoholics Anonymous, supportive psychotherapy (including for carers), cognitive-behavioural therapy, and marital and family therapy.
- After detoxification, only 20–50% of patients remain abstinent at one year. Predictors of relapse include poor motivation, lack of social support, and comorbid psychiatric illness.

Continued...

11

Drug misuse

- According to the 2001–02 British Crime Survey, 26% of 16–29 year olds in England had used illicit drugs in the previous year, and 5.1% had used heroin, methadone, cocaine, or crack.
- Social factors such as the availability of the drug and attitudes to drug taking in the peer group increase the likelihood of experimentation. About 10% of experimenters go on to develop problems, usually at a young age.
- Drug misuse is reinforced by sought-after effects such as euphoria. These effects are mediated by the midbrain dopamine system that projects from the ventral tegmental area to the forebrain, including the *nucleus accumbens* (the so-called 'craving centre').
- Drug misuse in general can lead to a number of medical, psychiatric, and social complications. Intravenous drug use carries a risk of local complications such as infection of the injection site and venous thrombosis, and systemic complications such as bacterial endocarditis, hepatitis B and C, and HIV. Drug misuse in early pregnancy can lead to foetal abnormalities, and in late pregnancy to dependence in the foetus. Psychiatric illness is common, especially depressive disorders, anxiety disorders, and personality disorders, and is often precipitated and/or perpetuated by drug misuse. An inability to fulfil social obligations results in unemployment, marital problems, and neglect of children. Other social consequences include motoring offences, accidents, and criminal activity.

Self-assessment

Simply answer with true or false. Answers on p. 219.

1. The recommended daily limits for alcohol consumption are 2–3 units a day in males.
2. A unit is about 12 g of alcohol, equivalent to half a pint of ordinary beer.
3. In alcohol dependence there is a compensatory upregulation of GABA to compensate for the CNS depressant effects of alcohol.
4. The average level of alcohol consumption in a population is influenced by three principal factors: price, availability, and social attitudes to alcohol.
5. Alcohol withdrawal symptoms are more likely to occur last thing before going to bed.
6. Wernicke's encephalopathy is a delirious disorder characterised by fear, agitation and restlessness, coarse tremor, nausea and vomiting, seizures, vivid hallucinations and delusions, insomnia, autonomic disturbances (tachycardia, hypertension, hyperthermia, sweating, dilated pupils), and dehydration and electrolyte imbalances.
7. Wernicke's encephalopathy results from a deficiency in vitamin B_{12}, most commonly secondary to alcohol dependence, and can therefore be prevented by vitamin B_{12} supplementation.
8. Korsakov's psychosis is a long-term syndrome characterised by severe memory impairment and confabulation. It is a misnomer in that it does not actually involve psychosis.
9. Gamma-glutamyltransferase (GGT) has the highest specificity for alcohol misuse, but is only raised in about 50% of cases.
10. An example of a detoxification regimen is chlordiazepoxide 20 mg QDS reducing daily over 7 days supplemented by thiamine 200 mg OD (usually in the form of a multivitamin preparation).
11. After detoxification, controlled drinking has a better prognosis than total abstention.
12. Disulfiram is an 'anticraving' drug that enhances GABA and therefore mimics the CNS depressant effects of alcohol.
13. Disulfiram is contraindicated in hypertension, coronary artery disease, and cardiac failure as it can cause cardiac arrhythmias.
14. Morphine and heroin are relatively selective for the δ-opioid receptor subtype.
15. Effects of opioids include euphoria, analgesia, constipation, anorexia, loss of libido, pruritus, and dilated pupils.
16. Recognised effects of amphetamines include over-activity, talkativeness, insomnia, anorexia, dry lips, mouth and nose (frequent lip licking), constricted pupils, tachycardia, hypertension, and hyperthermia.
17. Prolonged use of high doses of amphetamines may lead to stereotyped repetitive behaviour and paranoid psychosis.
18. Speed refers to a mixture of cocaine and heroin.
19. Cannabis use has not been linked with an increased risk of psychotic disorders.
20. Users of ecstasy should be educated to avoid hyperthermia by replacing fluids and taking breaks from dancing.

11

Eating, sleep, and sexual disorders

12

Key learning objectives

- Epidemiological and aetiological factors in anorexia and bulimia
- Clinical features and complications in anorexia and bulimia
- Management of eating disorders

- Definition of primary and secondary sleep disorders
- Causes of insomnia
- Principles of good sleep hygiene
- Assessment and management of sexual dysfunction

Eating disorders

Anorexia nervosa

Epidemiology

Anorexia nervosa is more common in females than in males by a ratio of more than 10:1. It is also more common in middle to upper socioeconomic groups, models, gymnasts, and dancers. The average age of onset is 15–16 years, and onset is rare after the age of 30 years. Interestingly, anorexia nervosa is far more common in occidental or occidentalised societies, in which the prevalence rate in adolescent females is about 1%. The disorder appears to be strongly related to occidental values such as individualism and the idealisation of thinness and 'beauty', for which reason it is sometimes considered to be a culture-bound syndrome (see Chapter 7).

Aetiology

The various aetiological factors in anorexia nervosa are summarised in Table 12.1. From a psychodynamic point

Psychiatry, 2e. By Neel Burton. Published 2010 by Blackwell Publishing.

of view, anorexia nervosa has sometimes been considered as a struggle for control and identity, or as a form of escape from the emotional problems of adolescence.

> *Addiction, obesity, starvation (anorexia nervosa) are political problems, not psychiatric: each condenses and expresses a contest between the individual and some other person and persons in his environment over the control of the individual's body.*
>
> Thomas Szasz

Clinical features and complications

DSM-IV diagnostic criteria for anorexia nervosa are:
A. Refusal to maintain normal body weight at more than 85% of expected body weight
B. Intense fear of gaining weight or becoming fat
C. Disturbed perception of body weight or shape
D. In postmenarchal females, amenorrhoea for at least three consecutive cycles (if not on the oral contraceptive pill).

DSM-IV specifies two types of anorexia nervosa: 'binge-eating/purging type' and 'restricting type'. In the

Table 12.1 Aetiological factors in anorexia nervosa.

	Biological	Psychological	Social
Precipitating factors			• Stressors such as failing an exam or changing schools
Predisposing factors	• Family history of eating disorder, mood disorder, or substance misuse • Chromosome 1p has been implicated in eating disorder susceptibility	• Altered body image characterised by a perception of fatness • Poor self-esteem, undue compliance, extreme perfectionism • Personality disorder, especially cluster C personality disorder • Premorbid anxiety and depressive disorder	• Pressure to diet in a society that emphasises individualism and idealises thinness and its concept of beauty • Family environment characterised by overprotection, rigidity, and lack of confliction resolution
Perpetuating factors	• Starvation leads to neuroendocrine changes that perpetuate anorexia		As above

binge-eating/purging type there is regular engagement in binge-eating and purging behaviour such as self-induced vomiting or the misuse of laxatives, diuretics, or enemas. In the restricting type there is no regular engagement in binge-eating or purging behaviour.

ICD-10 criteria are very similar to those of DSM-IV, but also specify delayed or arrested puberty in anorexia nervosa of prepubertal onset.

Figure 12.1 summarises the medical complications of anorexia nervosa.

Differential diagnosis

The differential diagnosis of anorexia nervosa is, firstly, from other psychiatric disorders – in particular, bulimia nervosa, body dysmorphic disorder, depressive disorder, obsessive–compulsive disorder, social phobia, conversion disorder, schizophrenia, and personality disorder. It is, secondly, from medical conditions – in particular, from endocrine disorders such as diabetes mellitus, diabetic ketoacidosis, hyperthyroidism, Graves' disease and Addison's disease; from gastrointestinal disorders such as gastroenteritis, inflammatory bowel disease, malabsorption and intestinal obstruction; and from other medical disorders such as chronic renal failure, chronic anaemia, chronic infections, neoplasms, and pregnancy.

Investigations

After the psychiatric history and mental state examination, a physical examination should be carried out to ascertain the degree of emaciation, to look for complications (see Figure 12.1), and to exclude other causes for the patient's symptoms (see above). Laboratory investigations to consider include FBC, U&Es, calcium, LFTs, TFTs, blood glucose, ESR, pregnancy test, urine drug screen, urinalysis, and faecal occult blood tests. Other investigations to consider include ECG, CXR, and AXR.

Management

- Educate the patient and family about the disorder and its treatment. In particular, carers should understand the need to be firm but supportive.
- Support the patient and alter disturbed perceptions of the body. Consider supportive psychotherapy and support groups, cognitive-behavioural therapy, and family therapy.
- Encourage refeeding. Establish a good therapeutic relationship with the patient and negotiate a realistic treatment plan. Aim for a balanced diet of about 3000 kcal a day provided as small meals and supplementary snacks.
- Monitor the patient's physical condition and treat any complications.
- Treat any associated psychiatric disorders.
- Consider hospitalisation in severe or intractable cases, especially if there are medical complications, associated psychiatric disorders, and/or poor social support. Day treatment may be an acceptable alternative to hospitalisation. If there is threat to life, compulsory admission and treatment may be necessary.

12

Metabolic:
Dehydration, hypoglycaemia, impaired glucose tolerance, hypoproteinaemia, hypokalaemia, hyponatraemia, hypocalcaemia, vitamin defiencies, hypercholesterolaemia, deranged LFTs

Endocrine:
- Decreased gonadotrophins, oestrogens, and testosterone leading to amenorrhoea in females and to loss of libido and impotence in males
- Increased GH and cortisol
- Decreased triiodothyronine

Cardiovascular:
- ECG abnormalities and arrhythmias
- Hypotension, bradycardia, peripheral oedema, congestive cardiac failure
- Mitral valve prolapse

Gastrointestinal:
- Parotid enlargement and erosion of tooth enamel from self-induced vomiting
- Delayed gastric emptying, constipation
- Peptic ulceration
- Acute pancreatitis

Renal:
Renal failure, partial diabetes insipidus, renal calculi

Neurological:
Enlarged ventricles, seizures, peripheral neuropathy, autonomic dysfunction

Haematological:
Iron-deficiency anaemia, leucopaenia, thrombocytopaenia

Musculoskeletal:
Osteoporosis, muscle cramps

Other:
Hypothermia, infections, dry skin, brittle hair and nails, lanugo hairs

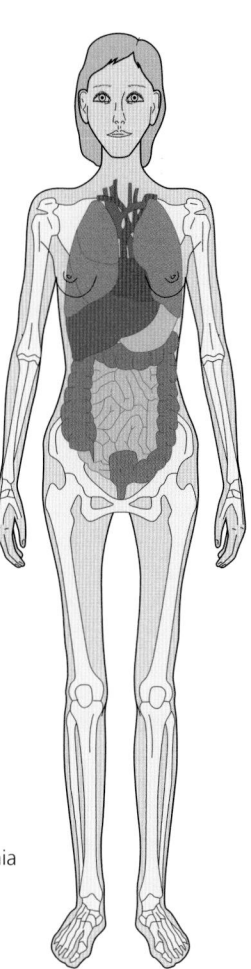

Figure 12.1 Medical complications of anorexia nervosa.

! Compulsory admission and treatment for anorexia nervosa (including force feeding) is sometimes possible under the Mental Health Act, but controversial because the patient's cognitive abilities may otherwise be fully intact and therefore he may not lack capacity in the legal sense. Furthermore, compulsory admission and treatment may serve to undermine the therapeutic relationship and further alienate the patient.

Prognosis

Prognosis is very variable, and a younger age of onset and a short history are important positive prognostic factors. One-fifth of sufferers recover completely but another fifth experience chronic, severe illness. The remainder make a recovery of sorts but retain abnormal eating habits and sometimes become bulimic. The long-term mortality from suicide and from the complications of starvation is about 15%, **higher than for any other mental disorder**.

12

Bulimia nervosa

Epidemiology

Bulimia nervosa is more common in females than in males by a ratio of about 10:1. It is also commoner in models, gymnasts, dancers, and male homosexuals. The typical age of onset is in teenagehood and the early 20s, and the disorder affects 1–3% of females in these age groups. Like anorexia nervosa, bulimia nervosa is far more common in occidental or occidentalised societies that promote individuality and idealise thinness and beauty. Many bulimia sufferers also have a history of anorexia nervosa.

Aetiology

There appears to be a dysfunction in the serotonin neurotransmitter system and other neurological and endocrine abnormalities. Generally speaking, aetiological factors are very similar to those involved in anorexia nervosa, and genetic factors play a similarly important role. Obesity is common and there may be a history of affective disorders, personality disorders, anxiety disorders, substance misuse, physical abuse, or childhood sexual abuse. There may also be a family history of obesity or psychiatric disorder.

Clinical features and complications

Bulimia nervosa was first described by the British psychiatrist Gerald Russell in 1979, and derives its name from the Greek *bous* (ox) and *limos* (hunger). It is characterised by recurrent episodes of binge-eating followed by attempts to counteract the 'fattening' effect of the food by such methods as prolonged fasting, excessive exercise, self-induced vomiting, laxative or diuretic misuse, and stimulant drug misuse. Unlike in anorexia nervosa, the patient is usually of normal weight.

DSM-IV diagnostic criteria for bulimia nervosa are:

A. Recurrent episodes of binge eating
B. Recurrent inappropriate compensatory behaviour to prevent weight gain
C. Episodes of binge eating and compensatory behaviour **occur at least twice a week for a period of three months**
D. Self-evaluation is unduly influenced by body shape and weight
E. The disturbance does not occur exclusively during periods of anorexia nervosa.

DSM-IV specifies two types of bulimia nervosa: 'purging type' and 'non-purging type'. In the non-purging type there is regular engagement in compensatory behaviours such as fasting and regular exercise, but no regular engagement in self-induced vomiting or misuse of laxatives, diuretics, or enemas; in the purging type there is also regular engagement in self-induced vomiting or misuse of laxatives, diuretics, or enemas. If there are no compensatory behaviours at all, the diagnosis is not one of bulimia nervosa but of **binge-eating disorder**.

The onset of bulimia nervosa is typically preceded by a period of dietary restriction. The patient often complains of fatigue, bloating, flatulence, constipation, abdominal pain, and menstrual irregularities. Depressive symptoms are more prominent than in anorexia nervosa, and a high proportion of patients also meet the criteria for depressive disorder.

Other clinical features and complications of bulimia nervosa include:

- From purging behaviour: dehydration, malnutrition, oedema, electrolyte abnormalities, cardiac arrhythmias, renal failure, urinary tract infection, muscle paralysis, tetany, seizures
- From induced vomiting specifically: dental erosion, enlargement of the parotid glands ('chipmunk facies'), oesophagitis, oesophageal tears, aspiration pneumonia. The Russell sign, named after Gerald Russell, refers to callosities, scarring, and abrasions on the dorsal surface of the index and long finger that form as a result of repeated self-induced vomiting
- Drug side-effects and overdose.

Differential diagnosis

- Anorexia nervosa
- Binge eating disorder
- Body dysmorphic disorder
- Obesity
- Depressive disorder
- Obsessive–compulsive disorder
- Personality disorder
- Medical disorders such as diabetic ketoacidosis or intestinal obstruction

Investigations

After the psychiatric history and mental state examination, a physical examination should be carried out to look for complications and to exclude other causes for the patient's symptoms. Laboratory investigations to consider include FBC, U&Es, calcium, blood glucose, preg-

12

nancy test, drug screen, and urinalysis. Other investigations to consider include ECG, CXR, and AXR.

Management

- Educate the patient and family about the disorder and its treatment.
- Support the patient and alter disturbed perceptions of the self. Consider supportive psychotherapy and support groups, cognitive–behavioural therapy, interpersonal therapy, and family therapy.
- Serotonin-selective reuptake inhibitors (SSRIs) have been demonstrated to have a specific antibulimic effect at higher doses, so consider prescribing an SSRI such as fluoxetine or sertraline.
- Monitor the patient's physical condition and treat any complications.
- Treat associated psychiatric disorders.
- Consider hospitalisation in severe or intractable cases, especially if there are medical complications or associated psychiatric disorders, or if the patient has poor social support.
- Prognosis is better than in anorexia nervosa, not least because bulimia sufferers are keener to seek and accept help.

Sleep disorders

Methought I heard a voice cry 'Sleep no more!
Macbeth does murder sleep', the innocent sleep,
Sleep that knits up the ravell'd sleeve of care,
The death of each day's life, sore labour's bath,
Balm of hurt minds, great nature's second course,
Chief nourisher in life's feast,

Shakespeare, *Macbeth*, Act II, Scene ii

Introduction and classification

Sleep disorders are very often related to other psychiatric disorders or to general medical conditions. Such 'secondary' sleep disorders should be distinguished from 'primary' sleep disorders on the basis of their

---

> **ICD-10 classification of primary sleep disorders**
>
> **F51** Non-organic sleep disorders
> | | F51.0 | Non-organic insomnia |
> | --- | --- | --- |
> | | F51.1 | Non-organic hypersomnia |
> | | F51.2 | Non-organic disorder of the sleep–wake schedule |
> | | F51.3 | Sleep-walking (somnambulism) |
> | | F51.4 | Sleep terrors (night terrors) |
> | | F51.4 | Nightmares |
> | | F51.8 | Other non-organic sleep disorders |

---

clinical presentation and course. Primary sleep disorders, the subject of this section, can be divided into dysomnias (insomnia and hypersomnia), disorders of the sleep–wake schedule (sleep delay, jet lag, and narcolepsy) and parasomnias (nightmares, night terrors, and somnambulism).

Dysomnias

Insomnia

Insomnia – difficulty in initiating or maintaining sleep – affects 30% of the population, and is more common in females and in the elderly. **It only becomes clinically significant if it causes distress or daytime effects (fatigue, poor concentration, poor memory, irritability), and should only be diagnosed if it dominates the clinical picture.**

Insomnia results from a variety of biological, psychological, physical, and environmental factors. Short-term insomnia more often results from a stressful life event or a poor sleep environment, and chronic insomnia from psychiatric and medical disorders and drug side-effects (Tables 12.2 and 12.3).

In assessing insomnia, it is important to take a detailed history and to enquire about sleep hygiene and the sleep environment. As part of the history, aim to cover the sleep disturbance and its daytime effects, as well as the psychiatric history, medical history, drug history, and social history. An informant history from the bed-partner may be especially useful. A clearer picture can be obtained by asking the patient to hold a sleep diary or, less commonly, by carrying out sleep studies (polysomnography).

12

Table 12.2 Psychiatric and medical disorders that can cause insomnia. (NB: This list is non-exhaustive.)

Psychiatric disorders	Medical disorders
Depressive disorder	Restless leg syndrome
Mania and bipolar affective disorder	Sleep apnoea (pauses in breathing during sleep)
Anxiety disorders	Chronic pain, e.g. from arthritis or cancer
Post-traumatic stress disorder	Chronic obstructive pulmonary disease
Schizophrenia	Chronic renal failure
Alcohol and drug misuse	Neurological disorders such as Parkinson's disease and other movement disorders
Chronic fatigue syndrome	
	Headaches
	Fibromyalgia

Table 12.3 Drugs that can cause insomnia. (NB: This list is non-exhaustive.)

- Benzodiazepines
- Alcohol*
- Stimulants such as caffeine, amphetamines, and cocaine
- Nicotine
- Serotonin-selective reuptake inhibitors
- Levodopa
- Phenytoin
- Beta-blockers
- Diuretics
- Theophylline
- Corticosteroids
- Thyroid hormone

* Note that alcohol may make it easier to fall asleep, but makes it more difficult to *remain* asleep, and also decreases the overall quality of sleep.

Management involves treatment of the cause (if any), advice on sleep hygiene (see clinical skills box), and behavioural strategies such as sleep restriction. Sedatives may be effective in the short-term but are best avoided in the longer term. Even if they are used, they should only play a minor role in overall management. Over-the-counter sleeping remedies often contain an antihistamine, whilst herbal alternatives are usually based on the herb valerian, a hardy perennial flowing plant with heads of sweetly scented pink or white flowers.

Clinical skills: Advice for patients with insomnia

- Have a strict routine involving regular and adequate sleeping times. Allocate a time for sleeping, e.g. 11 pm to 7 am, and do not use this time for any other activities. Avoid daytime naps, or make them short and regular. If you have a bad night, avoid 'sleeping in'.
- Have a relaxing bedtime routine that enables you to relax and 'wind down' before bedtime. This may involve doing breathing exercises or meditation or simply reading a book, listening to music, or watching TV.
- Many people find it helpful to have a hot drink: a herbal or malted or chocolate drink should be preferred to stimulant drinks such as tea or coffee.
- Sleep in a familiar, dark, and quiet room that is adequately ventilated and neither too hot nor too cold. Try to use this room for sleeping only, so that you come to associate it with sleeping.
- If you can't sleep, don't become anxious and try to force yourself to sleep. The more anxious you become, the less likely you are to fall asleep, and this is only likely to make you more anxious! Instead, get up and do something relaxing and enjoyable for about half an hour, and then try again.
- Take regular exercise during the daytime, but do not exercise in the evening or just before bedtime because the short-term alerting effects of exercise may make it more difficult for you to fall asleep.
- Eat an adequate evening meal containing a good balance of complex carbohydrates and protein. Eating too much can make it difficult to fall asleep; eating too little can disturb your sleep and decrease its quality.
- Avoid caffeine, alcohol, and tobacco, particularly in the evening. Also avoid stimulant drugs such as cocaine, amphetamines, and ecstasy. Alcohol may make you fall asleep more easily, but it decreases the quality of your sleep.

Adapted from *Master your Mind* (2009), by Neel Burton

Hypersomnia

In hypersomnia, patients complain of excessive daytime sleepiness, sleep attacks, or sleep drunkenness. **For a diagnosis of primary hypersomnia to be made these symptoms should not be better accounted for by a lack of sleep or by another sleep disorder or psychiatric or medical disorder, and should result in significant distress or impairment of functioning.** The condition often

Table 12.4 Causes of secondary hypersomnia.

Other sleep disorders	Insomnia
	Sleep apnoea
	Narcolepsy
Psychiatric disorders	Dysthymia
	Depressive disorder
	Bipolar affective disorder
	Neurasthenia (chronic fatigue syndrome)
Medical disorders	Chronic pain
	Urinary tract infection
	Brain tumour, etc
Drugs	
Other	E.g. head trauma, viral infection

responds to small doses of CNS stimulant drugs. The principal causes of secondary hypersomnia are listed in Table 12.4.

Kleine–Levin syndrome

Kleine–Levin syndrome is a rare, recurrent primary hypersomnia associated with behavioural and cognitive disturbances, overeating, and/or hypersexuality. Episodes last for days or weeks and are interspersed by long periods of normality. The condition most often presents in adolescent males and resolves in early adult life. Its aetiology is unclear.

Narcolepsy

Narcolepsy (Ancient Greek, 'seized by somnolence') is a relatively rare disorder that has its onset in adolescence or early adulthood, and results from a disruption in the pattern of rapid-eye-movement (REM) and non-REM sleep. Clinical features include daytime somnolence and sleep attacks, cataplexy (sudden loss of muscle tone), sleep paralysis, and hypnagogic hallucinations, although not all of these features need be present for a confident diagnosis to be made. Of Caucasian patients affected by narcolepsy, 85–98% are HLA-DR2 positive. The principal differential diagnosis is from hypersomnia and epilepsy, notably *petit mal* absence seizures. Management involves support and counselling (e.g. advice on the importance of sleep hygiene and daytime naps), and use of drugs including CNS stimulants such as methylphenidate, modafinil, and antidepressants.

Disorders of the sleep–wake schedule

Disorders of the sleep-wake schedule include sleep delay and jet lag.

In **sleep delay** there is chronic difficulty initiating sleep at socially accepted times, although once asleep there is no difficulty in maintaining sleep and total sleep time is normal. The disorder is commonest in adolescents and university students and tends not to present to medical attention. The differential diagnosis is from life-style choice, insomnia, and psychiatric and medical disorders.

Jet lag tends to be experienced after crossing three or more time zones, and results from a mismatch between body rhythms and environmental rhythms. Symptoms include disturbed sleep, tiredness, poor concentration, and irritability. The rate of adjustment to jet lag is 1.5 hours per day after a westward flight and 1 hour per day after an eastward flight. Management should aim at matching body rhythms and environmental rhythms (see clinical skills box). Melatonin has been reported to be effective in some cases in the prophylaxis and treatment of jet lag.

> **Clinical skills: Advice for patients at risk of jet lag**
>
> - If you are able to, choose a destination that involves flying westwards: evidence suggests that flying westwards causes less jetlag than flying eastwards.
> - Choose daytime flights to avoid losing sleep.
> - Use sleeping aids such as blindfolds, earplugs, and neck rests to help you sleep during the flight.
> - Before your departure, gradually adjust your sleep schedule so that it approximates to that at your destination. For example, if you are going to be flying eastwards, try to go to bed (and to wake up) earlier than you usually do.
> - When you arrive, immediately reset your watch and time givers to local time.
> - Do as the locals do in terms of eating and sleeping. Have your meals when they do and try not to have more than one short nap during the daytime.
> - Take exercise.
> - Avoid caffeine and alcohol.
> - Avoid sleeping tablets.

12

Parasomnias

Parasomnias are abnormal episodic events during sleep and include nightmares, night terrors, and somnambulism (sleep walking) (Table 12.5). They are part of normal development in children, but in adults they usually arise during times of stress. Important differentials are epilepsy, substance misuse, and psychiatric and medical disorders (e.g. anxiety disorders, post-traumatic stress disorder).

Sexual disorders

Sexual dysfunction

Sexual dysfunction can occur at any stage of sexual intercourse: initiation, arousal, penetration, and orgasm (Table 12.6). It can result from organic causes (such as diabetes, angina, prostate surgery, antihypertensives, antidepressants, antipsychotics) or from psychological

Table 12.5 Parasomnias.

Type	Incidence	Onset	Sleep stage	Behaviour	Recall	Treatment
Nightmares	Very frequent in children	Late in sleep	REM	Easily rousable, awareness	Usual	Support
Night terrors	3% of children, commonest in ages 4–7 There is often a family history	First 1–2 hours of sleep	Non-REM stage 4	Terrified, screaming, thrashing Cannot easily be aroused May last 10–20 minutes	None	Reassurance and practical advice for parents Behavioural waking schedule if persistent
Somnambulism	1–15% of 8–15 year olds, but also seen in adults Associated with night terrors	First 1–2 hours of sleep	Non-REM stage 4	May last minutes to one hour	None	Safety precautions Avoid sleep deprivation and alcohol

Jacob's dream and the significance of dreams

And Jacob went out from Beersheba, and went toward Haran.

And he lighted upon a certain place, and tarried there all night, because the sun was set; and he took of the stones of that place, and put them for his pillows, and lay down in that place to sleep.

And he dreamed, and behold a ladder set up on the earth, and the top of it reached to heaven: and behold the angels of God ascending and descending on it.

And, behold, the LORD stood above it, and said, I am the LORD God of Abraham thy father, and the God of Isaac: the land whereon thou liest, to thee will I give it, and to thy seed;

And thy seed shall be as the dust of the earth, and thou shalt spread abroad to the west, and to the east, and to the north, and to the south: and in thee and in thy seed shall all the families of the earth be blessed.

And, behold, I am with thee, and will keep thee in all places whither thou goest, and will bring thee again into this land;

for I will not leave thee, until I have done that which I have spoken to thee of.

And Jacob awaked out of his sleep, and he said, Surely the LORD is in this place; and I knew it not.

Genesis 28:10–16 (KJV)

Though dreams contribute to the self-regulation of the psyche by automatically bringing up everything that is repressed or neglected or unknown, their compensatory significance is often not immediately apparent because we still have only a very incomplete knowledge of the nature and the needs of the human psyche. There are psychological compensations that seem to be very remote from the problem on hand. In these cases one must always remember that every man, in a sense, represents the whole of humanity and its history. What was possible in the history of mankind at large is also possible on a small scale in every individual. What mankind has needed may eventually be needed by the individual too.

C. G. Jung, *General Aspects of Dream Psychology* (1916)

Figure 12.2 Freud called dreams the 'royal road to the unconscious'. Photo by Neel Burton.

Table 12.6 Types of sexual dysfunction (common types are in bold).

Type of sexual dysfunction	Male	Female
Sexual desire disorders	Hypoactive sexual desire Sexual aversion (rare)	**Hypoactive sexual desire** (F > M) Sexual aversion (rare)
Sexual arousal disorders	**Erectile dysfunction***	Failure of genital response
Sexual pain disorders	Dyspareunia	Dyspareunia (F > M)
Orgasm disorders	Ejaculatory impotence **Premature ejaculation****	Vaginismus§ **Anorgasmia** (F > M)

* Erectile dysfunction or impotence is more common in elderly males.
** Premature ejaculation is more common in young males engaging in their first sexual relationships.
§ Vaginismus describes involuntary vaginal contractions in response to attempts at penetration.

causes (such as depression, anxiety, sexual inexperience, traumatic sexual experience, relationship difficulties, stress), or from a combination of either. In secondary dysfunction there is a history of normal function, but in primary dysfunction such a history is lacking. The epidemiology of sexual dysfunction is difficult to establish, but erectile dysfunction and premature ejaculation are common in males, and anorgasmia and hypoactive sexual desire are common in females.

The sexual history is often omitted by embarrassed students, but is nevertheless an important part of the psychiatric history. This is not only because sexual problems are important *per se*, but also because they frequently result from psychiatric disorders and/or their medical treatments, and are themselves aetiological factors for psychiatric disorders. In the author's experience, the sexual history is best taken by direct but tactful questioning at or near the end of the psychiatric history. Remain professional and formal throughout, but do not persist in your questioning if the patient becomes uncomfortable.

12

12

Clinical skills/OSCE: Taking a sexual history

Presenting complaint

Ask about:

- The presenting problem (in detail). Ask specifically about erectile dysfunction and ejaculatory dysfunction in males, and about hypoactive sexual desire, anorgasmia, vaginismus, and dyspareunia in females
- The onset, course, and duration of the problem. Is the problem primary or secondary?
- The frequency and timing of the problem. Is the problem partial or situational? In situational erectile dysfunction the patient is still able to hold morning erections
- The effect that the problem is having on the patient's life.

Sexual history

If not already covered, ask about:

- Number of partners and nature and quality of relationships
- Frequency of sex
- Type of sex
- Sexual preferences and paraphilias (see later)
- Contraceptive methods
- Sexual development: age at puberty and first intercourse
- Sexual experience
- Attitudes to sex
- History of physical or sexual abuse (avoid suggestive questioning).

And also

Make sure you cover:

- The psychiatric history
- The medical history
- The drug history, including alcohol and illicit drugs

In sexual dysfunction resulting from an organic cause, treat the cause if at all possible. In sexual dysfunction resulting from psychological causes, treatment may involve simple reassurance and advice, sex therapy (Masters and Johnson techniques), and drugs and physical treatments.

In sex therapy the couple is usually seen together over a limited number of sessions and encouraged to discuss their sexual relationship openly. They are educated about sex and given a series of assignments to perform at home. These assignments progress from non-genital 'sensate focus technique' (that is, non-genital caressing) to full intercourse, and are designed to rebuild the couple's sexual relationship through the behavioural technique of graded exposure. In addition, specific exercises are taught for specific forms of dysfunction, such as Seman's technique for premature ejaculation (involves the partner squeezing the base of the penis as orgasm approaches so as to prevent ejaculation), and relaxation training and vaginal dilators for vaginismus. The outcome of sex therapy is generally good, except for disorders of sexual desire.

Drugs and physical treatments used in sexual dysfunction include phosphodiesterase type 5 inhibitors such as sildenafil (caution in heart disease), intracavernosal injections of alprostadil (prostaglandin E_1), testosterone replacement, vacuum erection devices, penile prosthetic implants, and penile microrevascularisation.

Paraphilias

Homo sum; humani nihil a me alienum puto.
(I am human, and consider nothing human to be alien to me.)

Terence (c.185–159BC), *Heauton Timorumenos*

In assessing sexual dysfunction, it is important to take a full sexual history (see clinical skills box), including details of the medical and psychiatric history. A physical examination emphasising the genitourinary, vascular, and neurological systems and some laboratory investigations may be required to exclude organic causes of sexual dysfunction. Laboratory investigations may include FBC, U&Es, glucose, LFTs, TFTs, urinalysis, and hormone levels.

Paraphilias are disorders of sexual preference that begin in late adolescence or early adulthood and most commonly affect males (Table 12.7). They are 'disorders' in that the principal object of sexual arousal or the principal method of achieving sexual arousal is abnormal (note that this circular definition is heavily values loaded). If there is a rapid change in sexual behaviour, particularly in middle or old age, it is important to exclude psychiatric disorders such as dementia, psychotic disorders, and affective disorders.

Table 12.7 Paraphilias.

Transvestism	Disturbance of gender role behaviour Transvestites intermittently or permanently assume the appearance, mannerisms, and interests of the opposite sex; unlike in transsexualism, there is no disturbance of core gender identity
Transsexualism	Transsexuals often describe themselves as being trapped inside a body of the opposite sex Not classified as a paraphilia but as a disturbance of core gender identity
Paedophilia	Sexually arousing fantasies, urges, or behaviours involving sexual activity with prepubescent children About 50% of victims of abuse are relatives or friends of the abuser
Exhibitionism	Sexually arousing fantasies, urges, or behaviours that involve exposing genitalia to unsuspecting strangers Offenders are typically young males and their victims, pubescent females
Voyeurism (scopophilia)	Sexually arousing fantasies, urges, or behaviours involving observing an unsuspecting person naked or undressing, or engaged in sexual activity
Frotteurism	Sexually arousing fantasies, urges, or behaviours involving rubbing against or touching a non-consenting person, typically in crowded places such as the Tube
Sexual sadism	Sexually arousing fantasies, urges, or behaviours involving humiliating, or causing suffering to, others (cf. sexual masochism). Sadism is named after the 18th century Marquis de Sade, author of *Justine ou les Malheurs de la Vertu* and other books. The film *Quills*, starring Geoffrey Rush, Kate Winslet, and Michael Caine is based on the story of his life
Sexual masochism	Sexually arousing fantasies, urges, or behaviours involving being humiliated or being made to suffer. Masochism is named after Leopold von Sacher–Masoch (1836–1895), author of *Venus in Furs*
Fetishism	Sexually arousing fantasies, urges, or behaviours involving non-living objects not limited to articles of clothing used in cross-dressing or to devices designated for genital stimulation
Other paraphilias	Incest (close relatives), zoophilia/bestiality (animals), necrophilia (dead bodies), coprophilia (faeces), urophilia (urine), klismaphilia (enemas), narratophilia (using obscene language), and telephone scatologia (making phone calls and using obscene language)
Homosexuality	Sexually arousing fantasies, urges, or behaviours involving sexual activity with members of the same sex to the exclusion of members of the opposite sex (this last clause differentiates homosexuality from bisexuality) Homosexuality is no longer classified as a paraphilia

How delightful are the pleasures of the imagination! In those delectable moments, the whole world is ours; not a single creature resists us, we devastate the world, we repopulate it with new objects which, in turn, we immolate. The means to every crime is ours, and we employ them all, we multiply the horror a hundredfold.

Marquis de Sade (1740–1814),
Belmor in *L'Histoire de Juliette, ou les Prospérités du Vice*

Man is the one who desires, woman the one who is desired. This is woman's entire but decisive advantage. Through man's passions, nature has given man into woman's hands, and the woman who does not know how to make him her subject, her slave, her toy, and how to betray him with a smile in the end is not wise.

Leopold von Sacher–Masoch (1836–1895),
Madame Venus in *Venus in Furs*

Recommended reading

Helping People with Eating Disorders: A Clinical Guide to Assessment and Treatment (2000) Bob Palmer. John Wiley & Sons.

Treating Eating Disorders: Ethical, Legal, and Personal Issues (1998) W. Vandereycken and P. J. V. Beumont (eds). New York University Press.

Masters and Johnson on Sex and Human Loving (1988) William H. Masters, Virginia E. Johnson and Robert C. Kolodny. Little, Brown & Co.

Conundrum (2002) Jan Morris. Faber & Faber. (An elegantly written narrative of a prize-winning author's gender dysphoria.)

Psychopathia Sexualis, Richard Von Krafft-Ebing.

Summary

Anorexia nervosa

- DSM-IV criteria for diagnosis include disturbed perception of body weight or shape, intense fear of gaining weight, refusal to maintain body weight above 85% of expected weight and, in postmenarchal females, amenorrhoea for at least three consecutive cycles.
- Epidemiology:
  - Commoner in females than in males by a ratio of greater than 10 : 1
  - Average age of onset is 15–16 years
  - Commoner in industrialised societies, in middle to upper socioeconomic groups, and in certain professional groups.
- Aetiology involves biological, psychological, and social factors.
- Principles of management include:
  - Educate the patient and family about the disorder and its treatment
  - Support the patient and alter disturbed perceptions of the body
  - Encourage refeeding, aiming for a balanced diet of about 3000 kcal a day
  - Monitor the patient's physical condition and treat any complications
  - Treat associated psychiatric disorders
  - Consider hospitalisation in severe or intractable cases.
- Prognosis is very variable. A short history and a younger age of onset are positive prognostic factors.

Bulimia nervosa

- Characterised by recurrent episodes of binge eating followed by attempts to counteract the 'fattening' effect of the food by such methods as self-induced vomiting, prolonged fasting, laxative or diuretic misuse, stimulant misuse, and excessive exercise. Unlike in anorexia nervosa, the patient is usually of normal weight.
- Depressive symptoms are more prominent than in anorexia nervosa, and a high proportion of patients meet the criteria for major depression. Other clinical features/complications

of bulimia nervosa result from purging behaviour, from induced vomiting, and from drug side-effects and overdose.
- Aetiological factors are very similar to those implicated in anorexia nervosa, although genetic factors play a lesser role.
- Epidemiology:
  - Commoner in females than in males by a ratio of about 10 : 1
  - Average age of onset is in teenagehood and early 20s years
  - Commoner in industrialised societies and in certain social groups.
- Principles of management include:
  - Educate the patient and family about the disorder and its treatment
  - Support the patient and alter disturbed perceptions of the self
  - Consider prescribing an SSRI such as fluoxetine or sertraline
  - Monitor physical condition and treat any complications
  - Treat associated psychiatric disorders
  - Consider hospitalisation in severe or intractable cases.
- Prognosis is better than in anorexia nervosa.

Sleep disorders

Insomnia

- Insomnia – difficulty in initiating or maintaining sleep – affects 30% of the population, and is more common in females and in the elderly. It only becomes clinically significant if it causes distress or daytime effects.

Hypersomnia

- In hypersomnia patients complain of excessive daytime sleepiness, sleep attacks, or sleep drunkenness. For a diagnosis of primary hypersomnia to be made, these symptoms should not be better accounted for by a lack of

Continued…

sleep or by another sleep disorder or psychiatric or medical disorder.

- Narcolepsy is a relatively rare disorder characterised by a tetrad of daytime somnolence and sleep attacks, cataplexy (sudden loss of muscle tone), sleep paralysis, and hypnagogic hallucinations.

Disorders of the sleep–wake schedule

- In sleep delay there is chronic difficulty initiating sleep at socially accepted times, although once asleep there is no difficulty in maintaining sleep and total sleep time is normal.

Parasomnias

- Parasomnias are abnormal episodic events during sleep and include nightmares, night terrors, and somnambulism. They are part of normal development in children but in adults usually arise during times of stress.

Sexual disorders

Sexual dysfunction

- Sexual dysfunction can be organic or psychological, primary or secondary, and can occur at any stage of sexual intercourse: initiation, arousal, penetration, and orgasm.

- Although the epidemiology of sexual dysfunction is difficult to establish, erectile dysfunction and premature ejaculation are common in males, and anorgasmia and hypoactive sexual desire are common in females.

- In assessing sexual dysfunction, it is important to take a full sexual history, including details of the medical and psychiatric history. A physical examination emphasising the genitourinary, vascular, and neurological systems, and laboratory investigations may be required to exclude organic causes of sexual dysfunction.

- In sexual dysfunction resulting from an organic cause, treat the cause if all possible. In psychological sexual dysfunction resulting from psychological causes, treatment may involve simple reassurance and advice, sex therapy (Masters and Johnson techniques), and/or drugs and physical treatments.

Paraphilias

- In a paraphilia the principal object of sexual arousal or the principal method of achieving sexual arousal is abnormal. Paraphilias begin in late adolescence or early adulthood and most commonly affect males.

Self-assessment

Simply answer with true or false. Answers on p. 220.

1. Eating disorders are more common in homosexual males than in heterosexual males.
2. Average age of onset for anorexia nervosa is the mid to late 20s.
3. One of the most important aetiological factors in anorexia nervosa is likely to be pressure to diet in a society that idealises thinness and beauty.
4. DSM-IV specifies two types of anorexia nervosa: purging type and non-purging type.
5. Depressive symptoms are more common in bulimia nervosa than in anorexia nervosa.
6. The Russell sign refers to the enlargement of the parotid glands that result from repeated induced vomiting.
7. SSRIs have been demonstrated to have a specific antibulimic effect at higher doses.
8. In refeeding, a balanced diet of about 3000 kcal a day should be aimed for.
9. Prognosis in bulimia nervosa is better than in anorexia nervosa.
10. Even after recovery, a majority of anorexics retain abnormal eating habits.
11. Insomnia is more common in males and in the elderly.
12. Sedatives should only play a minor role in the management of insomnia.
13. Narcolepsy is characterised by a tetrad of daytime somnolence and sleep attacks, cataplexy, sleep paralysis, and hypnopompic hallucinations, although not all of these features need be present.
14. In sleep delay, total sleep time is normal.
15. Nightmares, night terrors, and somnambulism are all more common in children.
16. Night terrors occur in non-REM stage 4 sleep.
17. Erectile dysfunction and ejaculatory impotence are common in males.
18. Vaginismus describes voluntary vaginal contractions in response to attempts at penetration.
19. Transsexuals intermittently or permanently assume the appearance, mannerisms, and interests of the opposite sex.
20. Voyeurism describes sexually arousing fantasies, urges, or behaviours that involve exposing genitalia to unsuspecting strangers.

12

Child and adolescent psychiatry

13

Key learning objectives

- Key milestones in the four areas of child development: motor skills, vision and fine movement, hearing and language, and social behaviour
- Theories of cognitive development of Freud, Piaget, and Erikson
- Overview of developmental disorders

- Overview of disorders specific to childhood and adolescence
- Overview of adult disorders presenting in childhood

Mental retardation is covered in Chapter 10 and childhood sleep disorders (parasomnias) are covered in Chapter 12.

What a distressing contrast there is between the radiant intelligence of the child and the feeble mentality of the average adult.

Sigmund Freud (1956–1939)

Someday, maybe, there will exist a well-informed, well considered, and yet fervent public convention that the most deadly of all possible sins is the mutilation of a child's spirit.

Erik Erikson (1902–1994)

The principal goal of education is to create men who are capable of doing new things, not simply of repeating what other generations have done – men who are creative, inventive, and discoverers.

Jean Piaget (1986–1980)

Psychiatry, 2e. By Neel Burton. Published 2010 by Blackwell Publishing.

Introduction

Like forensic psychiatry, child psychiatry is a subspecialty of psychiatry that most students receive only limited exposure to during their clinical attachments. There are basically three types or classes of childhood psychiatric disorders:

- Developmental disorders such as autism and Asperger's syndrome
- Disorders that are specific to childhood and adolescence such as attention-deficit hyperactivity disorder, conduct disorder, and tic disorders
- 'Adult' disorders occurring in childhood such as mood and anxiety disorders.

The practice of child psychiatry differs from that of adult psychiatry, not only in that the range of disorders is different, but also in that:

- Children's problems must be looked at in context of their developmental stage: some problems are normal at one stage but no longer so at a later one

- Children may not be able to express themselves as eloquently as (most) adults. This means that greater emphasis must be placed on their appearance and behaviour, and on informant histories taken from their carers, siblings, school teachers, social services, and other clinicians
- Children's distress is expressed more in terms of behavioural problems than in terms of clear-cut symptoms, so informant histories may differ significantly from one informant to another
- Carers must be closely involved in the management plan, not least because they may themselves be contributing to the child's presenting problem
- Medication should be used less often and more cautiously than in adult psychiatry.

Development

Children's problems must be looked at in the context of their development stage, as some problems are normal at one stage but no longer so at a later one. It is therefore necessary to have some knowledge of child development, and of the average ages at which key milestones are reached (Table 13.1).

Children are not just small versions of adults, but gradually develop into adults by progressing through various phases or stages of development. Stage theories of development include psychoanalytical development theories, cognitive development theories, and psychosocial development theories. Three of the most influential stage theories of development – those of Freud, Piaget, and Erikson – are summarised in Table 13.2.

Table 13.1 Average age for key milestones.

	Motor skills	Vision and fine movement	Hearing and language	Social behaviour
Newborn	Symmetrical movements, limbs flexed	Looks at light/faces in direct line of vision	Responds to noises/ voices	Responds to parents
Supine infant (2–3 months)	Raises head in prone position	Tracks objects	Cries, coos, grunts	Smiles at faces
Sitting infant (6–9 months)	6/12: Sits unsupported 9/12: Stands supported	6/12: 'Palmar grasp' 7/12: Transfers objects	Babbles	Develops stranger and separation anxiety Likes playing 'peek-a-boo'
Toddler (18–24 months)	12/12: Stands unsupported and makes first steps 24/12: Climbs stairs	12/12: 'Pincer grip' 16/12: Uses spoon or fork	12/12: Vocabulary of 1–3 words 24/12: Vocabulary of > 200 words; makes phrases	Is prone to temper tantrums
Communicating child (3–4 years)	Stands on one leg Jumps Pedals tricycle	Mature pencil grip Draws a circle and a cross	Makes complete sentences	Plays cooperatively with other children Imitates parents Achieves urinary continence

Adapted from *Clinical Skills for OSCEs*, 3e (2009), by Neel Burton, Scion Publishing.

13

Table 13.2 Three influential theories of development.

Age (years)	Sigmund Freud Psychosexual development	Jean Piaget Cognitive development	Erik Erikson Psychosocial development
1	**Oral stage (0–1.5)** Dependent for his/her needs. Focus is on sucking (mouth). Fixation leads to dependent and passive adults	**Sensorimotor stage (0–2)** Cognition limited to physical experiences and interactions Develops object permanence Lacks symbolic representation	**Trust *vs* mistrust (0–1.5)** Develops trust, security, and basic optimism
2	**Anal stage (1.5–3.5)** Issues of self-control and obedience. Focus is on anus Fixation leads to anal retentive (rigid) or anal expulsive (disorganised) adults	**Preoperational stage (2–7)** Increasing use of symbolic representation, principally language Thinking is intuitive, egocentric, and irreversible	**Autonomy *vs* doubt (1.5–3)** Learns to be self-sufficient and in control
3			
4	**Phallic stage (3.5–6)** Issues of morality and sexual identification. Focus is on penis and genital pleasure (Oedipus complex and castration anxiety). Fixation leads to amoral or puritanical adults		**Initiative *vs* guilt (3–6)** Inquisitive exploration of environment, e.g. through play situations, reinforces sense of purpose and independence
5			
6			
7	**Latency period (6–puberty)** Dormant sexuality Same-sex friendships	**Concrete operational stage (7–11)** Logical use of symbols related to concrete objects Develops conservation of numbers	**Industry *vs* inferiority (6–12)** Competence at certain tasks builds up self-esteem and leads to acceptance by the peer group
8			
9			
10			
11			
12		**Formal operational stage (11+)** Logical use of symbols related to abstract concepts Achieved by only 35% or so of high school graduates	**Identity *vs* role confusion (12–18)** Develops a sense of identity through thoughts and ideals, and peer group
13			
14			
15	**Genital stage (from puberty)** Resurgence in sexuality Successful resolution of conflicts from this and previous psychosexual stages leads to maturity		PLUS three other adult stages: • Intimacy *vs* isolation • Generativity *vs* stagnation • Integrity *vs* despair
16			
17			
18			

13

Attachment theory and the inheritance of loss

Inspired by the seminal work of John Bowlby (1907–1990) on attachment theory, Mary Ainsworth (1913–1999) devised a procedure called the 'Strange Situation' to observe patterns of attachment in human infants. In the Strange Situation, an infant is observed exploring toys for 20 minutes whilst his or her mother and a stranger enter and leave the room. Depending on the infant's behaviour upon being reunited with his or her mother, he or she is classified into one of three categories: secure attachment, anxious–ambivalent insecure attachment, and anxious–avoidant insecure attachment.

- In secure attachment, the infant explores freely and engages with the stranger whilst his or her mother is present. When his or her mother leaves, he or she is subdued but not distressed; and when she returns, he or she greets her positively. A pattern of secure attachment is thought to arise if the mother is generally available to the infant and able to meet his or her needs responsively and appropriately.
- In anxious–ambivalent insecure attachment, the infant is anxious of exploration and ambivalent towards the stranger, even in the presence of the mother. When the mother leaves, he or she is distressed; but when she returns he or she is ambivalent towards her. A pattern of anxious–ambivalent insecure attachment is thought to arise if the mother generally gives the infant attention, but inconsistently and according to her own needs rather than to his or hers.
- In anxious–avoidant insecure attachment, the infant explores the toys but seems unconcerned by the presence or absence of either the stranger or his or her mother, although he or she does not avoid the stranger as strongly as his or her mother. A pattern of anxious–avoidant insecure attachment is thought to arise if the mother generally disengages from the infant, such that the latter comes to believe that he or she has no influence over her.

An infant's pattern of attachment is important because it can lead to an internal model of the self as unlovable and inadequate, and of others as unresponsive and punitive. It can thus help to predict a person's response to loss or adversity, and his or her pattern of relating to peers, engaging in romantic relationships, and parenting children. Through parenting children, an insecure attachment can be passed on from parent to child, and in this manner one generation's loss can be inherited by the next.

Developmental disorders

Mental retardation

See Chapter 10.

Autism

First described by the Austrian–American psychiatrist Leo Kanner (1894–1981) in 1943, autism is a pervasive developmental disorder characterised by a triad of:

1. Impairments in social interactions despite a desire for them
2. Abnormalities in patterns of communication
3. A restricted, stereotyped, and repetitive repertoire of behaviours, interests, and activities.

In addition to these specific diagnostic features, there may be a range of non-specific problems such as phobias, abnormal movements, and behavioural problems (Table 13.3). Mental retardation is present in about three-quarters, and epilepsy in about one-quarter. 'Savant' skills such as calendar, mathematical, or musical skills may be present in a minority but are generally restricted to a specific area.

By definition, the onset of autism is before three years of age. Incidence is about 2 per 1000, but this figure masks a male-to-female ratio of about 4:1. All social classes are equally affected. Hypotheses about the aetiology of autism – a behavioural syndrome that may have several aetiologies – include genetics (the rate of autism in siblings is 2–6%), obstetric complications, and infections. However, theories about cold, rejecting parents ('refrigerator mothers') and the MMR vaccine have fallen out of favour. The differential diagnosis of autism is principally from other developmental disorders (mental retardation, developmental language disorder, Asperger's syndrome, Rett's syndrome, disintegrative psychosis), childhood-onset schizophrenia, and deafness. About 5% of children with autism have fragile X syndrome and about 3% have tuberous sclerosis. There is no specific treatment for autism. Management involves neuropsychological and psychiatric testing, patient and family education and support, speech and language therapy, behavioural modification, and treatment of associated medical and psychiatric conditions.

13

Table 13.3 Behavioural problems in autism.

- Difficulty interacting with others
- May avoid eye contact
- May not want cuddling
- May prefer to be alone
- Difficulty expressing needs; may use gestures
- Inappropriate response or no response to sound
- Inappropriate laughing or giggling
- Echoing of words or phrases
- Unusual or repetitive play
- Inappropriate attachment to objects
- Spinning of objects or of the self
- Insistence on sameness
- Apparent insensitivity to pain
- Lacks fear of danger

Asperger's syndrome

First described in 1944 by the Austrian paediatrician Hans Asperger, Asperger's syndrome is a pervasive developmental disorder characterised by:

- Qualitative impairments in social interaction
- A restricted, stereotyped, and repetitive repertoire of behaviours, interests, and activities.

Unlike in autism, there is no significant delay in language or cognitive development. As intelligence is normal, presentation may be later than in autism. Individuals may appear aloof, eccentric, and clumsy. Asperger's syndrome is thought to be closely related to autism. Although its prevalence is difficult to establish, it is more common than autism and, like autism, it is far more common in males (male-to-female ratio 6:1). The differential diagnosis is principally from schizoid and anankastic personality disorders. Prognosis is better than in autism and individuals are able to lead independent, successful lives. Referred to as 'my little professors' by Hans Asperger, some are even able to make valuable and important contributions to society, particularly in the fields of engineering, mathematics, and physics.

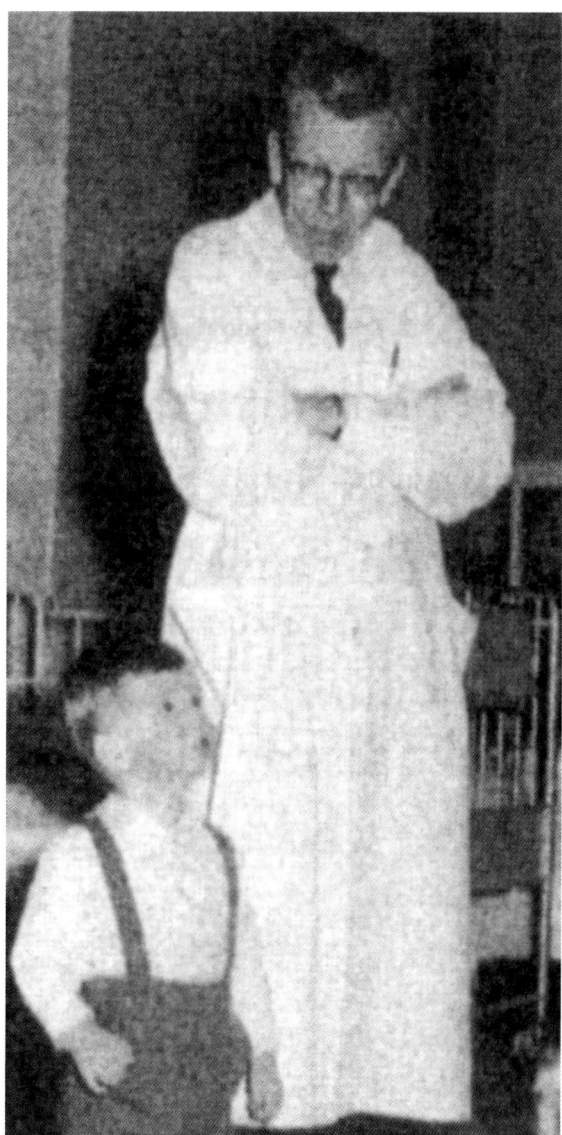

Figure 13.1 Hans Asperger (1906–1980). Asperger used to refer to his patients with Asperger's syndrome as 'my little professors'.

13

Behavioural disorders

Conduct disorder

Conduct disorder is characterised by a repetitive and persistent pattern of dissocial or aggressive behaviour to people and animals, destruction of property, deceitfulness or theft, and serious violation of rules. **Such conduct should amount to major violations of age-appropriate social expectations, and is therefore more severe than ordinary childish mischief or adolescent rebelliousness.** Duration should have been 6 months or more. Conduct disorder affects 5–10% of 8–16-year olds and is far more common in males. Environmental factors such as large families, poor parenting, deprivation, and abuse play an important aetiological role. In reaching a diagnosis, it is important to consider and rule out attention-deficit hyperactivity disorder, pervasive developmental disorders such as autism and Asperger's syndrome (see above), and mood and adjustment disorders.

Oppositional defiant disorder is a type of conduct disorder seen in younger children, and is thought to be a milder form of conduct disorder. It is defined by the presence of markedly defiant, disobedient, and provocative behaviour in the absence of the more severe dissocial or aggressive acts described above. Other subtypes of conduct disorder include conduct disorder confined to the family, unsocialised conduct disorder, and socialised conduct disorder (ICD-10).

Management of conduct disorder involves family therapy, parenting classes (for the parents), and social skills training (for the child). Prognosis is variable and depends in part on the severity of the conduct disorder. A fair number may progress to antisocial personality disorder, and substance abuse, violence, and criminality are common.

The Threat to Kill

Although a personality disorder cannot be diagnosed before adulthood, the presence of three types of behaviour in children is thought to predict the later development of antisocial personality disorder: bedwetting, cruelty to animals, and pyromania (impulsive fire setting for the purposes of gratification or relief). These three types of behaviour are collectively referred to as 'McDonald's triad', after the author of a 1963 paper entitled 'The Threat to Kill'.

Attention-deficit hyperactivity disorder (ADHD)

In the fifth century BC Hippocrates described patients with 'quickened responses to sensory experience, but also less tenaciousness because the soul moves on quickly to the next impression'. Today, the cardinal features of ADHD (referred to as 'hyperkinetic disorder' in ICD-10) are difficulty maintaining attention and hyperactivity. These features arise in early childhood, are pervasive over situations, and are persistent in time. Children are easily distracted, frequently shifting their attention from one task to another and unable to complete any. They appear fidgety and they are unable to sit still or be quiet. Associated features include impulsive and antisocial behaviour, learning difficulties, and soft neurological signs. ADHD is common and is diagnosed in 5–8% of school-age children in the USA, although this figure is substantially smaller in the UK (probably) due to more stringent diagnostic criteria and a greater reluctance to make the diagnosis. The disorder is three times more common in boys than in girls, but this may at least in part reflect a lesser likelihood of making the diagnosis in girls. The aetiology of ADHD has a strong genetic component, while environmental factors may modulate the expression of the disorder. Pathophysiology is thought to involve a deficiency of dopamine and noradrenaline neurotransmitters in frontal and prefrontal brain areas. Management is accordingly by psychostimulant drugs such as methylphenidate (Ritalin), amphetamines (Adderall), and dextroamphetamine (Dexedrine), or by noradrenaline reuptake inhibitors such as atomoxetine (Strattera). Other management strategies include behavioural modification and remedial education and, perhaps more controversially, dietary modifications such as the addition of omega-3 or the elimination of salicylates, artificial colours and flavours, and certain synthetic preservatives (the 'Feingold diet'). Prognosis is mitigated and in a majority of cases symptoms (especially attention-deficit) persist into adolescence and adult life.

Controversy surrounding ADHD

There is some debate as to whether ADHD constitutes a disability, an impairment, or simply a divergent or normal variant of human behaviour. David Neeleman, the founder and CEO of JetBlue Airways, has publicly stated that he considers his
Continued…

ADHD as one of his greatest assets, and it is the case that many people with ADHD are similarly creative, driven, and tenacious.

In a different vein, ADHD is sometimes criticised for being little more than a label for the consequences of poor parental attachment and childhood emotional trauma. A similar but more general criticism is that the diagnostic criteria for ADHD are unvalidated, socially and culturally biased, and sufficiently general or vague so as to include almost anyone with socially undesirable behaviour.

Emotional disorders

Affective disorders

Other than **depressive conduct disorder** in ICD-10, neither ICD-10 nor DSM-IV lists any specific childhood affective disorders. That having been said, adult-type depressive disorders are recognised to occur in adolescents, prepubertal children, and even preschool children. The point prevalence of depressive disorders in adolescents is about 4%, dropping to less than 1% in preschool children. Clinical features are similar to those in adults but recurrence is more common and prognosis is poorer. Hypomanic or manic episodes are very rare in prepubertal children, but 'masked symptoms' may include irritability, agitation, impulsiveness, and severe temper tantrums.

Anxiety disorders

Anxiety disorders of childhood (referred to as 'emotional disorders' to distinguish them from anxiety disorders of adulthood) must be distinguished from anxieties that are a normal part of child development by their timing, severity, and effect on social functioning. The prevalence of anxiety disorders of childhood is difficult to establish, but is probably around 5–10%. Unlike in adults, males and females are almost equally affected. In **separation anxiety disorder of childhood** the child fears that harm is going to befall his or her attachment figures and that he or she is going to lose them. This manifests itself as distress and physical symptoms on separation, fear of being alone, reluctance to go to school, reluctance to separate at night, and nightmares involving themes of separation. Other childhood anxiety disorders specifically recognised by ICD-10 include phobic anxiety disorder of childhood, social anxiety disorder of childhood, and sibling rivalry disorder. Management is along the lines of management of anxiety disorders of adulthood, except that drugs are seldom used. Prognosis is good.

Enuresis

Enuresis is the repeated involuntary voiding of urine in the absence of an organic cause **after the chronological and mental age of five years**. Organic causes include constipation, urinary tract infection, structural abnormalities of the urinary tract, diabetes, epilepsy, neurological abnormalities, and drugs such as diuretics. Enuresis can be:

- Nocturnal, diurnal, or both
- Primary (if continence has never been achieved) or secondary (if urinary incontinence has been preceded by a period of continence).

Enuresis (particularly nocturnal enuresis) is common and by age seven years still affects about 7% of boys and 3% of girls. In most cases it probably results from delayed maturation of the nervous system, although psychological factors may also play a role. Perhaps unexpectedly, a family history involving a first-degree relative can be found in as many as 70% of cases. Management involves exclusion of organic causes, reassurance and explanation, bladder training, 'bed and pad' or enuresis alarms, positive reinforcement systems such as star charts and, if appropriate, drugs such as desmopressin (a synthetic drug that mimics the action of antidiuretic hormone/vasopressin) and imipramine (a tricyclic antidepressant). In particular, parents must be explained that the condition is common, that it is rarely intentional, and that no one is to blame for it. Prognosis is good.

Encopresis

According to DSM-IV, encopresis is the 'repeated involuntary passage of faeces into places not appropriate for that purpose … the event must take place for at least three months, **the chronological age and mental age of the child must be at least four years …**'

Retentive encopresis is more common than non-retentive encopresis and results from both physical and psychological causes (Figure 13.2). Non-retentive encopresis, if it is primary, typically results from poor social training. If it is secondary, that is, preceded by a period of

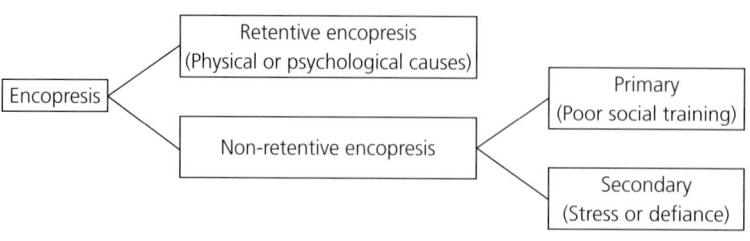

Figure 13.2 Types of encopresis and their causes. Mixed types are common.

faecal continence of one year or more, it typically results from emotional stress or defiance. Secondary non-retentive encopresis is therefore more commonly situational and/or accompanied by other regressive behaviours. Encopresis affects 1–2% of children under the age of 10 and is much more common in boys.

Management involves the exclusion of physical causes such as anal fissure, diarrhoea, constipation, and Hirschsprung's disease; explanation and reassurance; and, if appropriate, removal of stressors and retraining. Of particular note is the fact that children with encopresis are likely to suffer from hostile attitudes and behaviours on the part of parents and teachers, and as a result may come to feel undesired.

Elective mutism

In elective mutism or selective mutism, the child is unable to speak in certain defined situations (most commonly at school) but is able to do so normally in others. The child may also limit his or her participation in non-verbal activities such as playing. Elective mutism affects about one child in 1000 and is slightly more common in girls. Onset is usually at the time of entering school. Children tend to have an overprotective mother and to be confident and talkative inside the home but shy, anxious, and isolated outside. Other anxiety disorders and behavioural disorders are common. Parents and teachers need to be educated about the problem and reassured that, although it may last for months or years, it has a good longer-term prognosis.

Tic disorders

Tics are repetitive, stereotyped, and purposeless movements or vocalisations. They can be voluntarily suppressed, but this then leads to a build up in tension and anxiety (in this respect they are rather like compulsions). Tics affect up to 20% of all children in the first decade

of life and are three times more frequent in boys. The commonest tics are simple motor tics that involve a group of functionally related muscles, e.g. blinking, grimacing, and shoulder shrugging. Other types of tic include complex motor tics such as jumping, hitting oneself, and gesturing obscenities (copropraxia); simple vocal tics such as throat-clearing, sniffing, and barking; and complex vocal tics such as repeating one's utterances (palilalia), repeating others' utterances (echolalia), or shouting out obscenities (coprolalia). Tics are exacerbated by stress and attenuated by sustained concentration. Their differential diagnosis is essentially from other disorders of movement. In most cases they are mild and transient and do not require any treatment. If single or multiple motor and/or vocal tics last for less than 12 months, a diagnosis of transient tic disorder can be made. If single or multiple motor *or* vocal tics (but not both – see Gilles de la Tourette syndrome) last for more than 12 months, a diagnosis of chronic motor or vocal tic disorder can be made.

Gilles de la Tourette syndrome

Gilles de la Tourette syndrome or Tourette's syndrome is a tic disorder involving multiple motor tics *and* at least one vocal tic. First described by Jean Itard and then by George Gilles de la Tourette, Tourette's syndrome is thought to have affected such luminaries as Samuel Johnson and André Malraux. Both genetic and environmental factors play a role in its aetiology and symptoms are thought to result from dysfunction in the frontal cortex, thalamus, and basal ganglia. The syndrome can be mimicked by several conditions such as stroke, encephalitis, and carbon monoxide poisoning; and by drugs such as stimulants, levodopa, and carbamazepine ('tourettism'). Incidence is about 1 in 2000, but boys are more frequently affected than girls by a ratio of 3–4:1. Onset is before age 18 (mean 7 years for motor tics and 11 years for vocal tics). The number, location, and severity of the tics vary over time, and they often resolve by early adulthood. Coprolalia occurs in about 30% of cases and is largely responsible for the public notoriety of the syndrome. Comorbid psychiatric disorders, particularly obsessive–compulsive disorder and ADHD, are common and may eclipse and/or survive the tic disorder.

Management involves education of the patient and family, pharmacological treatment of the tic disorder if indicated (e.g. by clonidine, risperidone, or sulpiride), and treatment of comorbid psychiatric conditions such as obsessive–compulsive disorder and ADHD. Note that the use of stimulants, e.g. in the treatment of comorbid ADHD, is likely to aggravate any tic disorder.

Recommended reading

Child Psychiatry, 2e (2005) Goodman and Scott. Wiley-Blackwell.
The Uses of Enchantment – The Meaning and Importance of Fairy Tales (1991) Bruno Bettelheim. Penguin.

Summary

Autism
- Autism is a pervasive developmental disorder characterised by impairment in social interactions, abnormalities in patterns of communications, and a restricted, stereotyped, repetitive repertoire of behaviours, interests, and activities.
- In addition to these specific diagnostic features, a range of non-specific problems are common such as phobias, abnormal movements, and behavioural problems. About three-quarters are mentally retarded and one-quarter have epilepsy.

Asperger's syndrome
- Asperger's syndrome is a pervasive developmental disorder related to autism that is characterised by qualitative impairments in social interaction and a restricted, stereotyped, and repetitive repertoire of behaviours, interests, and activities. Unlike in autism, however, there is no significant delay in language or cognitive development. Individuals may appear aloof, eccentric, and clumsy but are able to lead independent, successful lives.

Conduct disorder
- Conduct disorder is characterised by a repetitive and persistent pattern of dissocial or aggressive conduct, including aggression to people and animals, destruction of property, deceitfulness or theft, and serious violation of rules.
- Oppositional defiant disorder is a type of conduct disorder seen in younger children, and is thought to be a milder form of conduct disorder. It is defined by the presence of markedly defiant, disobedient, and provocative behaviour in the absence of more severe dissocial or aggressive acts.

Attention-deficit hyperactivity disorder
- The cardinal features of ADHD (hyperkinetic disorder) are difficulty maintaining attention and overactivity. These features arise in early childhood, are pervasive over situations, and are persistent in time.

Affective disorders
- Adult-type depressive disorders occur even in very young children, but hypomanic or manic episodes are rare.

Anxiety disorders
- Anxiety (emotional) disorders in children must be distinguished from anxieties that are a normal part of child development by their timing, severity, and effect on social functioning. Childhood anxiety disorders specifically recognised in ICD-10 are separation anxiety disorder of childhood, phobic anxiety disorder of childhood, social anxiety disorder of childhood, and sibling rivalry disorder.

Enuresis
- Enuresis is the repeated involuntary voiding of urine in the absence of an organic cause after the chronological and mental age of five.

Encopresis
- Encopresis is the repeated involuntary passage of faeces into places not appropriate for that purpose in children of a chronological and mental age of four and over.

Elective mutism
- In elective mutism or selective mutism, the child is unable to speak in certain, defined situations (most commonly at Continued...

13

school) but is able to do so normally in others. The child may also limit his or her participation in non-verbal activities such as playing.

Tics

- Tics affect up to 20% of all children in the first decade of life and are three times more frequent in boys. The commonest tics are simple motor tics that involve a group of functionally related muscles, e.g. blinking. Other types of tics include complex motor tics, simple vocal tics, and complex vocal tics.

Gilles de la Tourette syndrome

- Gilles de la Tourette syndrome is a rare tic disorder involving multiple motor tics *and* at least one vocal tic.

Self-assessment

Simply answer with true or false. Answers on p. 220.

1. Stranger anxiety develops at around 6–9 months of age.
2. 'Pincer grip' develops at around 18 months of age.
3. According to Freud, fixation at the anal stage leads to amoral or puritanical adults.
4. Thinking in Piaget's preoperational stage is logical as opposed to intuitive.
5. 90% of high school graduates achieve Piaget's formal operational stage.
6. Erikson described eight stages of cognitive development.
7. In autism, the male-to-female ratio is about 10 : 1.
8. Autism principally differs from Asperger's syndrome in that there is no significant delay in language or cognitive development.
9. Environmental factors play a more important role in the aetiology of conduct disorder than in that of ADHD.
10. Pathophysiology in ADHD is thought to involve a deficiency of dopamine and noradrenaline neurotransmitters in the frontal and prefrontal brain areas.
11. Primary enuresis is diagnosed if incontinence is preceded by a period of urinary continence.
12. In enuresis, a family history can be found in 90% of cases.
13. Enuresis alarms are an example of operant conditioning.
14. Secondary non-retentive encopresis typically results from poor social training.
15. Elective mutism is a relatively rare disorder that is slightly more common in girls.
16. Gilles de la Tourette syndrome is characterised by multiple motor and at least one vocal tic.

So, why a career in psychiatry?

In 2008, just 6% of candidates sitting Paper 1 of the MRC-Psych exam were UK graduates, evidence if any were needed that recruitment into psychiatry is facing an unprecedented crisis.

In my experience, most medical students enjoy learning about mental illness and talking to mentally ill people, who often have a refreshing knack for saying things exactly how they are. In a fit of inspiration, some medical students tell me that psychiatry is the only specialty that enables them to think about themselves, about other people, and about life in general. They also like the lifestyle: an hour for each patient, 'special interest' days, protected time for teaching, light on calls from home, and guaranteed career progression. In medicine they might treat yet another anonymous case of asthma, chest pain, or pulmonary oedema. In surgery they might do one knee replacement after another, up until the day they retire or collapse. But in psychiatry there can be no factory line, no standard procedure, and no mindless protocol: each patient is unique and each patient has something unique to return to the psychiatrist. I often come across those same students again, months or sometimes years later. After the smiles and the niceties, it transpires that they are no longer so interested in psychiatry. So what happened?

The students are never too sure, but I think I have an idea. Whilst I was a medical student in London, an American firm offered me a highly paid job as a strategy consultant in their Paris office. So I gladly left medicine, and the many inconveniences of working in (and increasingly 'for') the NHS. I had a great time in Paris, but the job itself turned out to be more about dealing with personality disorders than about having good ideas. I quit after six months and freelanced as an English tutor to high-flying executives, bankers, venture capitalists, and such like. As my clients already spoke good English and merely wanted to improve their fluency, all I had to do was to make conversation with them. My lessons often turned into something akin to psychotherapy, as I realised that I could make my clients open their hearts and minds simply by listening to them speak. Although they seemed to have everything in life, they were actually deeply unhappy, and had rarely stopped to ask themselves why. I wanted to find out why, so I decided to go back to the UK, do my house jobs, and specialise in psychiatry. I had always been far too 'ambitious' to consider psychiatry, but by then it had become clear that I didn't want to pursue a career that didn't allow me to think and feel, and to relate to others and to the world in a genuine and meaningful way. There are not many such jobs, but psychiatry – along with general practice, teaching, academia, and the clergy – is certainly one of them, and is even, arguably, their archetypal form.

The following year whilst going about my house jobs I put up with all sorts of abuse from my colleagues in medicine and surgery. One of the other house officers, by then a good buddy, took me aside one day and said with an alcoholic mixture of concern and disdain, 'Why do you want to go into psychiatry? You're a good doctor. Can't you see you're wasting your talents?' It became very clear, first, that the stigma that people with a mental disorder are made to feel also extends to the doctors who look after them; and, second, that this stigma emanates most strongly from the medical profession itself, mired as it is in middle class preoccupations and prejudices and, as a whole, far too grounded in neurosis not to be terrified of psychosis.

Of course, it is simply not true that psychiatry is 'a waste of talent'. The term 'psychiatry' was first used 200 years ago in 1808, in a 188-page paper by Johann Christian Reil. He argued for the urgent creation of a medical specialty to be called 'psychiatry', and contended that only the very best physicians had the skills to join it. These physicians needed not only to have an understanding of the body, but also a much broader range of skills than standard physicians. Indeed, a psychiatrist can change a person's entire outlook with a single sentence, so long as he or she can find the right words at the right time. No protocols, no high-tech equipment or expensive drugs, no pain or side-effects, and no complications or follow-up. Now that *is* talent, and one so great that I can only ever aim at it. And each time I fail, I always have medicine to fall back upon.

Further information on careers in psychiatry can be found on the Royal College website.

Psychiatry, 2e. By Neel Burton. Published 2010 by Blackwell Publishing.

Know then thyself, presume not God to scan
The proper study of mankind is man
Placed on this isthmus of a middle state
A being darkly wise, and rudely great
With too much knowledge for the sceptic side
With too much weakness for the stoic's pride
He hangs between, in doubt to act, or rest
In doubt to deem himself a God, or Beast
In doubt his mind or body to prefer
Born but to die, and reasoning but to err
Alike in ignorance, his reason such
Whether he thinks too little, or too much
Chaos of thought and passion, all confused
Still by himself abuse, or disabuse
Created half to rise, and half to fall
Great lord of all things, yet a prey to all
Sole judge of truth, in endless error hurled
The glory, jest, and riddle of the world.

From *An Essay on Man*,
by Alexander Pope (1688–1744)

Self-assessment EMQs

EMQ 1: Descriptive psychopathology – disorders of perception

A. Hypnogogic hallucination
B. Hypnopompic hallucination
C. Thought echo
D. Extracampine hallucination
E. Pseudo-hallucination
F. Delusional perception
G. Synaesthesia
H. Derealisation
I. *Déjà vu*
J. Illusion

For each of the following situations, select the most appropriate term.

1. A teenager who has lost his way in the woods becomes anxious and, as night begins to fall, begins to see 'shapes' in the trees and bushes.
2. On further questioning, a 27-year-old woman with a mild-to-moderate depressive disorder reveals that she sometimes hears her name being called out just before falling asleep.
3. A 33-year-old woman with a personality disorder complains of hearing the voice of the devil telling her that she is going to join him in hell. On further questioning, she reveals that she experiences this voice inside her head, and is able to blot it out at any time.
4. A 26-year-old man with schizophrenia hears the voice of his dead grandmother coming from 'beyond the grave'.
5. A 19-year-old student with a first episode of psychosis is distressed because he saw the pattern on a medical student's belt buckle and thought it meant that the student was 'one of them' and 'out to get him'.

Psychiatry, 2e. By Neel Burton. Published 2010 by Blackwell Publishing.

EMQ 2: Descriptive psychopathology – delusional themes/types of delusion

A. Thought broadcasting
B. Thought echo
C. Delusional perception
D. Delusion of reference
E. Idea of reference
F. Capgras' syndrome
G. Fregoli syndrome
H. Cotard's syndrome
I. De Clérambault's syndrome
J. Othello syndrome
K. *Folie à deux*

1. A 45-year-old woman, who works as the secretary to the director of a large and successful company in the City, fixedly believes that she is secretly loved by her boss.
2. A 28-year-old man with schizophrenia refuses to see his psychiatrist, because he fixedly believes that the psychiatrist has been replaced by an identical looking imposter who is in fact a Russian secret agent.
3. After the sudden death of his parents in a car crash, a 21-year-old psychology student begins experiencing the feeling that people are talking about him behind his back, and that what he reads in textbooks and journals could have been written with him in mind.
4. The sister and long-term carer of a 38-year-old man with a long history of schizophrenia shares his delusion that the ghosts of their ancestors are trying to have them killed.
5. A patient who was admitted to a psychiatric hospital four weeks ago with features of a severe and treatment-resistant depressive disorder no longer wants to eat in the presence of the other patients. When asked about this, she says that her insides are rotting, as a result of which her breath is so bad that it puts the other patients off their food.

EMQ 3: Descriptive psychopathology – disorders of movement

A. Catalepsy
B. Catatonia
C. Cataplexy
D. Retardation
E. Stupor
F. Dystonia
G. Akathisia
H. Parkinsonism
I. Tardive dyskinesia
J. Negativitism

For each of the following situations, select the most appropriate term.

1. A 19-year-old man with new onset psychosis is started on a small dose of risperidone. After just a few hours, the on-call psychiatrist is called to see him because 'he can no longer move his eyeballs'. The on-call psychiatrist prescribes a small dose of procyclidine, to which the patient makes an excellent response.
2. A 19-year-old man with new onset psychosis is started on a small dose of risperidone. After just a few days, he is noted to be even more restless and agitated, and apparently unable to sit still. The on-call psychiatrist increases the dose of the risperidone, but this only seems to make him worse.
3. A patient with severe depression is admitted to a psychiatric hospital because he is immobile and mute. As he is not eating and drinking and is visibly dehydrated, he is started on a course of electroconvulsive therapy.
4. A 25-year-old man with schizophrenia is admitted to a psychiatric hospital after being found in the street, standing on one leg and immobile.
5. Once in hospital, the psychiatrist examining this man finds that his limbs can be placed in any posture, after which they are maintained in that posture for several minutes at a time.

EMQ 4: Mental healthcare services

A. CRHT
B. Liaison psychiatry
C. CMHT
D. EIS
E. GP practice and Accident and Emergency
F. Day hospital
G. Rehabilitation
H. AOT

For each of the following situations, select the most appropriate service.

1. Engages 'revolving door' patients in treatment and supports them in their daily activities.
2. Improves the short- and long-term outcomes of schizophrenia and other psychotic disorders through a three-pronged approach involving preventative measures, earlier detection of untreated cases, and intensive treatment and support in the early stages of illness.
3. Is at the centre of mental healthcare provision.
4. Provides psychiatric services in a general hospital setting, both for in- and out-patients.
5. Acts as a gatekeeper to a variety of psychiatric services, including admission to a psychiatric hospital.

EMQ 5: Psychiatric ethics

A. Competence
B. Capacity
C. *Bolam v Friern Hospital Management Committee (1957)*
D. *Tarasoff v Regents of the University of California (1976)*
E. *Gillick v West Norfolk and Wisbech Area Health Authority (1985)*
F. *Re F (1990)*
G. *Re C (1994)*

For each of the following situations, select the most appropriate term.

1. The legal presumption that adult persons have the ability to make decisions.
2. The clinical determination of a patient's ability to make decisions about his or her treatment.
3. Established that a patient with a severe mental disorder can retain the capacity to make certain decisions about his or her treatment.
4. Ruled that physicians have a duty to breach confidentiality if maintaining confidentiality may result in harm to the patient or to the community.

5. Ruled that a child can be competent to consent to treatment if he or she fully understands the treatment proposed.

EMQ 6: The Mental Health Act

A. Section 2
B. Section 3
C. Section 4
D. Section 5(2)
E. Section 5(4)
F. Section 17
G. Section 35
H. Section 36
I. Section 37
J. Section 41
K. Section 58
L. Section 117
M. Section 135
N. Section 136

For each of the following situations, select the most appropriate Section.

1. Emergency admission for assessment.
2. Doctor's emergency holding power.
3. Removal by the police of a person with a suspected mental disorder from a public place to a place of safety.
4. Detention and treatment of a person convicted of an imprisonable offence.
5. Restriction order.

EMQ 7: First rank symptoms of schizophrenia

A. Third person auditory hallucination
B. Running-commentary
C. *Gedankenlautwerden*
D. *Echo de la pensée*
E. Thought insertion
F. Thought withdrawal
G. Thought broadcasting
H. Passivity of affect
I. Passivity of volition
J. Passivity of impulse
K. Somatic passivity
L. Delusional perception
M. None of the above

For each of the following situations, select the most appropriate symptom.

1. A patient complains that his thoughts are being vaporised, and that people are catching them in butterfly nets and pinning them into photo albums.
2. A patient complains of hearing several voices telling him to slit his wrists.
3. A patient complains of hearing his own thoughts at the same time as he is having them.
4. A patient who tried to strangle himself with his shoelaces says that it was nothing to do with him.
5. A patient who sees you peering at your watch in yet another endless team meeting says that her time has come to leave this madhouse.

EMQ 8: Organic differentials of schizophrenia

A. Cannabis misuse
B. Hallucinogen misuse
C. Stimulant misuse
D. Head injury
E. Central nervous system infection
F. Brain tumour
G. Temporal lobe epilepsy
H. Delirium
I. Dementia
J. Cushing's syndrome
K. Porphyria
L. Systemic lupus erythematosus

For each of the following situations, select the most appropriate term.

1. An agitated 23-year-old student is brought to A&E with visual and auditory hallucinations, paranoid ideation, itching, and formication. On physical examination his pupils are noted to be dilated, his pulse rate is 110 beats per minute, his blood pressure is 170/140 mmHg, and his temperature is 37.9°C.
2. A 73-year-old woman is admitted to hospital following an overdose of eight tablets of temazepam 10 mg following the death of her dog three months ago. During the evening shift she becomes particularly agitated and claims that she is seeing spiders on the curtains. Urinary dipstick reveals a urinary tract infection.
3. A 28-year-old woman seen in psychiatry outpatients describes discrete episodes involving a sense of

jamais-vu, distortion of the shape and size of objects, and olfactory and gustatory hallucinations.

4. A 22-year-old woman presents to A&E with recent-onset severe abdominal pain, accompanied by hallucinations and paranoid delusions. A urine sample is noted to become dark on standing.

5. A 42-year-old woman develops paranoid delusions shortly after being started on prednisolone for the treatment of her rheumatoid arthritis.

EMQ 9: Psychiatric differential of schizophrenia

A. Schizophrenia
B. Manic psychosis
C. Depressive psychosis
D. Schizoaffective disorder
E. Drug-induced psychosis
F. Schizotypal disorder
G. Persistent delusional disorder
H. Brief psychotic disorder
I. Induced delusional disorder
J. Puerperal psychosis

For each of the following situations, select the most appropriate term.

1. After the death of her father in a car crash, a 26-year-old office worker quickly begins to experience florid psychotic symptoms which, however, completely resolve within the next 10 days.

2. Three years after losing the custody of her three-year-old son, a 42-year-old inpatient continues to believe that the government conspired to have the child removed from her. She further believes that the doctors are government agents who are preventing her from seeing her son by locking her up and drugging her under the pretext of a mental disorder.

3. A 19-year-old student who is in his first year at university and making the most of his new-found freedom is admitted to a psychiatric hospital on a Saturday night. By the ward round on Monday morning, he is back to his normal self and is discharged by the consultant psychiatrist.

4. After her husband leaves her, a 36-year-old GP is admitted with tearfulness and prominent psychomotor retardation. After a few days, she develops a

number of psychotic symptoms, some of which are first rank symptoms of schizophrenia.

5. A 17-year-old is referred to psychiatric services because his parents are concerned that he is a 'loner'. He remains guarded and suspicious throughout the interview, but reveals a number of odd beliefs, such as the belief that he must keep his hair long or else his parents will die.

EMQ 10: Differential diagnosis of depression

A. Bipolar I
B. Bipolar II
C. Cyclothymia
D. Mild depressive disorder
E. Moderate depressive disorder
F. Severe depressive disorder
G. Adjustment disorder
H. Bereavement reaction
I. Abnormal bereavement reaction
J. Dysthymia

For each of the following situations, select the most appropriate term.

1. A 32-year-old woman complains of low mood, poor concentration, fatigue with early-morning waking, and loss of appetite. In the last few days, her husband has had to do all the school runs.

2. A 26-year-old woman with prominent psychomotor retardation complains of low mood. Both her speech and her movements are retarded.

3. Three months after her husband's death, a 45-year-old woman with prominent psychomotor retardation says that she would rather be dead.

4. A 36-year-old man moved to the UK from the United States four months ago. Whilst succeeding at his new job, he complains of being unable to cope. His wife tells you that, since moving to the UK, he has been uncharacteristically irritable, and has on occasion had angry outbursts.

5. A 40-year-old man has a long history of recurrent depressive episodes and hypomania, but has never had a full-blown manic episode.

6. Three months after the death of her husband in a knife attack, a 32-year-old woman says that she has made plans to be with him.

EMQ 11: Antidepressant drugs

A. Citalopram
B. Fluoxetine
C. Paroxetine
D. Amitriptyline
E. Lofepramine
F. Venlafaxine
G. Reboxetine
H. Mirtazepine
I. Trazodone
J. Lamotrigine

For each of the following situations, select the most appropriate drug.

1. Discontinuation of this drug is most likely to result in the SSRI discontinuation syndrome.
2. This drug is so frequently prescribed that it has been found in trace quantities in tap water.
3. This drug is a good choice in a patient with moderate depression and prominent weight loss.
4. These two drugs are a good choice for the treatment of bipolar depression (two marks).
5. These three drugs are a good choice for a patient with moderate depression and prominent sleep disturbance (three marks).
6. These two drugs should be avoided in depressed patients who are at a high risk of suicide (two marks).
7. This drug is a secondary amine.
8. This drug is a NaSSa (noradrenaline and serotonin-specific antidepressant).
9. This drug is a NARI (noradrenaline reuptake inhibitor).
10. This drug requires blood pressure monitoring.

EMQ 12: Differential diagnosis of anxiety

A. Panic disorder
B. Agoraphobia
C. Social phobia
D. Post-traumatic stress disorder
E. Hyperthyroidism
F. Substance misuse
G. Obsessive-compulsive disorder
H. Anankastic personality disorder
I. Conversion disorder
J. Somatoform disorder (Briquet's syndrome)
K. Cerebrovascular accident
L. Hypochondriacal disorder
M. Factitious disorder
N. Malingering

For each of the following situations, select the most appropriate term.

1. After losing her mother in a car crash, a 25-year-old woman suddenly loses the function of her right arm.
2. A consultant cardiologist is increasingly frustrated by a 35-year-old woman with a long history of multiple and severe physical symptoms that cannot be accounted for by a physical disorder.
3. A 45-year-old businessman who frequently travels presents to his GP with anxiety, sweating, tremor, and nausea. He has no past psychiatric history.
4. A 35-year-old company director who is depressed complains of being overworked. During a follow-up appointment, he appears vexed that the psychiatrist is not adhering to the latest guidelines for the management of moderate depressive disorder.
5. A 29-year-old woman experiences palpitations about three or four times a month. As they come on unexpectedly, she feels unable to leave her home alone or go to places such as cinemas and crowded shopping centres where help may be difficult to obtain.
6. A 29-year-old woman brings her two-year-old son into A&E for the third time this month. Blood tests reveal that the toddler has a high sodium level, for which no cause is found.

EMQ 13: Ego defence mechanisms

A. Compensation
B. Denial
C. Displacement
D. Distortion
E. Idealisation
F. Intellectualisation
G. Manic defence
H. Projection
I. Rationalisation
J. Reaction formation
K. Repression
L. Sublimation

For each of the following situations, select the most appropriate term.

1. A woman whose husband has left her still continues sending him text messages as though he were only on a business trip.
2. After an especially bad year, a person organises a big party for New Year's Eve and parties like there was no tomorrow (or like it was 1999).
3. When asked about the banking crisis by the Leader of the Opposition, the Prime Minister replies, 'We saved the world … er, the banks'.
4. When summarising a psychiatric history, an SHO in psychiatry says, 'After being diagnosed with a mitotic lesion, the patient attempted to cessate her life'.
5. A young man makes advances on a pretty woman. He says she never called him back because 'she has issues with an ex'.
6. An abducted hostage develops a keen sympathy for and loyalty to her hostage-taker.

EMQ 14: Mental retardation

A. Mild mental retardation
B. Moderate mental retardation
C. Severe mental retardation
D. Schizophrenia
E. Hypomania
F. Depression
G. Attention-deficit hyperactivity disorder
H. Conduct disorder
I. Autism
J. Down's syndrome – trisomy 21
K. Down's syndrome – Robertsonian translocation
L. Fragile X syndrome
M. Phenylketonuria
N. Neurofibromatosis type I (Von Recklinghausen's syndrome)
O. Tuberous sclerosis

For each of the following situations, select the most appropriate term.

1. A 16-year-old boy with an IQ of 67 for which no specific cause can be found.
2. A 16-year-old boy with severe mental retardation suffers a progressive deterioration from his previous level of functioning. At times, he is noted to become very agitated and to bang his ears.
3. A 16-year-old boy with severe mental retardation is noted to suffer from prominent loss of appetite and sleep disturbance, and no longer enjoys interacting with his carers or listening to music like he used to.
4. A two-month-old boy with a karyotype 46, XY, t(12;21) has Brushfield spots on his irises.
5. A four-year-old boy with moderate mental retardation has an elongated face, large and protruding ears, prognathism, macroorchidism, and hypotonia. DNA testing reveals more than 200 CGG trinucleotide repeats in the *FMR* gene.

EMQ 15: Psychotropic drugs

A. Chlordiazepoxide
B. Chlormethiazole
C. Lorazepam
D. Diazepam
E. Temazepam
F. Haloperidol
G. Phenelzine
H. Moclobemide
I. Venlafaxine
J. Mirtazepine
K. Trazodone
L. Donepezil
M. Zopiclone

For each of the following situations, select the most appropriate drug.

1. A 73-year-old woman is seen in the dementia clinic. One week ago she got lost whilst out in her neighbourhood and almost got run over by a motorcycle. Her MMSE score is 19/30.
2. A 73-year-old man with a long history of binge drinking currently has six of the seven features of alcohol dependence syndrome. His GP prescribes thiamine and recommends that he should start a programme of detoxification.
3. A 24-year-old man with paranoid schizophrenia who has been admitted to hospital becomes extremely agitated, smashing windows and threatening members of staff and fellow patients. As he does not respond to de-escalation techniques, rapid tranquillisation is required.
4. A 49-year-old woman with a moderate to severe depressive episode and a history of hypertension has not responded to an adequate trial of an SSRI. She is

noted to have prominent sleep disturbance and appetite disturbances.

5. A 55-year-old man with a long history of moderate to severe depression has failed to respond to a variety of different antidepressants. His psychiatrist therefore decides to start him on a reversible monoamine oxidase inhibitor (RIMA).

6. The above man is asking for one of these two drugs to help him sleep (two marks).

EMQ 16: Side-effects of psychotropic drugs

A. Chlorpromazine
B. Risperidone
C. Olanzapine
D. Clozapine
E. Fluoxetine
F. Paroxetine
G. Venlafaxine
H. Amitriptyline
I. Lithium
J. Semisodium valproate
K. Lorazepam
L. Disulfiram
M. Acamprosate

For each of the following situations, select the most likely drug.

1. Dry mouth, blurred vision, glaucoma, constipation, urinary retention, sedation, weight gain, sexual dysfunction, cardiac arrhythmias, neurotoxic side-effects.

2. Weight gain, sedation, anticholinergic side-effects, orthostatic hypotension, increased risk of convulsions at higher doses, agranulocytosis.

3. Prominent hyperprolactinaemia.

4. Nausea, tremor, sedation, weight gain, alopecia, blood dyscrasias, hepatotoxicity, pancreatitis.

5. Long-term side-effects include weight gain, oedema, goitre and hypothyroidism, hyperparathyroidism, cardiotoxicity, irreversible renal damage, nephrogenic diabetes insipidus, and a raised leucocyte and platelet count.

6. Discontinuation syndrome consists of headache, dizziness, shock-like sensations and paraesthesiae, gastrointestinal symptoms, lethargy, insomnia, and changes in mood (depression, anxiety/agitation).

EMQ 17: Child psychiatry

A. Mental retardation
B. Autism
C. Asperger's syndrome
D. Conduct disorder
E. Oppositional-defiant disorder
F. Hyperkinetic disorder
G. Complex vocal tics
H. Tourette's syndrome
I. Childhood depressive disorder
J. Elective mutism
K. Enuresis
L. Encopresis
M. Part of normal development

For each of the following situations, select the most appropriate term.

1. A three-year-old girl regularly wets her bed, much to the frustration of her parents who take her to the GP to have her assessed.

2. An 11-year-old boy is bought to his GP after developing socially embarrassing vocal tics, sometimes involving the shouting out of obscenities. On further questioning, the GP uncovers an earlier history of multiple motor tics. He refers the child to a neurology clinic where he is started on clonidine.

3. A three-year-old girl is noted to be confident and talkative inside the home but shy, anxious, and isolated outside. After she starts school, her teacher reports that she does not speak in class.

4. A five-year-old boy's behaviour is consistently defiant, disobedient, and provocative, although he has never caused any serious destruction of property or harm to others. He is noted to be from a large single-parent family which depends on social benefits for its income.

5. A six-year-old boy is noted to be aloof, eccentric, and clumsy. His IQ is 112 and there are no significant delays in language or cognitive development.

Answers to self-assessment

Chapter 2

1. True. Strictly speaking, the mental state examination is a snapshot of the patient's mental state at or around that time.
2. True. The mental state examination is like a physical examination in that it elicits the signs of mental illness and like a functional enquiry in that it elicits the symptoms of mental illness.
3. False. One of the most important principles of descriptive psychopathology is *not* to make assumptions about the causes or consequences of signs and symptoms of mental illness.
4. False. Suicide should be asked about.
5. True.
6. True.
7. False. This describes a mannerism. A stereotypy is an odd, repetitive movement that is *not* of functional significance.
8. False. This describes dyspraxia. Apraxia is defined as an *inability* to carry out purposive movements in spite of intact comprehension and motor function.
9. False. *Mitgehen* is an extreme form of *mitmachen*.
10. True.
11. False. This describes dysphonia. Dysphasia describes impairment of the ability to comprehend or express language.
12. True.
13. False. This describes dissociation of affect. In incongruity of affect, affect is not appropriate to circumstances, e.g. laughter upon recounting the death of a loved one.
14. True.
15. True.
16. True.
17. True.
18. False. This describes Capgras' syndrome. Fregoli syndrome is the delusion that a familiar individual is disguising as various strangers.

Psychiatry, 2e. By Neel Burton. Published 2010 by Blackwell Publishing.

19. False. The opposite is true: a pseudo-hallucination differs from a hallucination in that it is perceived to come from the mind and not from the sense organs.
20. False. This describes a functional hallucination. A reflex hallucination is a hallucination triggered by an environmental stimulus in another modality, e.g. a visual hallucination triggered by the sound of music.
21. False.
22. True.
23. False. This describes the ICD-10 classification.
24. False. This describes the ICD-10 classification.
25. True.

Chapter 3

1. True.
2. True.
3. False. If a psychiatric referral is required, this is usually to the Community Mental Health Team or, in an emergency or at night, to the Crisis Resolution and Home Treatment Team.
4. False. This best describes the Assertive Outreach Team.
5. True.
6. False – *fully* understands.
7. True.
8. True.
9. False.
10. True.
11. False.
12. False.
13. False. Under common law perhaps.
14. False. Any doctor.
15. False. A patient can only be detained under Section 5(2) if he or she has been admitted to hospital.
16. True.
17. False.
18. False. Section 136.
19. True.
20. True.

Chapter 4

1. False. Bleuler.
2. False. Men.
3. False. It is, although to a lesser extent.
4. True.
5. False. Dopamine underactivity.
6. False.
7. False. The definition of a delusion is a fixed belief held in the face of evidence to the contrary, *and that cannot be explained by culture or religion.*
8. True.
9. True.
10. False.
11. True.
12. True.
13. True.
14. False. This is DSM-IV.
15. False. 25%.
16. True.
17. True. Extrapyramidal side-effects. Oculogyric crisis is an acute dystonia.
18. False. 20%.
19. False. They also include ejaculatory failure.
20. False. Risperidone.
21. False. Olanzapine.
22. False. Agranulocytosis.
23. False. Hyperthermia, rigidity, autonomic instability, and altered mental status.
24. False. They are used to treat other extrapyramidal side-effects, but may exacerbate tardive dyskinesia.
25. True.
26. False. ICD-10.
27. False. One month.
28. True.
29. True.
30. False.
31. False. This describes persistent delusional disorder.
32. True.
33. False. At least for the next six months.
34. False.
35. True.
36. False. Cardiovascular disease.
37. False. A risk factor.
38. False. A risk factor.

Chapter 5

1. False. Core symptoms of depression are low mood, loss of interest and enjoyment, and fatiguability.
2. True. In males, the peak prevalence of depressive disorders is in old age.
3. True.
4. False. Dopamine, noradrenaline, and serotonin.
5. False. 50%.
6. True.
7. True.
8. False. Less and less attributable.
9. False, loss of a mother only. Sorry for the trick question!
10. False. This is according to psychoanalytic theory.
11. False. The self, of the present, and of the future.
12. False.
13. True.
14. False.
15. True.
16. True.
17. False. Tricyclic antidepressants.
18. True.
19. True.
20. True.
21. False. Imipramine is a TCA, not an SSRI.
22. False.
23. True.
24. True.
25. True.
26. False.
27. False.
28. False. This is psychodynamic psychotherapy.
29. True.
30. False. Major depression and hypomania.
31. False. Four or more episodes of mania, hypomania, and/or depression in one year.
32. True.
33. True.
34. False. This is true of lithium, not of valproate.
35. False.
36. True.
37. False. Four months. Six months is the average length of a depressive episode.
38. True.

Chapter 6

1. True.
2. True.
3. True.
4. False. A small minority. The vast majority of suicides result from psychiatric illness.
5. False. Three times higher.
6. False. It has been increasing. Since 1976, the suicide rate in elderly males has been falling.
7. True.
8. True.
9. False. In spring only.
10. False. The statistics are not reliable.
11. True.
12. False. 50% of suicides had visited a GP in the month prior to killing themselves, but two-thirds had told someone of their intentions.
13. False. *Females* aged 15–19 are at the highest risk of deliberate self-harm.
14. True.
15. True. About 85%.
16. True.
17. True.
18. True.

Chapter 7

1. False. They often blur.
2. False. They are disorders of perception.
3. False.
4. False. In social phobia and obsessive-compulsive disorder the male-to-female ratio is closer to 1 : 1.
5. False. Noradrenergic neurones originate in the *locus coeruleus* and serotonergic neurones in the raphe nuclei.
6. False. This is according to psychoanalytical theory.
7. True.
8. True.
9. True.
10. False. Unlike other anxiety disorders, specific phobias most often have their onset in childhood.
11. False. Specific phobias.
12. True.
13. False. This describes agoraphobia. In social phobia there is a persistent irrational fear of being scrutinised by others and of being embarrassed or humiliated, either in most social situations or in specific social situations such as public speaking.

14. False. Sudden onset.
15. False. It fluctuates.
16. False.
17. True.
18. False. This described as PTSD.
19. False. This is *la belle indifférence*. Briquet's syndrome describes a long history of multiple and severe physical symptoms that cannot be accounted for by a physical disorder or other psychiatric disorder.
20. True.
21. False.
22. True.
23. True.
24. True.
25. True.
26. False.
27. True.
28. False. By half-life and potency. Side-effects are all similar.
29. True.
30. True.
31. True.
32. False. Flumazenil.

Chapter 8

1. True.
2. False. Cluster B is described as dramatic, erratic and includes antisocial, borderline, histrionic, and narcissistic personality disorders.
3. True. Cluster C is described as anxious, fearful and also includes avoidant and dependent personality disorders.
4. False.
5. False. Up to 50%.
6. True.
7. True.
8. False.
9. True.
10. False. This describes schizotypal personality disorder.
11. True.
12. False.
13. True.
14. False. This describes histrionic personality disorder.
15. False. The conditions are not related.
16. False. This describes dependent personality disorder.
17. False. Projection.
18. True.

Chapter 9

1. False. The commonest cause of delirium is drugs.
2. True. Delirium has a multitude of causes.
3. False. Consciousness is clouded. In dementia consciousness is not clouded.
4. False. Remote memory is relatively spared.
5. False. The reverse is true. The patient is typically most agitated at night and improves in the daytime.
6. True.
7. True.
8. True.
9. False. Mortality is high, both in hospital and after discharge, and one-year mortality has been estimated to be as high as 50%.
10. False. There should be evidence of a decline in *both* memory or thinking sufficient to impair activities of daily living.
11. False. Lesions in the non-dominant temporal lobe can lead to visuospatial difficulties, prosopagnosia, and hallucinations. Lesions in the dominant temporal lobe can lead to verbal agnosia, visual agnosia, receptive aphasia, and hallucinations.
12. True. Lesions in the dominant parietal lobe lead to receptive aphasia, agnosia, apraxia, and Gerstmann's syndrome (finger agnosia, dyscalculia, dysgraphia, left-right disorientation).
13. False. Female sex.
14. False. Inheritance of the ε4 allele of apolipoprotein E on chromosome 19 is a risk factor for the common sporadic, late-onset form of Alzheimer's disease. The ε2 allele is protective.
15. False. This describes senile plaques. Neurofibrillary tangles consist of coiled filaments of abnormally phosphorylated microtubule-associated protein tau.
16. True.
17. True.
18. False. This best describes vascular dementia.
19. True.
20. False. If capacity is lacking, the doctor in charge has the responsibility to act in the best interests of the patient, although it is good practice for him or her to involve the carers and relatives in the decision-making.

Chapter 10

1. False.
2. True.
3. True.
4. False. About 95%.
5. True.
6. True.
7. False. The prevalence rate of mental retardation is about 2–3%.
8. False. The male-to-female ratio in severe mental retardation is about 1.2 : 1 although it is higher in mild mental retardation.
9. False.
10. True.
11. False. Down's syndrome is the commonest cause of mental retardation.
12. False. 95%.
13. True.
14. False. Cri di chat syndrome results from deletion of the short arm of chromosome 5.
15. False.
16. True.
17. False. Type II neurofibromatosis.
18. False. This describes 'disability'. 'Handicap' is a disadvantage for a given individual, resulting from an impairment or disability that limits or prevents the fulfilment of a role that is normal for that individual.
19. True.
20. True.

Chapter 11

1. False. The recommended daily limits are 3–4 units a day in males and 2–3 units a day in females.
2. False. A unit is about 8 g of alcohol.
3. False. There is a compensatory upregulation of GABA.
4. True.
5. False. They are more likely to occur first thing in the morning as alcohol blood levels are at a trough.
6. False. This describes *delirium tremens*, not Wernicke's encephalopathy.
7. False. Wernicke's encephalopathy results from a deficiency in thiamine.
8. True.
9. False. Mean corpuscular volume has the highest specificity for alcohol misuse.
10. True.
11. False. Total abstention has a better prognosis than controlled drinking.
12. False. This describes acamprosate.

13. True.
14. False. The μ-opioid receptor subtype.
15. False. Constricted pupils.
16. False. Dilated pupils.
17. True.
18. False. This refers to speedball. Speed is dexamphetamine.
19. False.
20. True.

Chapter 12

1. True.
2. False. Age 15–16, rare after 30 years.
3. True. Anorexia is uncommon in countries that do not idealise thinness and beauty.
4. False. Binge-eating/purging type and restricting type.
5. True.
6. False. This describes 'chipmunk facies'. The Russell sign refers to callosities, scarring, and abrasions on the dorsal surface of the index and long finger that form as a result of repeated self-induced vomiting.
7. True.
8. True.
9. True.
10. True.
11. False. In females and the elderly.
12. True.
13. False. Hypnagogic hallucinations.
14. True.
15. True.
16. True.
17. False. Erectile dysfunction and premature ejaculation. Ejaculatory impotence is comparatively uncommon.

18. False. Involuntary vaginal contractions.
19. False. This describes transvestites.
20. False. This describes exhibitionism.

Chapter 13

1. True.
2. False. 12 months.
3. False. Fixation at the anal stage leads to anal retentive (rigid) or anal expulsive (disorganised) adults. Fixation at the phallic stage leads to amoral or puritanical adults.
4. False. Logical thinking develops in the concrete operational stage.
5. False. Only 35%!
6. True. Three are in adulthood.
7. False. The male-to-female ratio is about 4 : 1.
8. False. The other way round.
9. True. Genetic factors play an important role in the aetiology of ADHD.
10. True.
11. False. *Secondary* enuresis is diagnosed if incontinence is preceded by a period of urinary continence.
12. False. 70% of cases.
13. False. Classical conditioning.
14. False. Primary non-retentive encopresis usually results from poor social training. Secondary non-retentive encopresis typically results from emotional stress.
15. True. Incidence is about 1 in 1000.
16. True.

Answers to EMQs

EMQ 1

1. J
2. A
3. E
4. D
5. F

EMQ 2

1. I
2. F
3. E
4. K
5. H

EMQ 3

1. F*
2. G
3. E
4. B
5. A

EMQ 4

1. H
2. D
3. C
4. B
5. A

EMQ 5

1. B
2. A
3. G
4. D
5. E

EMQ 6

1. C
2. D
3. M
4. I
5. J

EMQ 7

1. G
2. M
3. C
4. J
5. L

EMQ 8

1. C
2. H
3. G
4. K
5. J

EMQ 9

1. H
2. G
3. E
4. C
5. F

EMQ 10

1. E
2. F
3. I
4. G

5. B
6. I

EMQ 11

1. C
2. B
3. H
4. G, J
5. D, E, I
6. D, E
7. E
8. H
9. G
10. F

EMQ 12

1. I
2. J
3. F
4. H
5. A
6. M

EMQ 13

1. B
2. G
3. D
4. F
5. I
6. J†

EMQ 14

1. A
2. D

3. F
4. K
5. L

EMQ 15

1. K
2. A
3. C
4. I
5. G
6. E, M

EMQ 16

1. H
2. D
3. B
4. J
5. I
6. F

EMQ 17

1. M
2. H
3. J
4. E
5. C

* A form of acute dystonia called 'oculogyric crisis'.
† This is known as Stockholm syndrome.

Psychiatry, 2e. By Neel Burton. Published 2010 by Blackwell Publishing.

Appendix: Some psychiatric questionnaires and rating scales

General instruments

General Health Questionnaire (GHQ)

A 12–60 (depending on the version) item self-report inventory designed for screening psychiatric disorders in community settings. For each question, the patient can choose from a list of options, each rated on a four-point severity scale.

Hopkins Symptom Checklist (SCL-90)

A 90 item self-rated inventory designed for the screening and monitoring of psychiatric symptoms in outpatient settings. 83 of the 90 items relate to nine sub-scales such as anxiety, depression, obsessive-compulsive symptoms, anger or hostility, and paranoid ideation. The remaining seven items assess disturbances of sleep and appetite.

Composite International Diagnostic Interview (CIDI)

A comprehensive and fully-structured yes/no interview used for the assessment of mental disorders coded in ICD-10 and DSM-IV. It can be used for clinical, research, or screening purposes. It is available in several languages and can be used in different cultures by both clinicians and trained lay people.

Structured Clinical Interview for DSM-IV (SCID)

A semi-structured interview covering nine separate modules used for making current and lifetime Axis I DSM-IV diagnoses. It can be used for clinical, research, and screening purposes. As the interview is conducted, a decision tree guides the clinician in testing diagnostic hypotheses.

Schedules for Clinical Assessment for Neuropsychiatry (SCAN)

A set of instruments and manuals aimed at assessing, measuring, and classifying symptoms associated with the principal adult mental disorders coded in ICD-10 and DSM-IV. It can be used for clinical, research, or training purposes. The method used is that of a semi-structured standardised clinical interview, although the order in which sections are completed is flexible.

Depression

Beck Depression Inventory (BDI-II)

A 21 item self-report inventory with cognitive and somatic subscales. Each item requires the patient to select one of four to six responses, each scored on a four-point scale. Reliance on physical symptoms may result in symptoms of physical illness inflating scores.

Hamilton Depression Rating Scale (HAM-D)

A 21 item clinician-rated inventory. The first 17 items contribute to the total score and items 18–21 are recorded to give further information about the depression such as if paranoid symptoms are present. HAM-D is useful for monitoring progress, rather than as a diagnostic or screening tool.

Montgomery-Asberg Depression Rating Scale (MADRS)

A clinician-rated inventory designed to be sensitive to change with treatment. The inventory has 10 items, each rated on a four-point scale. Comparative lack of emphasis on somatic symptoms makes it useful for the assessment and monitoring of depression in physical illness.

Anxiety disorders and obsessive-compulsive disorder

Hospital Anxiety Depression Scale (HAD)

A 14 item self-rated inventory of symptoms and functioning designed to assess the presence and severity of anxiety and depression in non-psychiatric hospital settings. Anxiety and depression are assessed on separate sub-scales, each with seven items scored on a four-point scale. The inventory can also be used in primary care or in the community.

Hamilton Anxiety Rating Scale (HAM-A)

A 14 item clinician-rated inventory. Items include anxious mood, tension, fears, autonomic symptoms, and cardiovascular, respiratory, gastrointestinal, and genitourinary symptoms, and each is scored on a five-point scale. HAM-A is useful for monitoring progress, rather than as a diagnostic or screening tool.

Yale–Brown Obsessive Compulsive Scale (Y-BOCS)

Using a symptom checklist, the clinician asks the patient to identify his or her three most distressing obsessions and compulsions and to focus on these during the ensuing Y-BOCS semi-structured interview. Y-BOCS is not a diagnostic instrument.

Schizophrenia

Brief Psychiatric Rating Scale (BPRS)

A semi-structured interview covering up to 18 items measuring positive symptoms, general psychopathology, and affective symptoms, each rated on a seven-point scale of severity ranging from 'not present' to 'extremely severe'. The BPRS is particularly useful for monitoring progress in patients with psychosis.

Positive and Negative Syndrome Scale (PANSS)

A 30 item clinician-rated inventory evaluating general psychopathology (16 items) and positive and negative symptoms (seven items each). Each item is rated on an eight-point scale of severity ranging from 'absent' to 'extreme'. The PANSS is not to be confused with the Scale for Assessment of Positive Symptoms (PANS) and the Scale for Assessment of Negative Symptoms (SANS).

Extrapyramidal Symptom Rating Scale (ESRS)

A clinician-rated scale designed for assessing extrapyramidal side-effects from antipsychotic medication. Involves six questions about the patient's subjective experience of extrapyramidal symptoms, a standardised physical examination, and seven clinician-assessed items relating to parkinsonian features. Another alternative for assessing EPSEs is the Simpson–Angus Scale (SAS).

Mania

Young Mania Rating Scale (YMRS)

An 11 item clinician-rated scale used to assess the severity of mania. Items include elevated mood, irritability, appearance, speech, sleep, and insight and are scored on a scale of 0–4 or 0–8.

Bech–Rafaelsen Mania Rating Scale (BRMRS)

An 11 item clinician-rated scale used to assess the severity of mania. Items include motor activity, verbal activity, loudness of voice, self-esteem, flight of ideas, and decrease in sleep, and are scored on a scale of 0 (normal) to 4 (extreme).

Intelligence testing

Wechsler Adult Intelligence Scale (WAIS III)

A general test of intelligence standardised for use in adults, with intelligence quantified as the global capacity of an individual to act purposefully, think rationally, and deal effectively with the environment. There are 14 sub-tests comprising of seven verbal sub-tests (information, comprehension, arithmetic, similarities/difference, vocabulary, digit span, letter-number sequencing) and seven performance sub-tests (picture completion, digit symbol, block design, matrix reasoning, picture arrangement, symbol search, object assembly), yielding a verbal IQ, a performance IQ and a composite full-scale IQ. The average full-scale IQ is 100, with a standard deviation of 15. The increase in average IQ over the course of the 20th century has been referred to as the 'Flynn effect'.

Index

Note: Page numbers in *italic* refer to figures and/or tables